Cerebrovascular Neurosurgery

NEUROSURGERY BY EXAMPLE

Key Cases and Fundamental Principles
Series edited by: Nathan R. Selden, MD, PhD, FACS, FAAP

Cerebrovascular Neurosurgery

Edited by

Peter Nakaji and Michael R. Levitt

OXFORD
UNIVERSITY PRESS

OXFORD
UNIVERSITY PRESS

Oxford University Press is a department of the University of Oxford. It furthers
the University's objective of excellence in research, scholarship, and education
by publishing worldwide. Oxford is a registered trade mark of Oxford University
Press in the UK and certain other countries.

Published in the United States of America by Oxford University Press
198 Madison Avenue, New York, NY 10016, United States of America.

CIP data is on file at the Library of Congress
ISBN 978–0–19–088772–8

9 8 7 6 5 4 3 2 1
Printed by Sheridan Books, Inc., United States of America

Contents

Series Editor's Preface

Dear Reader,

I am delighted to introduce this volume of *Neurosurgery by Example: Key Cases and Fundamental Principles*. Neurosurgical training and practice are based on managing a wide range of complex clinical cases with expert knowledge, sound judgment, and skilled technical execution. Our goal in this series is to present exemplary cases in the manner they are actually encountered in the neurosurgical clinic, hospital emergency department, and operating room.

For this volume, Drs. Peter Nakaji and Michael R. Levitt invited a broad range of expert contributors to share their extensive wisdom and experience in all major areas of vascular neurosurgery. Each chapter contains a classic presentation of an important clinical entity, guiding readers through the assessment and planning, decision-making, surgical procedure, aftercare, and complication management. "Pivot points" illuminate the changes required to manage patients in alternate or atypical situations.

Each chapter also presents lists of pearls for the accurate diagnosis, successful treatment, and effective complication management of each clinical problem. These three focus areas will be especially helpful to neurosurgeons preparing to sit for the American Board of Neurological Surgery oral examination, which bases scoring on these three topics.

Finally, each chapter contains focused reviews of medical evidence and expected outcomes, helpful for counseling patients and setting accurate expectations. Rather than exhaustive reference lists, chapter authors provide focused lists of high-priority additional reading recommended to deepen understanding.

The resulting volume should provide you with a dynamic tour through the practice of vascular neurosurgery, guided by some of the leading experts in North America. Additional volumes cover each subspecialty area of neurosurgery using the same case-based approach and board review features.

Nathan R. Selden, MD, PhD
Campagna Professor and Chair
Department of Neurological Surgery
Oregon Health and Science University
Portland, Oregon

Contributors

Adib A. Abla, MD
Associate Professor
Department of Neurological Surgery
University of California, San Francisco
San Francisco, CA

Pankaj Agarwalla, MD
Skull Base and Cerebrovascular Fellow
Department of Neurosurgery and
  Brain Repair
University of South Florida
Tampa, FL

Siviero Agazzi, MD, MBA
Professor
Department of Neurosurgery and
  Brain Repair
University of South Florida
Tampa, FL

Felipe C. Albuquerque, MD
Professor
Department of Neurosurgery
Barrow Neurological Institute
St. Joseph's Hospital and Medical Center
Phoenix, AZ

Rami O. Almefty, MD
Assistant Professor
Department of Neurosurgery
Lewis Katz School of Medicine at Temple
  University
Philadelphia, PA

Dorothea Altschul, MD
Interventional Neurologist
Neurosurgeons of New Jersey
Ridgewood, NJ

Sepideh Amin-Hanjani, MD
Professor
Department of Neurosurgery
University of Illinois at Chicago
Chicago, IL

Adam Arthur, MD, MPH
Professor
Department of Neurosurgery
University of Tennessee Health Sciences
  Center and Semmes–Murphey Clinic
Memphis, TN

Nicholas C. Bambakidis, MD
Vice President and Director, The
  Neurological Institute
University Hospitals of Cleveland
Professor of Neurological Surgery
Case Western Reserve University School
  of Medicine
Cleveland, OH

Jacob F. Baranoski, MD
Resident Physician
Department of Neurosurgery
Barrow Neurological Institute
St. Joseph's Hospital and Medical Center
Phoenix, AZ

Evgenii Belykh, MD
Department of Neurosurgery
Barrow Neurological Institute
St. Joseph's Hospital and Medical Center
Phoenix, AZ
Department of Neurosurgery
Irkutsk State Medical University
Irkutsk, Russia

Phillip A. Bonney, MD
Resident Physician
Department of Neurological Surgery
Keck School of Medicine
University of Southern California
Los Angeles, CA

Denise Brunozzi, MD
Fellow
Department of Neurosurgery
University of Illinois at Chicago
Chicago, IL

Jan-Karl Burkhardt, MD
Assistant Professor
Department of Neurosurgery
Baylor College of Medicine
Houston, TX

Brandon Burnsed, MD
Neurosurgeon
Raleigh Neurosurgical Clinic
Raleigh, NC

Claudio Cavallo, MD
Neurosurgery Research Fellow
Department of Neurosurgery
Barrow Neurological Institute
St. Joseph's Hospital and Medical Center
Phoenix, AZ

Fady T. Charbel, MD
Professor and Chair
Department of Neurosurgery
University of Illinois at Chicago
Chicago, IL

Vincent Cheung, MD
Resident Physician
Department of Neurosurgery
University of California, San Diego
La Jolla, CA

Tyler S. Cole, MD
Resident Physician
Department of Neurosurgery
Barrow Neurological Institute
St. Joseph's Hospital and Medical Center
Phoenix, AZ

E. Sander Connolly, Jr., MD
Professor and Vice Chairman
Department of Neurosurgery
Columbia University
New York, NY

Brian M. Corliss, MD
Resident Physician
Lillian S. Wells Department of
    Neurological Surgery
University of Florida
Gainesville, FL

William T. Couldwell, MD, PhD
Professor and Chair
Department of Neurosurgery
University of Utah
Salt Lake City, UT

Dale Ding, MD
Assistant Professor
Department of Neurosurgery
University of Louisville School of
    Medicine
Louisville, KY

David Dornbos III, MD
Resident Physician
Department of Neurological Surgery
The Ohio State University Wexner
    Medical Center
Columbus, OH

Andrew F. Ducruet, MD
Assistant Professor
Department of Neurosurgery
Barrow Neurological Institute
St. Joseph's Hospital and Medical Center
Phoenix, AZ

Ilyas Eli, MD
Resident Physician
Department of Neurosurgery
Clinical Neurosciences Center
University of Utah
Salt Lake City, UT

Basavaraj Ghodke, MBBS
Professor
Departments of Radiology and
  Neurological Surgery
University of Washington
Seattle, WA

Steven L. Giannotta, MD
Professor and Martin H. Weiss Chair
Department of Neurological Surgery
Keck School of Medicine
University of Southern California
Los Angeles, CA

Raghav Gupta, BS
Medical Student
Rutgers New Jersey Medical School
Rutgers, State University of New Jersey
Newark, NJ

Brian L. Hoh, MD
Professor and Chair
Lillian S. Wells Department of
  Neurological Surgery
University of Florida
Gainesville, FL

Adeel Ilyas, MD
Resident Physician
Department of Neurosurgery
University of Alabama at Birmingham
Birmingham, AL

Alexander A. Khalessi, MD, MS
Professor and Chair
Department of Neurosurgery
University of California, San Diego
La Jolla, CA

Louis Kim, MD
Professor and Vice Chair
Department of Neurological Surgery
Professor
Department of Radiology
Stroke and Applied Neuroscience Center
University of Washington
Seattle, WA

Robert Kim, MD
Resident Physician
Department of Neurosurgery
University of Utah
Salt Lake City, UT

Andrew L. Ko, MD
Assistant Professor
Department of Neurological Surgery
University of Washington
Seattle, WA

Sean D. Lavine, MD
Professor
Departments of Neurological Surgery
  and Radiology
Columbia University
New York, NY

Michael T. Lawton, MD
Professor and Chair
Department of Neurosurgery
Barrow Neurological Institute
St. Joseph's Hospital and Medical Center
Phoenix, AZ

Michaela H. Lee, MD
Neurosurgeon
Anacapa Surgical Associates
Ventura, CA

Michael R. Levitt, MD
Assistant Professor
Departments of Neurological
  Surgery, Radiology, and Mechanical
  Engineering; and Stroke and Applied
  Neuroscience Center
University of Washington
Seattle, WA

Elad I. Levy, MD, MBA
L. Nelson Hopkins III MD Chair of
  Neurosurgery
Professor of Neurosurgery and Radiology
Jacobs School of Medicine and
  Biomedical Sciences
Gates Vascular Institute at Kaleida Health
Canon Stroke and Vascular
  Research Center
University at Buffalo
Buffalo, NY

Brandon D. Liebelt, MD
Assistant Professor
Department of Neurosurgery
Larner College of Medicine
University of Vermont
Burlington, VT

Harry Van Loveren, MD
Associate Dean
College of Medicine
Professor and Chair
Department of Neurosurgery and
  Brain Repair
University of South Florida
Tampa, FL

Alex Lu, MD
Resident Physician
Department of Neurological Surgery
University of California, San Francisco
San Francisco, CA

William J. Mack, MD
Professor
Vice Chair, Academic Affairs
Department of Neurological Surgery
Keck School of Medicine
University of Southern California
Los Angeles, CA

Grace K. Mandigo, MD
Assistant Professor
Department of Neurological Surgery
Columbia University
New York, NY

Philip M. Meyers, MD
Professor
Departments of Neurological Surgery
  and Radiology
Columbia University
New York, NY

J. Mocco, MD, MS
Professor and Vice Chair
Department of Neurosurgery
Icahn School of Medicine at Mount Sinai
  Hospital
New York, NY

Jacques J. Morcos, MD
Professor
Departments of Neurosurgery and
  Otolaryngology
Miller School of Medicine
University of Miami
Miami, FL

John F. Morrison, MD
Resident Physician
Department of Neurosurgery
Brown University
Providence, RI

Stephan A. Munich, MD
Endovascular Neurosurgery Fellow
Jacobs School of Medicine and
    Biomedical Sciences
Gates Vascular Institute at Kaleida Health
University at Buffalo
Buffalo, NY

Peter Nakaji, MD
Professor
Department of Neurosurgery
Barrow Neurological Institute
St. Joseph's Hospital and Medical Center
Phoenix, AZ

Anil Nanda, MD, MPH
Professor and Chairman
Peter. W. Carmel M.D. Endowed Chair of
    Neurological Surgery
Rutgers–New Jersey Medical
    School, Newark
Rutgers–Robert Wood Johnson Medical
    School, New Brunswick
Senior Vice President of Neurosurgical
    Services, RWJBarnabas Health
New Brunswick, NJ

Vinayak Narayan, MD, MCh, DNB
Fellow
Department of Neurosurgery
Rutgers–Robert Wood Johnson
    Medical School
New Brunswick, NJ

Sabareesh K. Natarajan, MD, MS
Assistant Professor
Department of Neurological Surgery
University of Massachusetts
    Medical School
Worcester, MA

Jeffrey T. Nelson, MD
Resident Physician
Department of Neurological Surgery
Case Western Reserve University School
    of Medicine
Cleveland, OH

Christopher S. Ogilvy, MD
Professor
Department of Neurosurgery
Beth Israel Deaconess Medical Center
Harvard Medical School
Boston, MA

J. Scott Pannell, MD
Assistant Professor
Departments of Radiology and
    Neurosurgery
University of California, San Diego
La Jolla, CA

Colin J. Przybylowski, MD
Resident Physician
Department of Neurosurgery
Barrow Neurological Institute
St. Joseph's Hospital and Medical Center
Phoenix, AZ

Kristine Ravina, MD
Clinical Research Associate
Department of Neurological Surgery
Keck School of Medicine
University of Southern California
Los Angeles, CA

Zeguang Ren, MD, PhD
Assistant Professor
Department of Neurosurgery and
    Brain Repair
University of South Florida
Tampa, FL

Jonathan J. Russin, MD
Assistant Professor
Department of Neurological Surgery
Keck School of Medicine
University of Southern California
Los Angeles, CA

W. Caleb Rutledge, MD
Resident Physician
Department of Neurological Surgery
University of California, San Francisco
San Francisco, CA

David R. Santiago-Dieppa, MD
Resident Physician
Department of Neurosurgery
University of California, San Diego
La Jolla, CA

Ahsan Satar, MD
Interventional Neurologist
Neurosurgeons of New Jersey
Ridgewood, NJ

Philip G. R. Schmalz, MD
Resident Physician
Department of Neurosurgery
University of Alabama at Birmingham
Birmingham, AL

Richard H. Schmidt, MD, PhD
Associate Professor
Department of Neurosurgery
University of Utah
Salt Lake City, UT

Laligam N. Sekhar, MBBS
Professor and Vice Chair
Department of Neurological Surgery
University of Washington
Seattle, WA

Rajeev D. Sen, MD
Resident Physician
Department of Neurological Surgery
University of Washington
Seattle, WA

Hussain Shallwani, MD
Resident Physician
Department of Neurosurgery
Gates Vascular Institute at Kaleida Health
University at Buffalo
Buffalo, NY

Jason P. Sheehan, MD, PhD
Professor
Departments of Neurological Surgery
    and Neuroscience
University of Virginia
Charlottesville, VA

Matthew J. Shepard, MD
Resident Physician
Department of Neurological Surgery
University of Virginia
Charlottesville, VA

Adnan H. Siddiqui, MD, PhD
Professor
Departments of Neurosurgery and
    Radiology
Jacobs School of Medicine and
    Biomedical Sciences
Gates Vascular Institute at Kaleida Health
Canon Stroke and Vascular
    Research Center
University at Buffalo
Buffalo, NY

Parampreet Singh, MD
Fellow
Department of Neurological Surgery
Keck School of Medicine
University of Southern California
Los Angeles, CA

Robert A. Solomon, MD
Professor and Chair
Department of Neurosurgery
Columbia University
New York, NY

Robert F. Spetzler, MD
Emeritus Chair
Department of Neurosurgery
Barrow Neurological Institute
St. Joseph's Hospital and Medical Center
Phoenix, AZ

Philipp Taussky, MD
Associate Professor
Departments of Neurological Surgery
    and Radiology and Imaging Sciences
University of Utah
Salt Lake City, UT

Kunal Vakharia, MD
Resident Physician
Department of Neurosurgery
Gates Vascular Institute at Kaleida Health
University at Buffalo
Buffalo, NY

Arvin R. Wali, MD, MAS
Resident Physician
Department of Neurosurgery
University of California, San Diego
La Jolla, CA

Gabrielle A. White-Dzuro, MD
Resident Physician
Department of Anesthesia, Critical Care
  and Pain Medicine
Massachusetts General Hospital
Boston, MA

Robert T. Wicks, MD
Cerebrovascular and Skull Base Fellow
Department of Neurosurgery
Barrow Neurological Institute
St. Joseph's Hospital and Medical Center
Phoenix, AZ

John R. Williams, MD
Resident Physician
Department of Neurological Surgery
University of Washington
Seattle, WA

Ethan A. Winkler, MD, PhD
Resident Physician
Department of Neurological Surgery
University of California, San Francisco
San Francisco, CA

Kurt Yaeger, MD
Resident Physician
Department of Neurosurgery
Icahn School of Medicine at Mount Sinai
  Hospital
New York, NY

Benjamin Yim, MD, MS
Resident Physician
Department of Neurological Surgery
Keck School of Medicine
University of Southern California
Los Angeles, CA

Joseph M. Zabramski, MD
Emeritus Professor
Department of Neurosurgery
Barrow Neurological Institute
St. Joseph's Hospital and Medical Center
Phoenix, AZ

Xiaochun Zhao, MD
Fellow
Department of Neurosurgery
Barrow Neurological Institute
St. Joseph's Hospital and Medical Center
Phoenix, AZ

Nonaneurysmal Subarachnoid Hemorrhage

Peter Nakaji and Michael R. Levitt

Case Presentation

A 69-year-old male presented to the emergency department with the worst headache of his life that was sudden in onset and accompanied by nausea and vomiting. There was no loss of consciousness. He did not have a history of frequent or severe headaches. On neurological examination, the patient was alert and oriented to person, place, time, and situation, although slightly slower to respond to questions than baseline. He was otherwise fully intact on examination, including normal cranial nerve, motor, sensory, and cerebellar function.

A noncontrast computed tomography (CT) scan of the head was obtained in the emergency room (Figure 1.1), and consultation with the neurosurgeon was obtained.

Assessment and Planning

The neurosurgeon confronted with the classic pattern of subarachnoid hemorrhage must quickly determine the etiology of the bleed. Aneurysmal subarachnoid hemorrhage is most commonly suspected, although the differential diagnosis includes angiographically-negative subarachnoid hemorrhage either in a classic pattern or in a perimesencephalic prepontine pattern, as well as less common causes such as hemorrhage from an arteriovenous malformation, dural arteriovenous fistula, cavernous malformation, tumor, or a bleeding diathesis or other hypocoagulable condition. The last of these should be ruled out by taking a thorough history, performing a physical examination for other signs of hemorrhage such as petechiae, and ordering a routine coagulation panel and platelet count. Aneurysmal subarachnoid hemorrhage accounts for approximately 80–85% of nontraumatic subarachnoid hemorrhage, with nonaneurysmal angiographically-negative idiopathic hemorrhage accounting for 15–18% and the balance due to the other causes listed previously.

CT angiography has become standard of care in the acute setting to evaluate for the presence of a cerebral aneurysm. Frequently, an arteriovenous malformation or fistula can be diagnosed this way as well. It is believed that with current CT quality, CT misses a true aneurysmal source of bleeding in no more than 5% and possibly less than 1% of cases. If CT angiography is negative, a catheter angiogram should be performed. Catheter angiography should include injections of both carotid arteries and both vertebral arteries, as well as external carotid artery injections, for a total of 6 visualized vessels. Some angiographers will inject only one vertebral artery if reflux is seen down to the posterior inferior cerebral arteries. In general, a full examination is preferred. Each injection should be followed

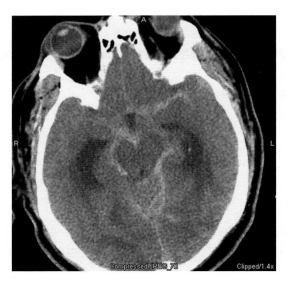

Figure 1.1 Noncontrast CT of the head demonstrates diffuse subarachnoid hemorrhage in the basal cisterns, with associated ventriculomegaly.

well into the venous phase to rule out the full range of abnormalities. The most common missed lesions include blister aneurysms of the internal carotid artery, small saccular anterior communicating artery and middle cerebral artery aneurysms, and small distal fusiform aneurysms beyond the usual circle of Willis locations.

Oral Boards Review—Diagnostic Pearls

1. Consider noncontrast CT, CT angiography, catheter angiography, magnetic resonance imaging (MRI) of the brain, and delayed repeat catheter angiography in that order if the diagnostic workup continues to be negative.
2. A high index of suspicion for an aneurysmal cause of subarachnoid hemorrhage should be maintained even if the initial CT angiography and even the catheter angiogram are negative.
3. A meticulous angiogram that includes all vessels, including the external carotid arteries, both vertebral arteries to their origins, and all vessels through the entire venous phase, is mandatory to avoid missing some lesions.
4. Angiographic three-dimensional reconstruction can help identify small lesions that could otherwise be overlooked.
5. A classic aneurysmal bleed pattern can still prove to be angiographically-negative subarachnoid hemorrhage and can have a benign course.

Surgical Procedure

In very rare cases, exploration of a possible but ill-defined source of bleeding is undertaken. This is usually in the setting of a classic pattern of subarachnoid hemorrhage when a possible bleeding source is identified on CT or catheter angiography. In this circumstance, the lesion of interest should be approached as if it is a true bleeding source, adhering to the usual vascular principles of proximal control, distal control, and dissection of the neck and dome. If a lesion such as a blister aneurysm is found, the surgeon must be prepared for clip-wrapping or bypass. For this reason, the neck is often prepped for access in case proximal control is needed. The superficial temporal artery is preserved during the opening. The forearm or leg may be prepped to have the radial artery or saphenous vein available, respectively.

Oral Boards Review—Management Pearls

1. In the setting of a perimesencephalic pattern of bleeding, a more conservative management strategy can be considered. The underlying cause of such hemorrhage remains unknown.
2. Angiographically-negative perimesencephalic hemorrhage rarely, if ever, recurs.
3. Transcranial Doppler ultrasonography can be used to screen for vasospasm.

Pivot Points

1. If the pattern of bleeding includes more cortical/convexity subarachnoid hemorrhage, occult trauma or vasculitis should be considered.
2. If a bleeding diathesis is suspected, dural venous thrombosis or another manifestation of a hypercoagulable state should be considered, including factor V Leiden, protein C or S deficiency, lupus anticoagulant, and others.

Aftercare

Most commonly, conservative management is undertaken in this setting. Most patients will be observed in the intensive care unit for other sequelae of subarachnoid hemorrhage, including hydrocephalus and vasospasm. Blood pressure is usually maintained in the 120–160 mmHg systolic range. If needed for vasospasm management, induced hypertension may still be used.

When initial catheter angiography is negative, practice varies. If the pattern of hemorrhage is classically perimesencephalic/prepontine, some surgeons advocate no further workup. In other cases that are more equivocal, a MRI with and without contrast of the brain may be performed to look for cavernous malformation or tumor. An MRI of the cervical spine or even the entire spinal canal may be performed to rule out rare causes, such as spinal ependymoma or a spinal vascular malformation.

In case of a classic pattern of bleeding, repeat angiography can be considered 7–14 days after the initial hemorrhage to look for missed sources of bleeding, as enumerated previously, and to assess for the presence of vasospasm.

Complications and Management

As mentioned previously, hydrocephalus and vasospasm are the most common issues that arise in the care of patients with angiographically-negative subarachnoid hemorrhage.

They are more common in patients with a classic aneurysmal pattern of bleeding than in those with the perimesencephalic prepontine form. Hydrocephalus in this setting can require placement of an external ventricular drain in the frontal horn of the lateral ventricle and even eventual ventriculoperitoneal shunting. Other medical problems that may supervene are the common problems found in intensive care unit patients in general, including pneumonia, urinary tract infection, myocardial infarction, and deep venous thrombosis.

Oral Boards Review—Complications Pearls

1. Patients with angiographically-negative subarachnoid hemorrhage should be managed as patients with aneurysm subarachnoid hemorrhage until it becomes clear that all tests are negative and the patients are showing a benign course.
2. Repeat hemorrhage should prompt immediate repeated diagnostic workup and evaluation of any missing imaging.
3. Hydrocephalus and vasospasm can still develop, requiring ventricular drainage and pharmacological/endovascular therapy, respectively.

Evidence and Outcomes

Although generally benign, angiographically-negative subarachnoid hemorrhage has a low but real chance of a poor outcome. Up to 11% of patients will not regain their premorbid level of function despite no cause of hemorrhage ever being found. However, the average outcome is still much better than that seen with aneurysmal subarachnoid hemorrhage.

Further Reading

Khan AA, Smith JD, Kirkman MA, et al. Angiogram negative subarachnoid haemorrhage: Outcomes and the role of repeat angiography. *Clin Neurol Neurosurg.* 2013;115(8):1470–1475. doi:10.1016/j.clineuro.2013.02.002.

Konczalla J, Schmitz J, Kashefiolasl S, Senft C, Seifert V, Platz J. Non-aneurysmal subarachnoid hemorrhage in 173 patients: A prospective study of long-term outcome. *Eur J Neurol.* 2015;22(10):1329–1336. doi:10.1111/ene.12762.

Moscovici S, Fraifeld S, Ramirez-de-Noriega F, et al. Clinical relevance of negative initial angiogram in spontaneous subarachnoid hemorrhage. *Neurol Res.* 2013;35(2):117–122. doi:10.1179/1743132812Y.0000000147.

Rinkel GJ, Wijdicks EF, Hasan D, et al. Outcome in patients with subarachnoid haemorrhage and negative angiography according to pattern of haemorrhage on computed tomography. *Lancet.* 1991;338(8773):964–968.

Blister Aneurysm of the Internal Carotid Artery

Peter Nakaji and Michael R. Levitt

2

Case Presentation

A 38-year-old male presented to the emergency department with sudden onset of the worst headache of his life. Initially, he had nausea and vomiting, and he collapsed but then regained consciousness. He stayed at home overnight before coming to the emergency department when his headache did not improve. He had previously been in good health and had no history of severe headaches. He was a nonsmoker, with no history of hypertension. On neurological examination, the patient was alert and oriented ×4 to person, place, time, and situation. He had normal cranial nerve, motor, sensory, and cerebellar function.

A noncontrast computed tomography (CT) scan of the head was obtained in the emergency department (Figure 2.1). A subsequent CT angiography (CTA) scan was interpreted as negative for vascular abnormality, and a consultation with a neurosurgeon was obtained.

Questions

1. What further workup should be pursued for a CTA-negative hemorrhage?
2. What medications should be investigated and what blood tests considered?
3. What constitutes a complete angiogram in a case such as this one? What lesions are most often missed on CTA or angiography?

Assessment and Planning

CTA can be falsely negative in 2–5% of patients. The neurosurgeon should inquire about the use of anticoagulant or antiplatelet medications, such as warfarin, heparin, aspirin, clopidogrel, and especially newer agents including apixaban (Eliquis) and dagibatran (Pradaxa). Testing should include blood coagulation studies (e.g., prothrombin time, partial thromboplastin time, international normalized ratio, platelet count, and aspirin response and P2Y12 inhibitor assays) and toxicology for stimulant drugs such as methamphetamine and cocaine. When patients present with the classic pattern of subarachnoid hemorrhage (SAH), the neurosurgeon should obtain a six-vessel catheter angiogram. A six-vessel study includes bilateral internal carotid arteries, bilateral external carotid arteries, and bilateral vertebral arteries. Alternatively, when only one vertebral artery is imaged, an angiogram is considered complete if contrast refluxes at least into the contralateral posterior inferior cerebellar artery. Both external carotid arteries should

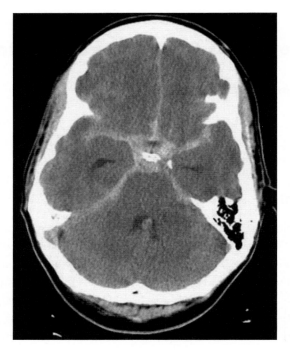

Figure 2.1 Noncontrast head CT demonstrates the pattern of subarachnoid hemorrhage classic for aneurysmal rupture, as well as enlarged temporal horns suggesting hydrocephalus.

Source: Used with permission from Barrow Neurological Institute, Phoenix, Arizona.

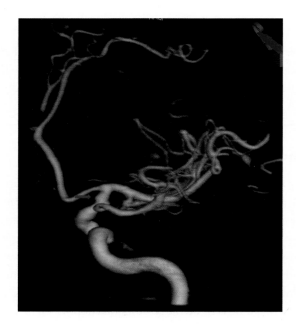

Figure 2.2 Three-dimensional rotational angiogram of the right internal carotid artery demonstrates a small, sessile, raised area (arrow) on the dorsal surface of the distal supraclinoid carotid artery.

Source: Used with permission from Barrow Neurological Institute, Phoenix, Arizona.

be studied to rule out a dural arteriovenous fistula. In this patient, the angiogram revealed an abnormality in the supraclinoid segment of the right internal carotid artery (Figure 2.2).

Questions

1. What is significant about the location of this vascular abnormality?
2. What is important about the anatomy in this particular patient? What additional anatomical information may be particularly noteworthy in planning the treatment of this disease?
3. What are the management options for this patient?

Oral Boards Review—Diagnostic Pearls

1. Blister aneurysms are inflammatory lesions without a true neck.
2. The diagnosis of a blister aneurysm should be considered in patients with SAH when no saccular aneurysm is readily apparent.
3. Three-dimensional rotational angiography helps locate and define aneurysmal anatomy.

Decision-Making

The neurosurgeon should suspect a blister aneurysm when the aneurysm is not associated with a normal arterial branching point (e.g., the dorsally located aneurysm in the supraclinoid internal carotid artery of the previously discussed patient). This kind of aneurysm is an inflammatory lesion that creates a fusiform, or patch-like, weakening in the layers of the arterial wall. Because of their small size and atypical location, blister aneurysms can easily be missed on diagnostic studies, and patients can be mistakenly diagnosed as having angiographically negative hemorrhages. However, patients with blister aneurysms usually have a classically extensive subarachnoid bleeding pattern (see Figure 2.1) rather than a perimesencephalic, prepontine-type SAH. They may present with any Hunt and Hess grade, and they may manifest a relatively benign clinical appearance. Catheter angiography, including three-dimensional rotational angiography, is often required to help make the diagnosis.

Blister aneurysms are particularly unstable and are prone to rebleeding, both spontaneously and during either surgical or endovascular treatment. In contrast, carotid aneurysms located more proximally (i.e., close to the ophthalmic artery) are usually saccular ophthalmic artery aneurysms. Carotid aneurysms that are located proximally and medially may be superior hypophyseal or carotid cave aneurysms. Aneurysms that are ventral are generally posterior communicating artery (PCOM) or anterior choroidal artery aneurysms. Those located at the carotid terminus, rather than dorsally, are also more likely to be saccular aneurysms. Saccular aneurysms are more amenable to traditional microsurgical clipping or endovascular coiling than are blister aneurysms, which are often small, broad-based, and fragile.

Assessment of the collateral circulation and options for vessel sacrifice are key considerations for internal carotid artery blister aneurysms. The anatomy of the aneurysm in this patient was complicated by the absence of an anterior communicating artery (ACOM) and the presence of a fetal-type PCOM directly opposite the aneurysm (Figure 2.3), which meant that in this patient the posterior cerebral artery distribution and the entire ipsilateral hemisphere were perfused only by the right carotid artery from which the blister aneurysm arose.

Options for intervention include surgical or endovascular treatment. Surgical clipping, clip-wrapping, or bypass and parent vessel sacrifice should all be considered. However, parent vessel sacrifice might be complicated in this patient because the blister aneurysm is located near the origin of key vessels (PCOM and anterior choroidal artery), which cannot be sacrificed without substantial risk of stroke and neurological deficit. These two arteries typically perfuse complementary vascular distributions. The sacrifice of either one is undesirable, and it is likely that the sacrifice of both would result in clinically significant neurological deficit.

The endovascular treatment of blister aneurysms (e.g., treatment with flow-diverting stents) is the focus of a growing number of published reports. In theory, endovascular treatment is appealing because it does not require much manipulation of the aneurysm. However, in patients with SAH, many surgeons are hesitant to start the dual antiplatelet therapy (most commonly aspirin and clopidogrel) required for stent placement because of the possibility of ventriculostomy-related complications. In addition, flow-diverting stent treatment of blister aneurysms does not always immediately occlude the aneurysm, which places the patient at risk of rebleeding during the immediate postoperative period. However, some endovascular therapists have documented success using this treatment strategy. In addition, hybrid strategies involving surgical clip-wrapping followed by

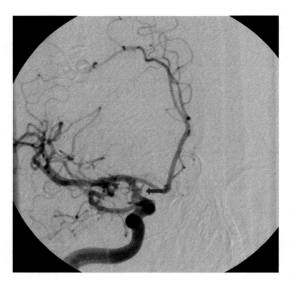

Figure 2.3 Anterior–posterior angiogram of the right internal carotid artery demonstrates blister aneurysm (arrow) close to the origin of the anterior choroidal artery and the origin of the fetal posterior communicating artery.

Source: Used with permission from Barrow Neurological Institute, Phoenix, Arizona.

delayed stenting have been reported. The optimal treatment for these aneurysms remains undefined. Any institution treating blister aneurysms should be proficient with all the necessary techniques, including direct clipping, bypass, and endovascular therapy.

Patients and their families should be informed about the risks associated with treatment. Such risks include the high likelihood of intraoperative rupture and/or the need for bypass. In this case, an open surgical approach was undertaken.

Questions

1. What special surgical considerations and preparations should go into planning for surgery in this case?
2. How should you plan for and manage intraoperative rupture?

Surgical Procedure

This patient underwent a right pterional craniotomy, with preservation of the superficial temporal artery. The right cervical internal carotid artery was also exposed in case proximal control was required. Parent vessel sacrifice would not be achieved by occluding the common carotid artery because there is collateral flow via branches of the external carotid artery. Closing the internal carotid artery in the neck alone would also not fully stop flow through the supraclinoid internal carotid artery because of collateral circulation from the ophthalmic artery, ethmoidal arteries, and small branches in the skull base that would still provide enough arterial flow to maintain vessel patency.

Sacrifice of the internal carotid artery and placement of a high-flow bypass can be considered in most patients with blister aneurysms. However, as mentioned previously, occlusion of the internal carotid artery sufficient to close the aneurysm in this patient would likely also occlude the fetal PCOM, resulting in a stroke and subsequent neurological deficit.

Therefore, clip-wrapping was performed with an expanded polytetrafluoroethylene sling (Gore-Tex), and the carotid artery was partially clipped. Intraoperative rupture occurred but was quickly controlled with temporary clips, and the blistered area was clipped with cotton reinforcement. Additional flow was provided by quickly performing a superficial temporal artery-to-middle cerebral artery bypass. The aneurysm was incorporated into the clip construct with only mild narrowing of the carotid artery (Figure 2.4).

When blister aneurysms are being explored, adequate exposure is essential to ensure that proximal control is available. For aneurysms located near the skull base, proximal control may require exposure of the cervical internal carotid artery. Proximal control should be obtained as quickly as possible in the intradural supraclinoid segment. Distal control should then be obtained. The superficial temporal artery should be preserved as a possible donor vessel for bypass, and the radial artery in the forearm and the saphenous vein in the leg should be considered when a high-flow bypass is anticipated.

Because of the propensity for intraoperative rupture, and the possibility of parent vessel sacrifice, proximal control should be obtained early in the operation, and the surgical team should prepare for a possible bypass before the final dissection of the blister

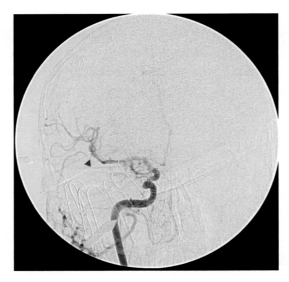

Figure 2.4 Intraoperative right common carotid artery angiogram shows good distal filling past a mild narrowing of the carotid artery associated with the aneurysm clip. Note superficial temporal artery–to–middle cerebral artery bypass (arrowhead).

Source: Used with permission from Barrow Neurological Institute, Phoenix, Arizona.

aneurysm. The aneurysm should be wrapped when primary clipping or complete sacrifice of the parent vessel is deemed inadvisable. Wrapping can be accomplished by placing a sling of Gore-Tex or Hemashield carotid patch circumferentially around the entire diseased segment of the vessel and then cinching it down with a clip to hold it in place over the aneurysm.

Oral Boards Review—Management Pearls

1. Surgery for internal carotid blister aneurysms involves the following steps:
   a. Prepare the ipsilateral neck for proximal control.
   b. Prepare a saphenous vein or a radial artery to serve as a bypass donor vessel (if needed).
   c. Have blood available for transfusion.
   d. Be prepared to use adenosine for temporary cardiac arrest, including placing cardioversion pads on the chest.
   e. Have available encircling (Sundt-type) clips and/or wrapping material (e.g., Gore-Tex).
   f. Achieve proximal and distal control early and before dissecting the blister aneurysm.
   g. Follow surgery with postoperative angiography to document the stability of the aneurysm because these lesions are known to progress after clipping more often than saccular aneurysms.

Pivot Points

1. If the patient does not have a fetal PCOM, there is a greater chance that the carotid artery can be sacrificed safely at the blister point. In this case, bypass would be more strongly considered.

2. If the ACOM was larger, the possibility of carotid sacrifice could also be considered. However, neither collateral circulation nor a bypass is likely to completely replace the blood flow formerly provided by the carotid artery. Thus, the patient is at greater risk of ischemia from subsequent vasospasm if blood flow is already compromised.

3. A patient who is an otherwise poor surgical candidate could be more strongly considered for endovascular treatment.

Aftercare

Careful management of blister aneurysm patients is necessary to achieve a good outcome. Blister aneurysms are known to re-rupture after clipping more often than saccular aneurysms. Induced hypertension, which is used to treat clinical or radiographic vasospasm, may be used with more caution in patients with blister aneurysms than in patients with saccular aneurysms that have been clipped. Patients with blister aneurysms, like patients with saccular aneurysms, have a risk of vasospasm that remains proportionate to the amount of SAH at presentation.

When the neurosurgeon is looking for propagation of the blister aneurysm along the wall of the internal carotid artery, postoperative angiography should be performed more frequently than it usually is performed for saccular aneurysms. Longer term follow-up angiograms are also necessary after the acute phase has passed because late progression of the aneurysm has been observed in some patients weeks to months later (Figure 2.5).

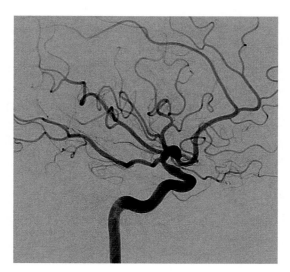

Figure 2.5 Lateral projection angiogram of the right internal carotid artery at follow-up shows mild narrowing of the carotid artery at the former location of the blister aneurysm, without progression.

Source: Used with permission from Barrow Neurological Institute, Phoenix, Arizona.

However, the process that drives these aneurysms seems to be self-limited. The wall often appears to heal, and further progression is typically not seen.

Complications and Management

The most feared complication of the blister aneurysm is uncontrollable intraoperative rupture because the "dome" of the aneurysm is just a weak portion of the dorsal carotid wall. Early proximal and distal control helps minimize the effect of such hemorrhages. The surgeon should consider preparation for clip reconstruction, carotid sacrifice with bypass, and direct or endoluminal balloon temporary occlusion of the carotid artery.

Vasospasm can present a special problem in cases of blister aneurysms because the patient will be reliant on the compromised parent vessel segment when it is preserved or on the bypass when it is not. In either scenario, the patient with a blister aneurysm is often more reliant on the preservation of single vessels than is the average SAH patient.

Oral Boards Review—Complications Pearls

1. At surgery, be prepared for intraoperative rupture with the possibility that carotid artery sacrifice may be necessary.
2. Follow-up catheter angiography or CTA is required to document the stability of the aneurysm because these lesions are known to progress after clipping more often than saccular aneurysms.
3. Careful dissection of the intradural carotid artery proximal and distal to the suspected blister aneurysm before the final dissection will allow for fast temporary clipping if intraoperative rupture occurs.
4. Patients and their families should be informed about the risks associated with treatment, including the possibility of the need for a bypass.

Evidence and Outcomes

Good outcomes can be obtained with the treatment of blister aneurysms. Select series show that with optimal management, patients with blister aneurysms will have outcomes similar to those of patients with other ruptured aneurysms. Nonetheless, patients with blister aneurysms, on average, historically do worse than patients with saccular aneurysms. To achieve the best results, the neurosurgeon should be experienced in using all the necessary management techniques.

Acknowledgment

We thank the staff of Neuroscience Publications at Barrow Neurological Institute for assistance with manuscript preparation.

Further Reading

Kalani MY, Albuquerque FC, Levitt M, Nakaji P, Spetzler RF, McDougall C. Pipeline embolization for definitive endoluminal reconstruction of blister-type carotid aneurysms after clip wrapping. *J Neurointerv Surg.* 2016;8(5):495–500.

Kalani MY, Zabramski JM, Kim LJ, et al. Long-term follow-up of blister aneurysms of the internal carotid artery. *Neurosurgery.* 2013;73(6):1026–1033.

Kung DK, Policeni BA, Capuano AW, et al. Risk of ventriculostomy-related hemorrhage in patients with acutely ruptured aneurysms treated using stent-assisted coiling. *J Neurosurg.* 2011;114(4):1021–1027.

Nerva JD, Morton RP, Levitt MR, et al. Pipeline embolization device as primary treatment for blister aneurysms and iatrogenic pseudoaneurysms of the internal carotid artery. *J Neurointerv Surg.* 2015;7(3):210–216.

Peschillo S, Cannizzaro D, Caporlingua A, Missori P. A systematic review and meta-analysis of treatment and outcome of blister-like aneurysms. *AJNR Am J Neuroradiol.* 2016;37(5):856–861.

Rouchaud A, Brinjikji W, Cloft HJ, Kallmes DF. Endovascular treatment of ruptured blister-like aneurysms: A systematic review and meta-analysis with focus on deconstructive versus reconstructive and flow-diverter treatments. *AJNR Am J Neuroradiol.* 2015;36(12):2331–2339.

Shah SS, Gersey ZC, Nuh M, Ghonim HT, Elhammady MS, Peterson EC. Microsurgical versus endovascular interventions for blood-blister aneurysms of the internal carotid artery: Systematic review of literature and meta-analysis on safety and efficacy. *J Neurosurg.* 2017;127(6):1361–1373.

Posterior Communicating Artery Aneurysm Presenting with and without Third Nerve Palsy

Brian M. Corliss and Brian L. Hoh

3

Case Presentation

An otherwise healthy 62-year-old female presents with sudden, severe, holocephalic headache, nuchal rigidity, and double vision. She denies any significant prior history of headaches. She has a history of hypertension, and her blood pressure on arrival is markedly elevated at 180/100 mmHg. The remainder of her vital signs are within normal limits. She is a chronic cigarette smoker. On physical examination, she has drowsiness and photophobia. Her right pupil is dilated, does not react to either direct or consensual light, and is abducted and depressed. The remainder of her neurological exam is nonfocal. During the assessment, she begins vomiting and is increasingly difficult to arouse. She is transported to a stroke center for urgent neurological assessment.

Questions

1. What is (are) the most likely diagnosis(es)? List a differential diagnosis.
2. What is your next step in management?
3. What is the most appropriate imaging modality to obtain for assessment in the emergency department?

Assessment and Planning

The differential diagnosis of sudden-onset neurological impairment in the absence of trauma should include cerebrovascular disease. Spontaneous intracerebral hemorrhage, subarachnoid hemorrhage (SAH), ischemic stroke, or rupture of a vascular malformation can all lead to sudden focal neurological deficits. Alternatively, seizures may result in sudden neurological deficit and may arise from mass lesions, such as tumors, abscesses, and hemorrhages; metabolic derangements such as hypoglycemia or hyponatremia; or secondary to toxins as in alcohol or benzodiazepine withdrawal.

The differential diagnosis of oculomotor nerve palsy (ONP) is broad. The oculomotor nucleus is located in the dorsal midbrain tegmentum, with fascicles exiting the midbrain through the cerebral peduncle. Ischemia affecting midbrain perforator vessels can result in infarction of the third nerve nucleus or fascicles. Usually, third nerve palsy from this etiology is associated with contralateral hemiataxia and tremor (Benedikt syndrome) or hemiplegia (Weber syndrome).

Outside of the brainstem, the third nerve travels through the interpeduncular cistern between the posterior cerebral artery and superior cerebellar artery, before approaching the medial border of the tentorium and entering the cavernous sinus. Compression of the nerve at any of these locations may result in ONP. The differential for ONP includes herniation of the uncus over the tentorium from a mass lesion in the supratentorial space; masses arising at that skull base near the cavernous sinus, such as meningiomas, sellar tumors, or cavernous aneurysms; inflammation or thrombosis in the cavernous sinus, such as in Tolosa–Hunt syndrome; and mass lesions at the orbital apex, such as lymphoma or hematoma after trauma. All of these disease processes, however, generally lead to multiple cranial neuropathies—due to the close proximity of the other cranial nerves—or other localizing signs. An isolated, painless ONP should immediately suggest compression from an unruptured posterior communicating artery (PCOM) aneurysm, whereas SAH must be excluded when ONP presents with severe headache. Initial imaging should include computed tomography (CT) and CT angiography (CTA) of the head to evaluate for SAH and aneurysm.

Oral Boards Review—Diagnostic Pearls

1. CT is the study of choice for identifying SAH, and CTA is superior to magnetic resonance angiography (MRA) for identification of aneurysms. In a setting in which the suspicion for SAH is high (e.g., patients presenting with severe headache, depressed mental status, and ONP) and no SAH is seen on CT, lumbar puncture (LP) should be obtained to rule out SAH.
   a. The normal ratio of red:white blood cells is less than 700:1, depending on whether the LP was traumatic. A higher ratio, or an increasing red blood cell count from the first tube to the last tube, suggests SAH.
   b. The presence of xanthochromia in the supernatant of spun cerebrospinal fluid is the most sensitive test for SAH on LP.
2. The most sensitive magnetic resonance imaging (MRI) sequence for SAH in the acute setting is fluid-attenuated inversion recovery. The proximity of the skull base to the basal cisterns and the presence of oxyhemoglobin in acute hemorrhage make susceptibility imaging less useful, although this sequence may detect trace amounts of intraventricular hemorrhage. Acute blood products also restrict diffusion, but artifact from the skull base decreases the sensitivity of this sequence.
3. The differential diagnosis of isolated ONP in the absence of other focal neurological findings or altered mental status is as follows:
   a. Aneurysm with third nerve compression (painless, unless aneurysm is ruptured)
   b. Diabetic mononeuropathy (painful)
   c. Lesion at the superior orbital fissure or cavernous sinus (usually associated with other cranial neuropathies)
4. ONP should be distinguished from Horner's syndrome and other forms of ptosis.

a. Horner's syndrome is the triad of mild ptosis (unlike the complete ptosis seen in third nerve palsy), miosis (in contrast to mydriasis in third nerve palsy), and anhydrosis on the affected hemiface. Headache with Horner's syndrome is highly suggestive of carotid artery dissection.

b. Thyroid disease is the most common cause of extraocular muscle weakness, including ptosis, and is not associated with pupillary abnormalities. Myasthenia gravis and Lambert–Eaton myasthenic syndrome do not involve the pupil.

c. Mydriasis in the absence of extraocular motor dysfunction is unlikely to be related to physical compression of the nerve by a mass lesion, such as an aneurysm. Elevated intracranial pressure, however, may cause this finding.

Decision-Making

The decision to treat any aneurysm is based on preventing future hemorrhage. Only occasionally does relief of mass effect play a significant role in decision-making. In the case of ruptured aneurysms, re-rupture of the aneurysm carries a dismal prognosis with rare exceptions. The risk of early re-rupture of untreated ruptured aneurysms ranges from 10% to 30%. It is therefore advisable to treat the aneurysm as quickly as reasonably possible, generally within 24 hours of presentation, unless the patient's neurological exam is extremely poor.

For unruptured aneurysms, there is controversy regarding published natural history studies; however, the International Study on Unruptured Intracranial Aneurysms (ISUIA) trial provides widely cited estimates of the rupture risk. For posterior circulation aneurysms, including PCOM aneurysms, in patients with no history of SAH, the 5-year cumulative risks of rupture per ISUIA data are 2.5% for aneurysms <7 mm in diameter, 14.5% for those 7–12 mm in diameter, 18.4% for those 13–24 mm in diameter, and 50% for those >25 mm in diameter. The PCOM location, in particular, appears to carry the highest risk of rupture in other studies, such as the Japanese Unruptured Cerebral Aneurysm Study. The size ratio (the ratio of maximum aneurysm diameter to parent vessel diameter) is correlated to aneurysm rupture risk, with higher size ratio conferring increased rupture risk even of small aneurysms. Family history of aneurysm increases the incidence of intracranial aneurysms, but data on whether this impacts the risk of aneurysmal rupture are conflicting. Tobacco use increases the incidence of aneurysm rupture from 1.5- up to 8-fold in very heavy smokers. Abnormal aneurysm morphology, such as irregular shape and the presence of a daughter sac, is another commonly cited factor for increased risk of rupture.

The approximate risk of rupture compared to the approximate risk of treatment is central to the decision to treat or to observe. If the decision is made to observe an unruptured aneurysm, follow-up imaging should be obtained and the risk of rupture versus treatment should be estimated with each set of follow-up images.

PCOM aneurysms presenting with ONP, whether ruptured or unruptured, should be treated urgently. Treatment may improve the symptoms from third nerve compression, but more important, the development of ONP may be an indication of rapid enlargement of the aneurysm and a harbinger of impending rupture. Whether the presence of ONP should play a role in the choice of management strategies (microsurgical clipping vs. endovascular coiling) for patients with PCOM aneurysms has been extensively debated, and results of studies have been conflicting. Large meta-analyses found no overall difference in ONP recovery between clipping and coiling, with a benefit of clipping seen only in ruptured PCOM aneurysms. No prospective or randomized trials have been undertaken to study this question; therefore, the decision regarding how to best treat an aneurysm causing ONP should be left to the treating surgeon's discretion.

Questions

1. What are some features of the clinical history and physical exam that increase the risk of aneurysm rupture?
2. What role does observation play in the management of unruptured intracranial aneurysms?
3. How does the presence of ONP affect the management of unruptured aneurysms? Ruptured aneurysms?

Surgical Procedure

Microsurgical Clipping

The patient is positioned supine on a standard surgical table. The bed is rotated 90 degrees to the side of the aneurysm. A shoulder bump is placed behind the scapula ipsilateral to the aneurysm. The patient's head is then pinned using a radiolucent Mayfield head clamp if the surgeon plans to perform intraoperative angiography following clip application; if not, then a metallic head clamp is used. The patient's head should be rotated away from the aneurysm side and extended slightly, equating to approximately 20 degrees of both rotation and extension for a standard pterional craniotomy. A curvilinear incision is planned from one fingerbreadth anterior to the tragus at the level of the zygoma, curving smoothly up to the midline, ending just behind the hairline. Neuromonitoring leads are placed if intraoperative evoked potentials are to be used.

Just prior to skin incision, prophylactic antibiotics, 0.5–1.0 g/kg mannitol, and (in most cases) prophylactic antiepileptic medications are administered. The patient may be gently hyperventilated to assist with brain relaxation. Sharp dissection is carried down through the scalp to the skull. Once exposed, subperiosteal dissection technique should be used to elevate anteriorly a myocutaneous flap containing the full thickness of the temporalis muscle and its superficial fascial planes. Elevating this myocutaneous flap as a single unit prevents injury to the frontalis branch of the facial nerve. If possible, the superficial temporal artery should be preserved during the exposure in case it is needed for a bypass.

With the skull exposed and skin flap retracted, a burr hole is placed at the keyhole. A second burr hole may be placed in the thin temporal squama, if desired. This burr hole makes crossing the sphenoid ridge easier and often is needed if the bone flap is to be fractured rather than cut using a craniotome. The dura is dissected and the bone flap turned with a craniotome.

Once the bone flap is removed, Leksell rongeurs, Kerrison punches, or the high-speed drill can be used to further take down the remaining lesser sphenoid wing, allowing better visualization of the internal carotid artery (ICA) and associated cisterns.

With this done, the dura is opened in a curvilinear fashion paralleling the medial and posterior borders of the craniotomy, allowing dura to be reflected forward toward the myocutaneous flap.

Exposure of the aneurysm begins anterior to the Sylvian fissure. Handheld instruments are used to retract brain to expose the chiasmatic cistern and optic nerve. It is not necessary to use static retractors to maintain this exposure. An arachnoid knife may then be used to open the arachnoid membrane overlying the optic nerve to release cerebrospinal fluid, and arachnoid dissection is extended posteriorly and laterally to expose the superior surface of the communicating segment of the ICA. If this maneuver does not expose the proximal M1 middle cerebral artery (MCA) segment, the proximal Sylvian fissure may be split to gain this exposure. Care should be taken to avoid temporal lobe retraction, especially in ruptured PCOM aneurysms, because the aneurysm dome may be adherent to the uncus, and aggressive temporal lobe retraction can result in intraoperative aneurysm rupture.

With the supraclinoid ICA exposed up to the M1 MCA segment, the falciform ligament (a dural fold spanning the dorsal surface of the optic nerve) may be opened sharply to augment the exposure of the proximal supraclinoid ICA and facilitate temporary clipping. At this point, the surgeon should be comfortable identifying the ICA from its proximal entry point into the field under the anterior clinoid process and optic nerve to its bifurcation. If the supraclinoid segment of the ICA is short, an anterior clinoidectomy may be performed to permit future temporary clip placement. The M1 MCA segment and the A1 anterior cerebral artery should be identifiable for temporary clipping. The anterior choroidal artery (AChA) and PCOM should be identified for temporary clipping and for protection during permanent clipping. The PCOM may be difficult to directly observe; it arises from the dorsal wall of the ICA and only a small knuckle may be visible adjacent to the aneurysm at its proximal junction with the ICA. The superior surfaces of the M1 MCA segment and the PCOM should not be dissected because numerous small perforating branches arise from these surfaces and enter the basal frontal lobe.

Depending on patient anatomy, temporary clips may be placed individually on the A1, M1, proximal ICA, AChA, and PCOM. Many PCOM aneurysms may be clipped using a single straight clip applied with the proximal blade immediately adjacent to the visible knuckle of the PCOM and the distal blade insinuated between the AChA and the aneurysm dome. In patients with aneurysm-related ONP, the aneurysm dome need not be dissected completely free of the oculomotor nerve because manipulation of the nerve may worsen ONP. Once clipped, indocyanine green angiography and micro-Doppler ultrasound may be used to confirm that the aneurysm is no longer filling and that all the adjacent branch vessels are filling appropriately. Changes in neurophysiologic monitoring may indicate ischemia, and they should prompt clip repositioning if present. Intraoperative catheter angiography may be performed to confirm obliteration of the aneurysm and filling of the adjacent normal vessels.

Once the aneurysm is satisfactorily clipped, hemostasis is obtained, the dura is closed, the bone flap is replaced, and the scalp is closed in appropriate layers. In the case of unruptured aneurysms or good grade ruptured aneurysms, the patient should be awakened and extubated in the operating room for neurological assessment. New focal neurological deficits such as hemiplegia may be associated with anterior choroidal artery ischemia and can be corrected with clip repositioning if caught early and addressed promptly.

Endovascular Approach

Endovascular embolization of PCOM aneurysms is usually done under general endotracheal anesthesia, although monitored anesthesia can also be used. A modified Seldinger technique is used to place a 6 Fr hemostatic vascular sheath in the common femoral artery, usually on the right. Balloon assistance may be employed in cases of ruptured wide-necked aneurysms to prevent herniation of coils into the parent vessel without the use of antiplatelet agents. If stent-assisted coiling is planned, patients should be started on dual antiplatelet therapy with aspirin and clopidogrel ideally 5 or more days prior to the procedure.

Once vascular access is obtained, systemic heparin is administered for a goal activated clotting time (ACT) of 250–300 seconds or approximately 1.5–2 times the patient's baseline ACT. ACTs are then checked periodically during the procedure, and heparin is re-dosed accordingly throughout the case. Some practitioners do not heparinize patients with ruptured aneurysms until the first coil is placed, to minimize the chance of aneurysmal re-rupture.

Angiography begins with a complete diagnostic cerebral angiogram (if not already performed) using a 4 or 5 Fr diagnostic catheter, with the plan to exchange for a more suitable catheter prior to the intervention. Generally, a 6 Fr guide catheter with an inner diameter of at least 0.070 in. is used for intervention to allow for the simultaneous positioning of two microcatheters within the same guide catheter. This is necessary in case the need arises to perform stenting or to use a balloon catheter, either for aneurysm neck remodeling during coiling or for hemostasis in the event of intraoperative rupture. For very tortuous vascular anatomy, a 6 Fr long guide sheath may be used to provide the support necessary to safely navigate the intracranial arteries.

After completion of the diagnostic portion of the case, the interventional guide catheter is positioned as distal in the cervical portion of the aneurysm's parent artery as safely possible. If planning to perform balloon- or stent-assisted coiling, the balloon microcatheter or the stenting microcatheter can then be positioned across the neck of the aneurysm with the aid of a microwire. Although most stents can be crossed with the coiling microcatheter after deployment, it is easier to access the aneurysm with the coiling microcatheter prior to stent deployment. Therefore, with the stent in position but housed inside of the microcatheter, a separate coiling microcatheter can be navigated into the aneurysm dome. The stent or balloon can then be deployed to "jail" the coiling microcatheter in the aneurysm. Alternatively, coiling may begin without deploying the stent or inflating a balloon, and these can be held in reserve until it becomes clear that they will be necessary.

Parent vessel angiograms may be performed intermittently as coiling proceeds to confirm obliteration of the aneurysm and rule out thromboembolic or hemorrhagic complications. In the case of PCOM aneurysms associated with a fetal-type posterior communicating artery, intermittent angiograms can be used to monitor the position of the coil mass relative to the PCOM and prevent occlusion of this vessel. Once the aneurysm is satisfactorily occluded, the microcatheters are removed and a final angiogram is performed once more to examine the distal vessels for thrombus or other complications. If none are evident, the catheters and sheath can be removed and either a closure device placed or manual pressure held at the arteriotomy site.

Oral Boards Review—Management Pearls

1. Observation of intracranial aneurysms is a mainstay of aneurysm treatment. Follow-up imaging is most helpful if the following apply:
   a. The imaging modality is uniform, usually CTA, so that accurate comparisons can be made.
   b. The follow-up interval is short initially (and extends over time).
   c. There is a conceivable trigger for ending observation and proceeding with treatment (i.e., no follow-up is needed if the aneurysm would never be treated, although the surgeon may consider referral to another surgeon if he or she is not comfortable treating an aneurysm).
2. Endovascular therapy is effective and has a lower rate of short-term significant morbidity compared to clipping. However, coiling is frequently less durable than surgical clipping with respect to aneurysm recurrence. More durable results are obtained with stent-assisted coiling or flow diversion; however, these are less useful for ruptured aneurysms because they necessitate the use of dual antiplatelet therapy.
3. There is evidence that ONP from PCOM aneurysms is more likely to resolve with surgical clipping rather than endovascular treatment, but the data are not high-quality.
4. Smoking cessation and control of hypertension are important modifiable medical risk factors for aneurysm enlargement and rupture.
5. Many patients present with SAH and multiple intracranial aneurysms. The pattern of hemorrhage, aneurysm morphology, and the presence of localizable neurological deficits should be used to identify the ruptured aneurysm, and therapy should focus on this aneurysm. Therapeutic hypertension is safe after securing the ruptured aneurysm, even in the face of multiple untreated aneurysms.

Pivot Points

1. Aneurysm enlargement, change in morphology, sentinel headache, and development of a neurological deficit are all signs that should trigger consideration of treatment of a previously observed aneurysm.
2. For patients with aneurysmal SAH, emergent treatment should be pursued in any salvageable patient with history concerning for rebleeding (e.g., development of new or worsening neurological deficit not attributable to hydrocephalus; recurrent severe headache similar to the presenting ictus; and new hemorrhage from ventriculostomy). Other SAH patients can be managed urgently, usually within 24 hours of presentation.

3. The decision between endovascular and open surgical treatment of an aneurysm should hinge on surgeon comfort; however, in the case of mass lesions such as subdural or intraparenchymal hemorrhage with evidence of herniation, emergent surgical decompression is mandatory. Preparations should be made to clip the aneurysm at the same time, although occasionally decompression can be achieved without disturbing the aneurysm, and endovascular therapies can be considered postoperatively.

Aftercare

Patients having undergone aneurysm clipping are generally observed in the intensive care unit (ICU) at least overnight. In the case of SAH patients, ICU stays are significantly longer because patients are observed for delayed cerebral ischemia. Patients who develop recalcitrant vasospasm despite aggressive medical measures such as induced hypertension or who cannot tolerate aggressive medical therapy may benefit from endovascular therapy for treatment of their vasospasm.

Repeat imaging should be obtained 6 months after aneurysm treatment to assess for early recanalization, with serial imaging follow-up thereafter. In the case of clipped aneurysms, imaging follow-up is in the form of CTA or catheter angiography, due to clip-related artifact on MRI. For coiled aneurysms, metallic streak artifact on CT generally precludes accurate appraisal of the aneurysm and may obscure other portions of the circle of Willis; therefore, catheter angiography or MRA is used.

Complications and Management

Complications of aneurysm treatment include ischemic stroke and aneurysm re-rupture. Inadvertent injury or temporary or permanent clipping of the anterior choroidal artery, which is distal to the posterior communicating artery, can result in contralateral hemiplegia, hemianesthesia, and hemianopsia secondary to infarction of the genu and posterior limb of the internal capsule, as well as the lateral geniculate nucleus of the thalamus. The use of neurophysiologic monitoring may alert the surgeon to this complication, as ischemia in the internal capsule can be detected. In addition, intraoperative indocyanine green angiography, micro-Doppler ultrasonography, and catheter angiography can all be used to confirm the patency of the anterior choroidal artery during surgery.

Intraoperative rupture can complicate both surgical and endovascular aneurysm treatment. In general, judicious use of temporary clip occlusion, obtaining both proximal and distal control, prevents or mitigates this complication. If rupture occurs prior to temporary clip placement, a large-bore emergency suction should be introduced into the field immediately for vessel visualization (this should always be made available at the beginning of the operation). Temporary clips can then be placed to improve visualization, or a permanent clip can be placed without temporary clipping to obtain immediate hemostasis if suction provides sufficient visualization. Caution should be taken, however, because clips placed this way are less likely to completely occlude the aneurysm and more likely to incorporate adjacent vessels or the oculomotor nerve, resulting in postoperative ONP. If intraoperative rupture occurs during placement of the permanent clip, the clip blades should be allowed to close and the aneurysm complex can be inspected after placement of the clip to confirm placement. In the event of intraoperative catastrophe, such as avulsion of the aneurysm from the ICA, clip ligation and distal vessel bypass can be performed. Cross-matched blood products should be available prior to any attempted clipping.

Intraprocedural aneurysm rupture during endovascular aneurysm treatment can be avoided by careful placement of the coiling microcatheter in the mid-position of the aneurysm dome prior to coiling to prevent coil herniation through the fragile aneurysm wall. Selection of coil sizes with diameters approximately the same size as the average diameter of the aneurysm dome will also prevent coil-related rupture. Should intraprocedural rupture occur, heparin should be immediately reversed with intravenous protamine infusion. If a balloon microcatheter is in place, it should be inflated across the aneurysm neck to temporarily halt blood flow into the aneurysm and permit further coil embolization. Should the rupture continue despite coiling due to injury of the aneurysm neck or parent vessel, then parent vessel sacrifice must be performed.

Antiepileptic drugs can be used prophylactically prior to any intradural procedure. In the case of aneurysm clipping, especially ruptured aneurysms, postoperative seizures can result in significant morbidity. The incidence of nonconvulsive status epilepticus in ruptured aneurysm patients is sufficiently high to warrant liberal use of electroencephalogram monitoring for patients who do not return to their neurological baseline rapidly following emergence from anesthesia and who do not have a postoperative mass lesion or stroke on CT or MRI. However, long-term prophylactic antiepileptic medication use in patients with ruptured aneurysms without seizures should be avoided.

Further complications related to SAH include delayed cerebral ischemic deficits, hydrocephalus, respiratory failure, cardiomyopathy, systemic infections, and thromboembolic complications such as deep venous thrombosis and pulmonary embolus (especially in patients receiving aminocaproic acid). These are best managed with the assistance of a multidisciplinary ICU team including neurosurgeons, intensivists, and neurologists, if needed.

Oral Boards Review—Complications Pearls

1. Intraoperative rupture should be avoided at all costs. Should intraoperative rupture occur, rapid tamponade with suction and a cotton patty can usually control aneurysmal bleeding and permit temporary parent vessel clipping or permanent aneurysm clipping.
2. Care should be taken to avoid undue retraction on the temporal lobe during sylvian fissure dissection, especially in ruptured aneurysm cases, to avoid avulsing an aneurysm that is stuck to the temporal lobe.
3. The use of neurophysiological monitoring (somatosensory and motor evoked potentials) can alert the surgeon to ischemic complications during aneurysm clipping, and changes should prompt immediate evaluation of parent and daughter vessels with possible revision of the aneurysm clip(s).

Evidence and Outcomes

The outcomes from both open surgical and endovascular treatment of unruptured aneurysms are good. ISUIA data indicate that the overall risk of death or significant disability (modified Rankin >3 or impaired cognition) for open clipping is approximately 10% at 1 year; endovascular treatments are slightly safer. These rates are lower for anterior circulation aneurysms than for posterior circulation aneurysms and generally are better for younger patients with smaller aneurysms. Data obtained from the United States National Inpatient Sample Database demonstrate a benefit to treatment of unruptured aneurysms using clipping for patients up to age 70 years and for coiling up to age 81 years. Outcomes for ruptured aneurysms are closely tied to the patient's clinical status on presentation. Long-term follow-up data from the International Subarachnoid Aneurysm Trial indicate that clipping and coiling are equivalent in this population, although short-term data do favor endovascular therapy with respect to mortality.

Further Reading

Gaberel T, Borha A, di Palma C, Emery E. Clipping versus coiling in the management of posterior communicating artery aneurysms with third nerve palsy: A systematic review and meta-analysis. *World Neurosurg.* 2016;87:498–506.

Lawson MF, Neal DW, Mocco J, Hoh BL. Rationale for treating unruptured intracranial aneurysms: Actuarial analysis of natural history risk versus treatment risk for coiling or clipping based on 14,050 patients in the National Inpatient Sample Database. *World Neurosurg.* 2013;79:472–478.

Molyneux A, Kerr R, Stratton I, et al. for the ISAT Collaborative Group. International Subarachnoid Aneurysm Trial (ISAT) of neurosurgical clipping versus endovascular coiling in 2,143 patients with ruptured intracranial aneurysms: A randomized trial. *J Stroke Cerebrovasc Dis.* 2002;11(6):304–314.

Morita A, Kirino T, Hashi K, et al. for the UCAS Japan Investigators. The natural course of unruptured cerebral aneurysms in a Japanese cohort. *N Engl J Med.* 2012;366(26):2474–2482.

Wiebers DO, Whisnant JP, Huston J, et al. Unruptured intracranial aneurysms: Natural history, clinical outcome, and risks of surgical and endovascular treatment. *Lancet.* 2003;362(9378):103–110.

Zheng F, Dong Y, Xia P, et al. Is clipping better than coiling in the treatment of patients with oculomotor nerve palsies induced by posterior communicating artery aneurysms? A systematic review and meta-analysis. *Clin Neurol Neurosurg.* 2017;153:20–26.

Incidental Anterior Communicating Artery Aneurysm

Kurt Yaeger and J. Mocco

4

Case Presentations

Case A is a 45 year-old female with no significant past medical history other than chronic headaches. A magnetic resonance imaging (MRI) scan obtained for the headaches showed what the radiologist interpreted to be an abnormality in the anterior communicating artery (ACoA). On further vascular imaging, there appeared to be a 7-mm saccular aneurysm arising from the ACoA. Aside from intermittent headaches, the patient is neurologically intact on exam, without any functional deficits. On further probing, she acknowledges that her sister died several years ago from a stroke, although she does not know further details.

Case B is a 68 year-old male with hypertension and coronary artery disease, requiring coronary artery stenting several years prior, but still on daily aspirin. Two weeks ago, he was brought to the emergency room after an episode of confusion, and his workup found an unruptured ACoA aneurysm measuring 7 mm. After his symptoms improved with intravenous hydration, he was discharged with plans for outpatient follow-up. On neurological exam, he has no deficits.

Questions

1. What is the next step in the workup?
2. What is the appropriate timing of the workup?
3. What are the potential treatment options for these patients?
4. Are there any precautions these patients should take prior to undergoing treatment?
5. Are there any indications for emergent treatment in these patients?

Assessment and Planning

The global prevalence of unruptured aneurysms is approximately 3.2%. In general, risk factors for aneurysm formation include female gender, older age, family history, and smoking history. Risk factors for aneurysm rupture include aneurysm size (>7–10 mm), location (posterior circulation), prior aneurysm rupture, interval aneurysm growth, female gender, hypertension, and smoking status. According to the International Study of Unruptured Intracranial Aneurysms study, published in 2003, the 5-year cumulative rupture rate for patients with anterior circulation aneurysms was 0%, 2.6%, 14.5%, and 40% for aneurysms sized <7, 7–12, 13–24, and ≥25 mm, respectively.

For patients with unruptured, incidental ACoA aneurysms, it is imperative to better understand their overall risk of rupture prior to making treatment decisions. A focused history is required, including discussion on modifiable risk factors. Subsequently, a diagnostic cerebral angiogram should be performed to better quantify aneurysm size, location, and morphology. This can be performed electively as long as there is no suspicion for previous rupture (e.g., neurological deficit or the presence of stereotypical thunderclap headache).

Oral Boards Review—Diagnostic Pearls

1. Not all aneurysms rupture. It is important to risk stratify prior to offering treatment to patients with incidental, unruptured ACoA aneurysms. High-risk features include size ≥7 mm, previous rupture, interval growth, female gender, hypertension, and smoking.
2. For patients with an extra-axial mass of the anterior skull base or near the internal carotid artery on noncontrast-enhanced imaging, consider aneurysm on the differential diagnosis, and obtain noninvasive vascular imaging.
3. For patients with a newly diagnosed aneurysm on noninvasive vascular imaging, a diagnostic cerebral angiogram is highly recommended, especially for young patients or those at high risk of rupture.
4. Diagnostic angiography should be used to quantify aneurysm size and morphology, assess blood flow around the aneurysm, and observe its anatomical relationship relative to proximal and distal vessels and perforator arteries. Aneurysmal dome projection should be used to guide a safe treatment approach.
5. Both clinical and radiographic features should be used to determine ultimate treatment modality.

Unruptured intracranial aneurysms are not typically diagnosed on noncontrast-enhanced imaging such as computed tomography (CT) or MRI. If large enough, they may appear as an extra-axial, hypodense mass on CT or a hypointense flow void on MRI. If the suspicion for aneurysm is high, noninvasive vascular imaging can be performed (CT or MR angiogram). These modalities will typically show an aneurysmal outpouching in the region of the ACoA, and gross estimates of size and morphology can be made. However, the gold standard diagnostic modality is cerebral angiography because it has the highest imaging quality and provides temporal resolution with circulatory flow. Cerebral angiography should be considered in patients in whom treatment is being considered or who have risk factors for aneurysm growth or rupture.

When performing a diagnostic cerebral angiogram for a patient with an ACoA aneurysm, it is essential to document several specific features to facilitate future decision-making. First, perform accurate aneurysm measurements in all three planes. Include

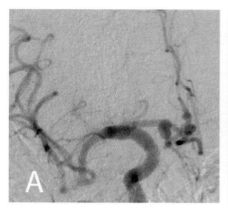
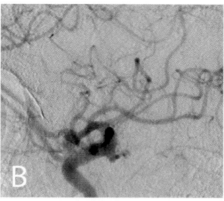
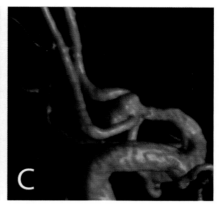

Figure 4.1 Case A was found to have an incidental ACoA aneurysm on noninvasive vascular imaging performed for chronic headaches. She subsequently underwent diagnostic cerebral angiogram, anteroposterior (A) and lateral (B), which showed a 7-mm wide-neck saccular aneurysm with anteriorly projecting dome. (C) A three-dimensional reconstruction shows the aneurysm in relation to the proximal A1 and distal bilateral A2 ACA segments.

measurements of the neck width, the maximal diameter, and the caliber of the ACoA artery and bilateral A1 and A2 segments. This information can be used to assess feasibility of either endovascular or microsurgical treatment modalities. Calculating the dome-to-neck ratio (greatest width ÷ neck width) or aspect ratio (maximal height ÷ neck width) can provide insight on whether the aneurysm can be coil embolized (with or without balloon or stent assistance) or if it requires microsurgical clipping.

Second, determine the aneurysm morphology in three dimensions. Does it have high-risk features such as a daughter sac or multiple lobes? Assess the relationship of the distal A2 segments as they transition from the A1 segments. Ensure that there are no vessels originating from the aneurysm dome. Importantly, determine the optimal anatomical approach corridor for either clipping or coiling. The trajectory of the aneurysm dome is the traditional target. For example, if the dome projects laterally to the right, the surgeon may decide to perform a right-sided craniotomy, whereas the interventionalist may approach the aneurysm from the left ACA to access the ostium.

Third, assess the vascular anatomy around the aneurysm. Observe the bilateral anterior cerebral artery (ACA) complexes. Are there two A1 and two A2 segments? Is there an azygous ACA? Determine the likely location of essential perforating arteries (i.e., bilateral arteries of Heubner and lenticulostriate arteries). Obtaining a global understanding of the vascular relationships is essential in both clipping and coiling the ACoA aneurysm.

As the next step in the workup, both patients undergo diagnostic cerebral angiography. The angiogram for Case A shows a 7-mm saccular aneurysm in the mid ACoA (Figure 4.1). The right A1 segment appears to be dominant, and the dome projects anteriorly. The angiogram for Case B shows a 7-mm saccular aneurysm, fed predominantly from the left A1 segment (Figure 4.2). The aneurysm dome projects superiorly.

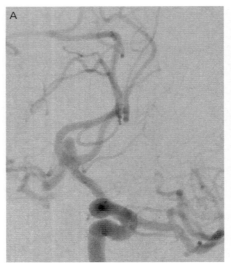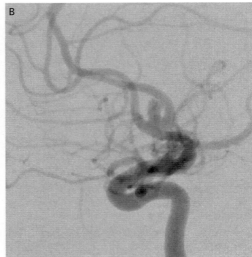

Figure 4.2 Case B was found to have an unruptured ACoA aneurysm after workup for confusion. He underwent diagnostic cerebral angiogram, anteroposterior (A) and lateral (B), which show a 6.9-mm wide-neck aneurysm with a superiorly projecting dome.

Questions

1. When deciding treatment modality options, what are the important clinical considerations?
2. When planning the treatment approach, what are some important anatomical considerations?
3. What is the appropriate timing for treatment?
4. How should patients with low-risk aneurysms be managed?

Decision-Making

Categorically, there are three management options for patients with ACoA aneurysms: microsurgical, endovascular, and observational. The decision should be determined based on clinical history, imaging characteristics, and, ultimately, patient preference. Although surgical clipping had long been the standard curative treatment modality, the development of endovascular techniques prompted a debate between surgeons and interventionalists on the efficacy and safety of the different options. However, several conclusions can be made from the existing body of published literature. Generally, microsurgical techniques are associated with improved rates of aneurysm occlusion on long-term follow-up but are associated with higher short-term (periprocedural) morbidity. In contrast, endovascular techniques are lower risk procedures but are associated with higher rates of incomplete occlusion and aneurysm recurrence. For both treatment options, long-term functional outcomes are comparable.

Given this trade-off between procedural morbidity and occlusion rates, the patient's clinical history is essential in determining options. Younger, healthy patients may prefer the curative option with microsurgical clipping. Older patients or those with comorbid conditions may not be surgical candidates; therefore, endovascular coiling may be ideal.

In patients for whom either treatment option is viable, aneurysm anatomical characteristics may ultimately determine treatment strategy. For example, a large ACoA aneurysm with a small neck may perfectly accommodate endovascular coils for complete occlusion. However, a smaller wide-neck aneurysm may not be able to hold coils without prolapse; therefore, surgical clipping may be preferred. This decision is ultimately made by the operating surgeon or interventionalist, drawing upon previous experience and comfort level.

Last, expectant management is reasonable for some patients with an ACoA aneurysm and low-risk features, including small size (<7 mm) and lack of growth on interval imaging. After size and morphological stability are proven on a subsequent cerebral angiogram, annual or semi-annual noninvasive vascular imaging (magnetic resonance angiography [MRA]) can be used in further long-term follow-up.

As with any treatment decision, the patient should be advised on the risks, benefits, and alternatives to all treatment options, including observation. Given these competing modalities, patient input is essential in determining a final treatment strategy. There is a balance between short-term (procedural) and long-term (residual aneurysm) risks, and it is up to the individual patient to decide his or her tolerance to these risks.

After a complete discussion of all treatment options, Case A decided to undergo surgery for microsurgical aneurysm clipping, whereas Case B decided to pursue endovascular coiling of his ACoA aneurysm.

Questions

1. Why is Case A a better candidate for surgical clipping?
2. Why is Case B a better candidate for endovascular coiling?
3. What are the risks of surgical clipping?
4. What are the risks of endovascular coiling?

Surgical Procedures

Microsurgical Technique

The patient is brought to the operating room and induced under general anesthesia. Clipping of ACoA aneurysms is typically performed via a pterional craniotomy. As such, the patient is positioned supine with head turned 15–20 degrees in approximately 20 degree extension. This positioning allows the frontal lobes to fall away from the anterior cranial fossa and the sylvian fissure to be positioned vertically, such that the frontal and temporal separate with gravity during dissection. Neuromonitoring (somatosensory evoked potential [SSEP], electroencephalogram [EEG], and motor evoked potential [MEP]) can be used to detect any early ischemic changes due to inadvertent vessel compromise. Laterality of craniotomy is determined by ACA dominance. If the vessels are symmetric, a right-sided approach can avoid unnecessary complications in the dominant hemisphere and may be easier for a right-handed surgeon. If the vessels are asymmetric, the craniotomy should be performed on the dominant side so as to have immediate access to proximal control, the aneurysm dome, and vital perforators.

After dural opening, the sylvian fissure is dissected, and the frontal and temporal lobes are retracted to enable visualization of the opticocarotid cistern. The bilateral A1 and A2 segments are dissected and skeletonized to ensure proximal and distal vascular control in the case of intraoperative aneurysm rupture.

The aneurysm should then be dissected from the surrounding brain parenchyma and normal vasculature. Inspection of the proximate vessels on all sides of the aneurysm dome should be performed to prevent inadvertent clipping. Of note, exquisite care should be taken to identify the recurrent artery of Heubner, which supplies the ipsilateral caudate head and internal capsule. Occlusion of the artery of Heuber can cause contralateral hemiplegia and sensory loss, as well as expressive aphasia on the dominant side. Given the aneurysm size, an appropriate aneurysm clip should be selected and applied across the aneurysm neck. Again, inspection is performed to ensure the normal vasculature is not being affected by clip placement. Doppler again confirms flow in the bilateral A1 and A2 segments. In many cases, fluoroscopy with indocyanine green allows visual confirmation of aneurysm occlusion and parent vessel preservation. If necessary, other surgical techniques can be utilized, including aneurysm bypass, aneurysm wrapping, and ACoA sacrifice.

Once the aneurysm is properly secured, care should be taken to ensure complete hemostasis, dural closure, craniotomy plating, and skin closure. Provided there are no major intraoperative complications, the patient should be extubated and monitored postoperatively in an intensive care unit.

Case A undergoes a right-sided modified mini-pterional craniotomy and clipping of her ACoA aneurysm (Figures 4.3 and 4.4). The procedure is uncomplicated, and she recovers well postoperatively.

Endovascular Technique

The patient is brought to the angiography suite. The type of anesthesia depends on operator preference. Typically, the patient is intubated under general anesthesia to prevent movement during intervention. However, some cases can be performed with local anesthesia and monitored sedation. Similarly, the choice of vascular access is operator dependent. Traditionally, the approach is from the femoral artery; however, the radial artery can be used in patients with a tortuous aortic arch.

Once vascular access is obtained, a large-bore support catheter is navigated to the distal internal carotid artery. Initial, single-vessel angiographic runs are performed to establish the aneurysm baseline characteristics and optimal biplanar views, ideally providing clear visualization of the proximal and distal aneurysm neck. Laterality for intervention is determined by optimizing microcatheter placement in the aneurysm ostium, typically the dominant proximal A1. If the aneurysm is wide-necked or has an unfavorable neck-to-dome ratio, then a stent or balloon can be used to help prevent coil prolapse out of the aneurysm. Given the anatomy of the ACoA, aneurysms in this location typically have relatively wide necks, and balloon or stent assistance is frequently required. A microcatheter is then carefully navigated into the aneurysm. The first coil is partially deployed, and then, if necessary, the stent or balloon is deployed. Subsequently, embolic coils are deployed in sequence to fill the aneurysm. The first coil is usually a large, three-dimensional framing coil, such that subsequent smaller coils fall into place

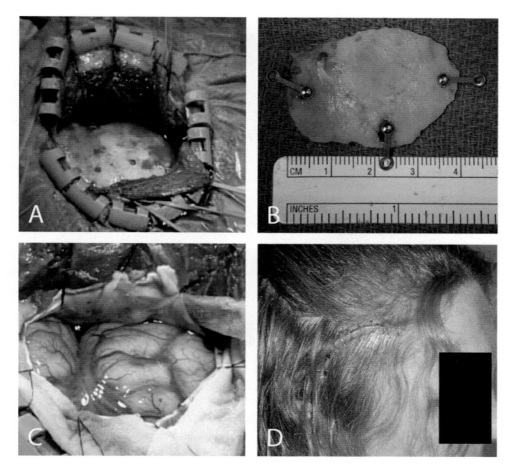

Figure 4.3 Case A underwent a right-sided modified pterional craniotomy for microsurgical clipping. (A and B) For this procedure, only a small skin incision and craniotomy are required. (C) After craniotomy and dural opening, the sylvian fissure is exposed and dissected. (D) The resulting exposure provides all that is necessary for ACoA aneurysm clipping, and it allows for faster recovery and improved cosmetic result.

within. Once completed, a final angiographic run is performed to confirm the degree of aneurysm occlusion and rule out vascular complications, such as distal vessel occlusion or vasospasm. The catheters are removed, and the access point is secured with manual compression or a closure device. The patient should be monitored postoperatively in an intensive care unit.

Case B undergoes endovascular treatment of his ACoA aneurysm. Given its wide neck, stent-assisted coiling is performed. He is started on dual antiplatelet therapy pre-procedurally. Given the location of the aneurysm ostium, the catheter is navigated from the left internal carotid artery. A stent is deployed from the right A2 to the left A1 (Figure 4.5A). Embolic coils are released into the aneurysm dome in succession. On final angiographic run, the aneurysm appears to be 95% occluded (Figures 4.5B and 4.5C). Postoperatively, he recovers well and is discharged home in stable condition.

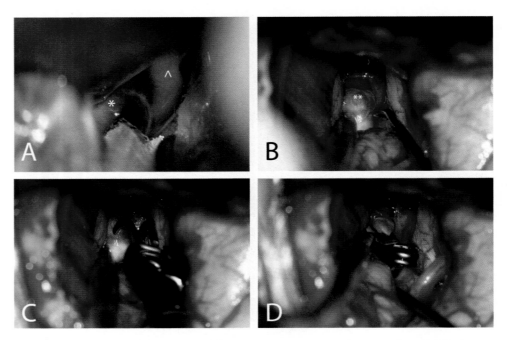

Figure 4.4 Intraoperative views of the Case A microsurgical approach and ACoA aneurysm clipping. (A) After modified mini-pterional craniotomy and sylvian fissure dissection, it is essential to identify the opticocarotid triangle. The ipsilateral carotid artery is denoted by the asterisk and the optic nerve by the caret symbol. (B) Careful microsurgical dissection exposes the ACoA aneurysm. (C) An aneurysm clip is advanced into position, ensuring no perforating vessels are entrapped. (D) After clipping, fastidious inspection of the aneurysm and collateral vessel ensures no occlusion or compression by aneurysm clip. Subsequently, Doppler and indocyanine green fluoroscopy can be performed to ensure appropriate collateral flow.

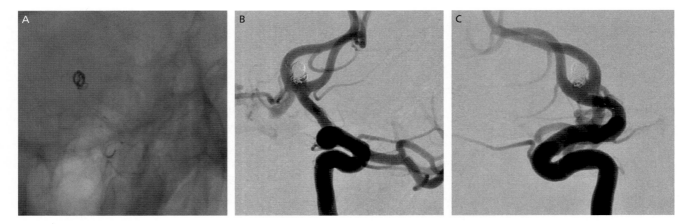

Figure 4.5 Case B underwent endovascular treatment of his ACoA aneurysm. Given the wide neck, the coil embolization required stent buttressing. (A) The stent was deployed from the left A1 into the right A2. After coiling, anteroposterior (B) and lateral (C) angiographic runs demonstrate 95% aneurysm occlusion.

Oral Boards Review—Management Pearls

1. Laterality of approach to an ACoA aneurysm, either surgical or endovascular, requires special consideration. Use preoperative imaging to envision the optimal clipping angle or microcatheter placement. Assess the recurrent blood supply to determine proximal and distal control.

2. In surgery, utilize multimodality, intraoperative monitoring to prevent compromise to distal vasculature. Obtain baseline SSEP, EEG, and MEP to which to compare during surgery. Use Doppler to assess collateral supply before and after clipping. Visually and fluoroscopically inspect the normal vasculature to ensure no arterial compromise.

3. Properly plan the endovascular strategy, including the need for balloon or stent assistance. Given the predisposition for ACoA aneurysms with wide necks, a balloon, stent, or both may be required. Have all the devices in the room, ready to deploy.

Pivot Points

1. Regardless of aneurysm size, morphology, or patient clinical status, if the patient experiences rupture of the aneurysm prior to elective treatment, the aneurysm must be emergently secured. Furthermore, if there is an intraparenchymal hematoma causing cerebral herniation, the patient must undergo emergent surgical decompression and likely concurrent aneurysm clipping.

2. If during the course of an endovascular treatment, all possibilities for intervention are exhausted (balloon, stenting, etc.), the patient must be considered for surgical treatment.

3. Even if an ACoA aneurysm is anatomically more suitable for clipping, patients with medical comorbidities that increase the risk of microsurgical treatment (e.g., cardiovascular problems, existing antiplatelet usage for cardiac stents, or systemic anticoagulation) should be considered first for endovascular aneurysm treatment.

Aftercare

Microsurgical Technique

For an uncomplicated craniotomy for ACoA aneurysm coiling, the patient should be observed in the intensive care unit overnight. Some practitioners favor a postoperative CT head to rule out insidious pathology, such as extra-axial hematoma or small subclinical infarct. An immediate postoperative angiogram can be considered but is not required, especially for straightforward surgeries in patients who remain at their neurological baseline. Given the typical length and invasiveness of the surgery, patients are typically discharged home 48–72 hours after admission.

Endovascular Technique

For an uncomplicated aneurysm coiling, the patient should be observed in the intensive care unit overnight. Given that a post-interventional angiographic run is obtained, there is no need for short-term follow-up imaging, as long as the patient remains at his or her neurologic baseline. Given the procedure's minimal invasiveness, the patient is typically discharged home the following day.

Follow-Up

All patients are seen in follow-up 2–4 weeks postoperatively to assess neurologic functioning and surgical/vascular access site. Subsequent diagnostic angiography is performed in delayed fashion, typically 6–12 months post-procedurally. If aneurysm occlusion remains stable on delayed angiography and there is no need for retreatment, further follow-up can be performed with noninvasive vascular imaging (CT angiography in the case of surgical clipping; MRA in the case of endovascular treatment). If there is residual aneurysm, further treatment can be considered in an elective manner. All patients should be further counseled on the risks of hemorrhage and to seek emergent medical attention if they experience signs or symptoms of aneurysmal rupture.

Complications and Management

Prior to reviewing the potential complications in treating ACoA aneurysms, it is essential to consider the neurological deficits commonly associated with this vascular territory. Proximal occlusions of the ipsilateral internal carotid artery or middle cerebral artery can cause hemiplegia, hemisensory loss, and aphasia when the dominant side is affected. Occlusion of the recurrent artery of Heubner can also cause a similar syndrome, although the stroke burden will appear much different on imaging. Ischemia of the distal ACA territory can cause abulia and isolated lower extremity weakness. Given the proximity of the bilateral ACA to the ACoA aneurysm, any focal deficit on neurological exam may be of concern.

Microsurgical Complications

The general risks of craniotomy include infection (from superficial skin to deep encephalitis) and bleeding (postoperative extra-axial hematoma). The management of these complications depends entirely on the patient's clinical status. Superficial infection may resolve with oral antibiotics, whereas a deep surgical site empyema may require re-exploration, washout, debridement, and long-term parenteral antibiotics. If the patient is neurologically stable with mild systemic signs of infection, a trial of antibiotics may be reasonable in both cases. However, with any neurological deterioration, surgical exploration should be strongly considered. Of important note, in the case of a deep infection, the vasculature may be friable, and any residual aneurysm may be prone to rupture. Management of a postoperative hematoma similarly depends on the patient's clinical status. Observation alone may be reasonable for small collections without mass effect in a patient at his or her neurological baseline. However, any deterioration in exam should prompt re-imaging or urgent re-exploration and decompression.

In craniotomy for clipping of ACoA aneurysm, several important considerations should be made with regard to unique complications. The first and most concerning complication is intraoperative aneurysmal rupture, in which the initial objective is to maintain visualization of the surgical field. This can be intensely difficult and often requires exchanging to a larger bore suction tip and flooding the field with saline. If possible, tamponade should be applied to the exact site or rupture, such that proximal and distal control can be obtained by applying temporary clips on the appropriate vessels. For an ACoA aneurysm, this may include bilateral A1 and A2 segments, the ipsilateral A1 and A2 and contralateral ACoA, or simply the ipsilateral A1 and A2, depending on aneurysm location along the ACoA. Once temporary clipping is applied, the aneurysm dome can be secured, and it can be subsequently tested by unclamping the proximal A1 segment. With no further hemorrhage, all temporary clips can be removed, and the procedure can proceed. If, however, no temporary clips can be applied, or rupture occurs prior to dissection of the collateral vessels, the rupture site should be isolated and clipped first, prior to clip application at the aneurysm neck.

Another complication specific to aneurysm clipping is inadvertent occlusion of normal vasculature by the clip. This can occur by either direct clipping or from external compression of the artery by the clip. The ischemic sequelae of this may be prevented by utilizing intraoperative monitoring (SSEP, EEG, and MEP) or by assessing post-clipping Doppler signal or fluoroscopic angiography. Unintended clipping of small perforating arteries may not be readily apparent intraoperatively.

In a patient with new neurological deficits postoperatively, emergent CT imaging should be obtained to rule out compressive hematoma or edema. CT angiogram can be performed to rapidly assess patency of large vessels or asymmetric hemispheric collaterals. However, cerebral angiography is the definitive study, able to assess patency, compression, or occlusion of ACA vessels and perforators. Furthermore, if something consequential is observed on angiography, treatment can be rapidly initiated. Vasospasm can be treated with angioplasty or intra-arterial infusion of a calcium channel blocker. Vessel thrombi can be aspirated or treated with intra-arterial fibrinolytic agents. However, if aneurysm clip placement is limiting distal flow, ultimately it may be required to return to the operating room for clip repositioning. Finally, if no causative factor is found on workup, empiric treatment with blood pressure augmentation may improve perfusion to ischemic regions.

Endovascular Complications

The general risks of angiography include access site complications (deep hematoma, compartment hemorrhage, and superficial infection), arterial dissection, and occlusion. Complication management depends on its impact on patient functioning and neurologic status. Clinical observation is reasonable for small groin hematomas and small femoral artery dissections. However, large access site hematomas, especially with continued hemorrhage into the thigh or intra-abdominal compartment, may require fibrin glue injection or covered stent placement at the site of arteriotomy. A cervical or cerebral arterial dissection can be treated with antiplatelet therapy, provided it is non-flow-limiting. However, flow-limiting or symptomatic dissections may necessitate stent placement.

Risks specific to interventional procedures for ACoA aneurysms include intraoperative aneurysm perforation, vasospasm, and distal vessel occlusion. Iatrogenic aneurysm rupture may occur with guidewire navigation or coil deployment into the aneurysm. Angiographically, this appears as contrast extravasation from the aneurysm dome into the subarachnoid space. In this circumstance, a balloon catheter must immediately be inflated over the aneurysm ostium to prevent massive subarachnoid hemorrhage. With the balloon inflated, the aneurysm rupture point should be rapidly secured with embolic coils. Aneurysm status is intermittently assessed by deflating the balloon and performing an angiographic run to observe further contrast extravasation. When secured, the procedure can proceed. However, if the rupture point cannot be secured, open craniotomy and aneurysm clipping may need to be considered, especially for cases with large subarachnoid hemorrhage and compressive hematoma.

Spontaneous vasospasm typically occurs in younger, female patients and affects areas in frequent contact with catheters. Typically, this does not require intervention. However, if the vasospasm is flow-limiting, then intra-arterial calcium channel blockers can be injected; if it is severe and pharmacologically refractory, balloon angioplasty can be considered.

Distal vessel occlusions are typically due to stasis around a catheter, guidewire, or balloon. An angiographic run is typically performed at the end of the procedure to rule out territorial perfusion deficits or vessel occlusion. However, if visualized, thrombectomy may be required for revascularization. Similarly, parent vessel occlusion can be caused from thrombus formation at the coil–vessel interface or by herniation of coils into the parent vessel. Thrombus formation may be addressed by further heparinization or administration of antiplatelet agents such as abciximab or eptifibatide. Mechanical obstruction of the parent vessel by coil loops may require removal of the coil (if it has not yet been detached), balloon remodeling, or stent placement.

Oral Boards Review—Complications Pearls

1. It is important to recognize subtle neurological changes postoperatively, such that rapid imaging can be obtained and potential reversible neurological deficits can be identified. For ACoA aneurysms, mild mental status change or onset of abulia should not be neglected.
2. The variety of complications depends on choice of treatment modality. Overall rates of surgical risks are higher than those of endovascular therapy, but both modalities can have devastating consequence.
3. Complication prevention with a fastidious surgical technique is of utmost importance.

Evidence and Outcomes

As the literature suggests, outcomes after elective treatment for incidental, unruptured intracranial aneurysms are good. A meta-analysis of studies assessing patients with incidental aneurysms treated with either clipping or coiling observed complete or near-complete occlusion rates of 95% and 82%, respectively; disability rates (modified Rankin

Scale ≥3) of 8% and 5%, respectively; and mortality rates of 1% for both modalities. However, there was no significant difference between any outcome measures between clipping and coiling. Similar results have been observed in recent direct head-to-head randomized trials.

As the neurointerventional field advances, both in technique and in device armamentarium, aneurysm occlusion rates continue to improve. However, a multimodal approach to care is required for all patients with intracranial aneurysms. It is therefore essential to be well versed in all treatment options, both surgical and endovascular, and recognize the benefits and limitations of each.

Further Reading

Brown RD Jr, Broderick JP. Unruptured intracranial aneurysms: Epidemiology, natural history, management options, and familial screening. *Lancet Neurol.* 2014;13(4):393–404.

Cai W, Hu C, Gong J, Lan Q. Anterior communicating artery aneurysm morphology and the risk of rupture. *World Neurosurg.* 2018;109:119–126.

Fang S, Brinjikji W, Murad MH, Kallmes DF, Cloft HJ, Lanzino G. Endovascular treatment of anterior communicating artery aneurysms: A systematic review and meta-analysis. *AJNR Am J Neuroradiol.* 2014;35(5):943–947.

Hernesniemi J, Dashti R, Lehecka M, et al. Microneurosurgical management of anterior communicating artery aneurysms. *Surg Neurol.* 2008;70(1):8–29.

O'Neill AH, Chandra RV, Lai LT. Safety and effectiveness of microsurgical clipping, endovascular coiling, and stent assisted coiling for unruptured anterior communicating artery aneurysms: A systematic analysis of observational studies. *J Neurointerv Surg.* 2017;9(8):761–765.

Ruan C, Long H, Sun H, et al. Endovascular coiling vs. surgical clipping for unruptured intracranial aneurysm: A meta-analysis. *Br J Neurosurg.* 2015;29(4):485–492.

Wiebers DO, Whisnant JP, Huston J 3rd, et al.; International Study of Unruptured Intracranial Aneurysms Investigators. Unruptured intracranial aneurysms: Natural history, clinical outcome, and risks of surgical and endovascular treatment. *Lancet.* 2003;362(9378):103–110.

Ruptured Anterior Communicating Artery Aneurysm

*E. Sander Connolly, Jr., Sean D. Lavine, Grace K. Mandigo,
Dorothea Altschul, Ahsan Satar, Robert A. Solomon, and
Philip M. Meyers*

5

Case Presentation

A 58-year-old right-handed female with past medical history notable for hypertension, non–insulin-dependent diabetes mellitus, and diverticular disease with recurrent lower gastrointestinal (GI) tract bleeding requiring transfusion presented with the worst headache of her life followed by lethargy and confusion. Neurological assessment was remarkable for intact cranial nerves, normal motor and sensory exam but orientation only to self, and somnolence. The patient underwent noncontrast computed tomography (CT) of the brain followed immediately thereafter by CT angiography (CTA). CT (Figure 5.1A) showed Fisher grade 4 subarachnoid hemorrhage (SAH), and the CTA demonstrated a 2.5-mm anterior communicating artery (ACoA) aneurysm pointing up into the hemorrhage cavity and filling preferentially from the left anterior cerebral artery A1 segment (Figures 5.1B–5.1D).

Questions

1. What are the presenting clinical symptoms of patients with ruptured cerebral aneurysms?
2. When is CTA sufficient for acute management of patients with aneurysmal SAH?
3. What additional benefits does digital subtraction catheter angiography provide?

Assessment and Planning

Given the small size of the aneurysm and the patient's previous GI bleeding (a relative contraindication to long-term antiplatelet use should a stent be required), it was believed that this aneurysm was best repaired via a microsurgical approach. Small aneurysms pose an increased endovascular treatment risk, especially in the ruptured setting. The very small landing zone for even ultrasoft coils, and the unfavorable neck-to-dome ratio is

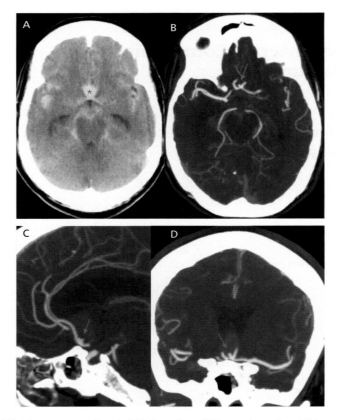

Figure 5.1 (A) Noncontrast head CT showing diffuse subarachnoid hemorrhage with focal clot in the inner hemispheric fissure (asterisk) just above the ACoA complex. (B–D) CTA (B, axial; C, magnified sagittal; and D, coronal) demonstrates a 2.5-mm ACoA aneurysm projecting superiorly to the right side with mild early hydrocephalus (arrows).

associated with a higher intraoperative rupture rate and a lower complete obliteration rate often requiring re-treatment with stent assistance. In this case, the need for a stent would be problematic given the history of recurrent symptomatic GI bleeding. Because clipping was deemed to be reasonable from a technical perspective, a decision was made to proceed to the operating room without a diagnostic digital subtraction angiogram (DSA). Although it is widely recognized that CTA is less sensitive than DSA, which remains the gold standard, it is also generally accepted that when the CTA is high quality and the aneurysm discovered is associated with a clot cavity, CTA alone is a reasonable course of management.

Questions

1. From what side does one generally approach a ruptured ACoA aneurysm and why?
2. What type of anterior cranial fossa craniotomy is best for which type of ACoA aneurysm?

Decision-Making

Ruptured aneurysms have a high risk for repeat hemorrhage and require urgent treatment. Currently, the treatments of choice for ruptured ACoA aneurysm are either microsurgical clipping or endovascular occlusion with coils, stents, or both. Surgery is generally associated with more definitive occlusion and a comparable risk of stroke and death, but this depends on institutional factors including surgeon experience. If intracranial pressure might be improved by removal of an associated hemorrhage, this would also favor microsurgery. Endovascular approaches have many advantages, especially when surgery is risky. Examples include a large superiorly and posteriorly projected ACoA aneurysm that is associated with a poor grade clinical status in an elderly patient and ruptured blister aneurysms in which clipping presents a higher incidence of intraoperative rupture.

Questions:

1. Which ACoA aneurysm is most difficult for microsurgical clipping?
2. What are some relative benefits to microsurgical clipping of ruptured ACoA aneurysms compared to endovascular coiling?
3. When is clipping most likely to result in a catastrophic disintegration of the parent artery?

Surgical Procedure

Plans were therefore made for a left frontal craniotomy via pterional incision for clipping of the aneurysm. This is a modification of the standard pterional craniotomy in that the sphenoid wing is not removed and the temporalis muscle is exposed but not taken down, providing cosmetic benefits and less postoperative pain. It is appropriate for a small aneurysm where a temporal angle to the lesion is not needed. With this approach, cerebrospinal fluid (CSF) drainage is essential in the setting of SAH because early access to the cisterns and fissures without retraction is compromised. Some have advocated this approach through an eyebrow incision, but we prefer to use the standard incision with exposure of the temporalis beneath the deep fascia as is done for an orbitozygomatic craniotomy for two reasons. First, it protects the frontalis branch of the facial nerve and keeps the incision in the hair, which if done in a hair-sparing manner is cosmetically superior. Second, should brain swelling become problematic, the larger incision permits expansion of the craniotomy.

The patient is placed in the supine position with head extended to facilitate brain retraction by gravity and placed in pins. To obtain CSF drainage and brain relaxation, a lumbar drain or ventriculostomy is placed preoperatively. Neuromonitoring such as somatosensory and motor evoked potentials may be used.

With the skin flap raised, the craniotomy is fashioned to avoid the left frontal sinus. This can be defined using neuronavigation or simply estimated in the case of a small sinus. A craniotomy is created, and the dura is opened in a C-shaped fashion, reflected inferiorly, and held in place with 4–0 silk suture. Under the operative microscope, the frontal lobe is retracted laterally to gain a view of the sylvian fissure. An arachnoid knife and microscissors are used to release the frontal lobe and drain additional CSF. As the dissection proceeds, the internal carotid artery and A1 are identified and prepared for temporary clipping. The olfactory nerve and optic nerve are identified, and the gyrus rectus is resected to expose the entire length of the A1 and protect the recurrent artery of Heubner. Once the ipsilateral left A1–A2 junction is identified, an arachnoid knife is used to open the most inferior frontal part of the inner hemispheric fissure and complete the gyrus rectus removal. The contralateral A1 is then identified along with the proximal neck of the aneurysm. The contralateral A1 is prepared for a temporary clipping as well. If there is substantial intraparenchymal or subarachnoid hematoma, it can be removed in a manner as to not disturb the aneurysm dome, until the contralateral A2 is identified. With both A1s and both A2s now dissected, and the ipsilateral artery of Hubner protected, the plane connecting the superior aspect of both A2s and the anterior communicating artery is dissected. The ipsilateral proximal A2 must be completely freed from the aneurysm prior to clipping.

In the current case, it was evident that the small aneurysm's neck involved the top two-thirds of the circumference of the communicator and proximal left A2. This was reconstructed using a pair of fenestrated clips with the ipsilateral A2 transmitted by fenestration. It is important to ensure the posterior clip blades close in front of the posteriorly directed contralateral A2. Doppler ultrasound is used to confirm parent and daughter vessel patency, and intraoperative indocyanine green videoangiography or DSA can be used for further confirmation of the repair (Figure 5.2). The craniotomy is then closed and the patient transferred to the intensive care unit for further management.

Oral Boards Review—Management Pearls

1. A detailed understanding of the anatomy is important for surgical planning.
   a. Most ACoA aneurysms can be approached via a standard pterional craniotomy. If this craniotomy is sizable and the patient's head is extended, this approach can help facilitate exposure with minimal or no retraction, especially if a lumbar or ventricular drain is used and the gyrus rectus is resected.
   b. Small aneurysms can also be approached via a mini-frontal craniotomy, but brain edema after SAH may limit exposure.

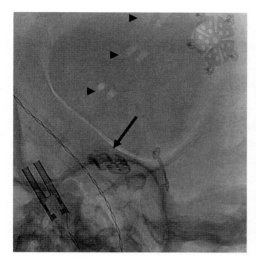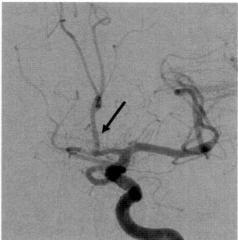

Figure 5.2 (A) Intraoperative left internal carotid angiogram showing the frontal craniotomy and the two fenestrated aneurysm clips (arrow); note the three paired cuts in the flap used to suspend the temporalis muscle beneath the fascia (arrowheads). (B) Digital subtraction angiogram showing the lack of aneurysm residual and preserved flow in the ipsilateral A2 (arrow).

> c. Aneurysms that are quite high might benefit from a more inferior to superior trajectory, which can be obtained via removal of the orbital rim.
> 2. Surgical clipping of wide-necked ACoA aneurysms often requires a fenestrated clip repair to avoid aneurysm recurrence and parent vessel compromise.

Pivot Points

1. If the aneurysm is superiorly directed and larger sized, endovascular coiling should be considered.
2. Ruptured anterior communicating artery aneurysms are generally approached from the side of the dominant A1 in order to obtain early proximal control. However, in situations of equal-sized A1s, most right-handed surgeons prefer a right-sided approach.
3. If the hemorrhage is associated with a large intraparenchymal hematoma, a longer course of anti-seizure medication is recommended.

Aftercare

The aftercare of aneurysmal SAH is quite complicated, and a complete review can be found in the published literature. Briefly, observation in the intensive care unit for 10–14 days is typical, with careful monitoring for vasospasm, hydrocephalus, and electrolyte disturbances.

Complications and Management

Intraoperative Surgical Complications and Management

The most common complications that occur and require specific maneuvers to avoid include retraction injury, premature aneurysm rupture (during either neck dissection or clip placement), vessel compromise due to clip construct impingement, subdural or epidural hematoma, and insufficient management of intracranial pressure. Retraction injury is best avoided by the judicious use of fixed retractors and the avoidance of their use whenever possible. These retractors should be moved as frequently as possible and placed after intracranial pressure has been reduced by cranial decompression, CSF drainage, anesthetic maneuvers, or some combination thereof. Retractors should be placed to avoid direct compression of cortical vessels (arteries and veins) when possible and to avoid stretching or kinking of these vessels. Premature aneurysm rupture, which occurs between the time of anesthetic induction and before the final exposure of the aneurysm, may be the result of unintended elevations in blood pressure or brain shift that disturbs an unstable aneurysm thrombus. If premature aneurysm rupture occurs, increasing anesthetic depth with neuroprotective agents followed by proximal vessel control and, if possible, distal vessel control will aid identification of the bleeding site, which can often be tamponaded prior to definitive and safe reconstruction. In general, blind clipping should be avoided except in the most extreme circumstances because this may lead to unrecoverable vessel injury. Adenosine arrest can also be used, but this is generally most effective with intact aneurysms where proximal control or trapping with suction decompression is difficult. Rupture of the aneurysm during dissection of the neck or placement of the clip is best avoided by avoiding the rupture site if obvious; full release of adherent tissues including small unimportant arteries; and, if possible, full release of the aneurysm dome. When freeing adherent vessels for preservation, temporary occlusion of the inflow is generally advisable and can be done either for multiple short periods with intervening reperfusion or for longer periods with neuromonitoring and neuroprotection. When intraoperative rupture of the dome occurs, the aneurysm may be partially clipped, packed, or trapped and completely clipped. If the neck is torn, cotton, Gore-Tex, or muscle can be placed within the clips to reinforce these areas. This is much more difficult if it occurs on the blind side of a vessel that cannot be fully mobilized; therefore, clearing the blind side of the aneurysm should be the last aspect of dissection and should performed with great care and patience. Vessel compromise due to clip constructs occurs due to overaggressive clipping; intravascular pathology such as atheroma, calcium, or thrombus; or constructs that kink or foreshorten efferent branches. Careful review of the preoperative imaging, as well as a combination of Doppler ultrasonography, indocyanine green, and DSA, is most helpful to avoid or diagnose this, permitting clip repositioning. Rarely, bypass may be necessary to provide distal revascularization to branch vessels that are involved in the aneurysm neck or dome. Subdurals and epidurals are best avoided by careful dissection technique, which includes the avoidance of draining veins and the use of dural tack-up sutures. Finally, in some cases, perioperative and intraoperative maneuvers fail to adequately manage intracranial pressure even with craniectomy. In these instances, it may be wisest to forestall clipping efforts and re-explore either endovascular options or a few days of intensive care unit management with anti-fibrinolytic support.

Postoperative Complications and Management

The most common postoperative complications related purely to the microsurgical clipping are wound infections, subdural hygromas, CSF leaks, deep venous thrombosis or pulmonary embolism, seizures, and cerebral sag. Wound infections are best avoided by meticulous technique and the appropriate use of perioperative antibiotics. When they do occur, most can be managed without discarding the bone flap. Due to the fact that some degree of communicating hydrocephalus usually accompanies, at least temporarily, SAH, it is not uncommon for CSF to enter the subdural space. Attempts to expand the ventricles and compress the subdural space early in the postoperative period may help, as might a short course of postoperative steroids. Eventually, shunting either the subdural or the ventricular space may be necessary. CSF leaks are best avoided by avoiding sinus entry, sinus exenteration when it occurs, careful waxing of the bone, and watertight dural closures. The use of dural substitutes in the epidural space and hydroxyapatite in drill grooves may also help. When leaks occur, oversewing the wound and CSF diversion (e.g., lumbar drainage) usually resolve the issue, but permanent CSF diversion with or without repeat dural closure may be needed. Deep venous thrombosis is best avoided by compression stockings, early mobilization, and early use of subcutaneous low-dose heparinoids. Seizures are best prevented by avoiding brain manipulation and the use of anticonvulsants in the perioperative period, although this is controversial. Avoiding CSF hypotension and cerebral sag is best accomplished by avoiding the concomitant use of spinal drainage and lamina terminalis fenestration. It is best treated by Trendelenburg positioning and 100% oxygen face tents; rarely, a blood patch is needed.

Oral Boards Review—Complications Pearls

1. Intraoperative rupture is best avoided by complete exposure of the aneurysm, often with temporary clipping of the inflow. It is best managed by careful suction and tamponade of the bleeding point, as well as temporary parent vessel clipping prior to definitive aneurysm clipping.
2. Cerebral hypotension can occur with spinal drainage and lamina terminalis fenestration and is best treated with Trendelenburg positioning.

Evidence and Outcomes

Anterior communicating artery aneurysm microsurgery is well established as a potential first-line treatment for many ruptured and unruptured aneurysms. Evidence from several randomized trials suggests advantages such as durability and lack of retreatment, whereas disadvantages include higher rates of short-term functional disability. Outcomes depend on the center and surgeon involved.

Further Reading

Chiappini A, Marchi F, Reinert M, Robert T. Supraorbital approach through eyebrow skin incision for aneurysm clipping: How I do it. *Acta Neurochir (Wien).* 2018;160(6):1155–1158. PubMed PMID:29654409.

Connolly ES Jr, Kader AA, Frazzini VI, Winfree CJ, Solomon RA. The safety of intraoperative lumbar subarachnoid drainage for acutely ruptured intracranial aneurysm: Technical note. *Surg Neurol.* 1997;48(4):338–344. PubMed PMID:9315129.

Lindgren A, Vergouwen MD, van der Schaaf I, et al. Endovascular coiling versus neurosurgical clipping for people with aneurysmal subarachnoid haemorrhage. *Cochrane Database Syst Rev.* 2018;2018(8):CD003085. PubMed PMID:30110521.

Molyneux A, Kerr R, Stratton I, et al. International Subarachnoid Aneurysm Trial (ISAT) of neurosurgical clipping versus endovascular coiling in 2143 patients with ruptured intracranial aneurysms: A randomised trial. *Lancet.* 2002;360(9342):1267–1274. PubMed PMID:12414200.

Naidech AM, Janjua N, Kreiter KT, et al. Predictors and impact of aneurysm rebleeding after subarachnoid hemorrhage. *Arch Neurol.* 2005;62(3):410–416. PubMed PMID:15767506.

Raper DM, Starke RM, Komotar RJ, Allan R, Connolly ES Jr. Seizures after aneurysmal subarachnoid hemorrhage: A systematic review of outcomes. *World Neurosurg.* 2013;79(5–6):682–690. PubMed PMID:23022642.

Spetzler RF, Zabramski JM, McDougall CG, et al. Analysis of saccular aneurysms in the Barrow Ruptured Aneurysm Trial. *J Neurosurg.* 2018;128(1):120–125. PubMed PMID:28298031.

Washington CW, Zipfel GJ, Chicoine MR, et al. Comparing indocyanine green videoangiography to the gold standard of intraoperative digital subtraction angiography used in aneurysm surgery. *J Neurosurg.* 2013;118(2):420–427. PubMed PMID:23157184.

Zacharia BE, Bruce SS, Carpenter AM, et al. Variability in outcome after elective cerebral aneurysm repair in high-volume academic medical centers. *Stroke.* 2014;45(5):1447–1452. PubMed PMID:24668204.

Ruptured Middle Cerebral Artery Aneurysm Presenting with Hematoma

Joseph M. Zabramski

6

Case Presentation

A 58-year-old female was brought to the emergency department after she was found lethargic and confused. Her partner reported that the patient had suffered the sudden onset of a severe headache approximately 1 week earlier but did not seek medical evaluation. She complained of continued headache and neck pain during the next 7 days. Soon after the patient arrived in the emergency department, her condition suddenly deteriorated. On repeat neurological examination, she was found to have a Glasgow Coma Scale score of 8 (E2, M5, V1).

Questions

1. What is the differential diagnosis?
2. What is the most likely cause of the patient's sudden deterioration?
3. What is the most critical issue requiring management?
4. What is the most appropriate imaging modality?

Assessment and Planning

The patient's history and computed tomography (CT) imaging study are most consistent with an aneurysmal subarachnoid hemorrhage (SAH). The sudden onset of severe headache 1 week before presentation, followed by persistent headache, neck pain, and photophobia, is consistent with a sentinel headache. Her sudden deterioration soon after presentation was most likely caused by aneurysm rebleeding.

The most critical issue requiring treatment following the patient's deterioration is the management of her airway to ensure adequate oxygenation. Although it is important to secure the airway, intubation should be performed with adequate sedation and analgesia to avoid hypertension and the risk of further rebleeding. Intravenous propofol is a good option for the management of these patients.

After intubation, a head CT was immediately performed (Figure 6.1). The CT demonstrates acute SAH consistent with a ruptured aneurysm. The distribution of blood is strongly suggestive of a ruptured left middle cerebral artery (MCA) aneurysm. In addition, the CT demonstrates the presence of blood in the third, fourth, and both lateral ventricles, placing the patient at high risk of developing acute hydrocephalus.

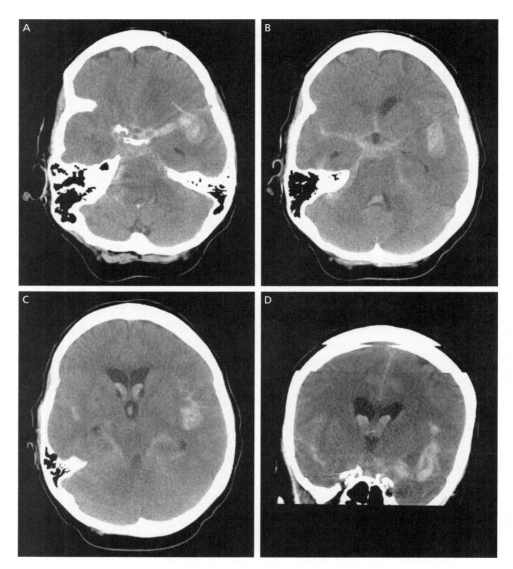

Figure 6.1 Noncontrast CT images of the head. (A–C) Axial and (D) coronal views demonstrating a large modified Fisher grade 4 subarachnoid hemorrhage in the left temporal lobe and sylvian fissure, as well as diffuse intraventricular hemorrhage. This pattern is most consistent with rupture of a left middle cerebral artery aneurysm.

Source: Used with permission from Barrow Neurological Institute, Phoenix, Arizona.

Before further evaluation, the patient should be transferred to the intensive care unit (ICU) to undergo emergency placement of an external ventricular drain (EVD). If an ICU bed is not immediately available, the EVD can be placed while the patient is in the emergency department. Again, management should include appropriate sedation, with care taken to avoid hypertension during any procedures or evaluations. Additional diagnostic workup includes cerebral angiography to confirm the cause of hemorrhage and to allow appropriate planning for treatment.

The decision to use digital subtraction angiography (DSA) or computed tomography angiography (CTA) varies from institution to institution. CTA has the advantage of being readily available at nearly all tertiary treatment centers and is preferable unless the endovascular team is immediately available to perform angiography.

CTA performed on modern multidetector helical CT scanners allows submillimeter slice thickness, multiplanar reformats, and three-dimensional reconstructions (Figure 6.2). Several investigators have demonstrated that current multidetector scanners have a spatial resolution that can reliably diagnose aneurysms greater than 4 mm with nearly 100% sensitivity. However, for aneurysms 3 mm or smaller, DSA provides higher resolution. DSA is indicated in all cases of nontraumatic SAH when the CTA study is negative.

After placement of an EVD, our patient underwent angiographic evaluation with an immediate CTA (see Figure 6.2).

Questions

1. How do the clinical and radiographic findings in this case influence treatment options?
2. What is the most appropriate timing for intervention?

Oral Boards Review—Diagnostic Pearls

1. The history of sudden onset of severe headache and neck pain, often described by the patient as "the worst headache of my life," is considered nearly diagnostic of SAH.
   a. Sentinel headache: Episodes of sudden onset of severe headache that occur up to 4 weeks before a major hemorrhage and that are either ignored by the patient or misdiagnosed by a physician are called *sentinel headaches*. Sentinel headaches have been reported in up to 50% of patients before the index hemorrhage, but in most recent studies the incidence of a sentinel headache is in the range of 20–30%. Some evidence suggests that patients with a history of a sentinel headache have an increased risk of recurrent bleeding episodes, which supports more urgent management.
2. The initial diagnostic test of choice to confirm SAH is a noncontrast head CT. The sensitivity of CT for detecting subarachnoid blood ranges from 90% to 100% when the CT is performed within the first 24 hours after symptom onset. At 5 days after symptom onset, the sensitivity of CT decreases to approximately 85%, and at 1 week it decreases to approximately 50%.
   a. If the patient's history indicates a possible SAH and the CT is negative, a lumbar puncture is indicated. The presence of xanthochromic cerebrospinal fluid (CSF) is considered diagnostic of SAH and necessitates further evaluation for an aneurysm or other vascular abnormality.
   b. CTA has been recommended by some authors for patients who present with severe headache when the basic head CT is negative. However, note

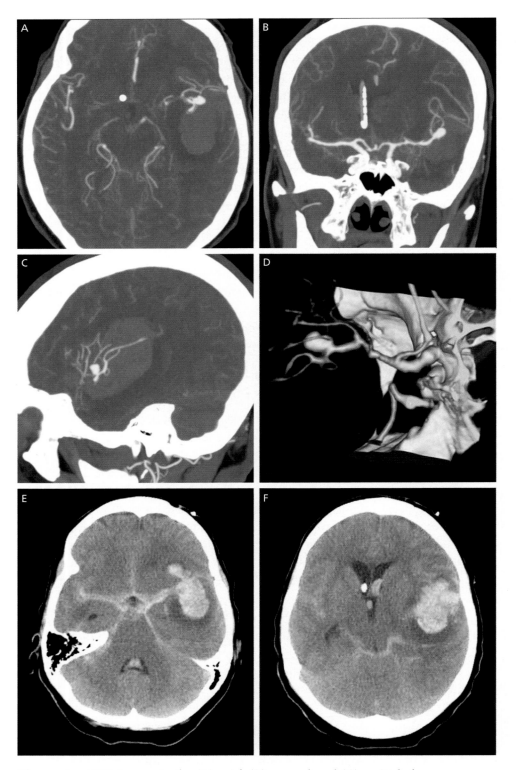

Figure 6.2 CTA images in the (A) axial, (B) coronal, and (C) sagittal planes demonstrating filling of the left middle cerebral bifurcation aneurysm. (D) A three-dimensional reconstruction of the aneurysm illustrates the broad-based neck. (E and F) Repeat basic CT images in the axial view performed immediately prior to the CTA demonstrate an increase in the size of the temporal lobe hematoma compared to that seen in Figures 6.1A–6.1C.

Source: Used with permission from Barrow Neurological Institute, Phoenix, Arizona.

that approximately 2% or 3% of the adult population harbors an incidental intracranial aneurysm. Thus, the presence of an aneurysm is suggestive, but not conclusive, of SAH. Several recent publications support the cost-effectiveness and clinical utility of lumbar puncture compared to CTA in this population.

c. Magnetic resonance imaging and magnetic resonance angiography are other alternatives when initial diagnostic tests are negative for SAH. Fluid-attenuated inversion recovery sequences can be particularly useful for detecting SAH, especially in the subacute period, when CT is negative.

3. Evidence of hydrocephalus is a common finding in patients with SAH, particularly those who present with a depressed level of consciousness. It occurs in 3–5% of patients with a good grade (Hunt and Hess grades 1 and 2) and in 30–50% of patients with higher grades (Hunt and Hess grades 3–5).

Decision-Making

The CTA in our patient demonstrates a large (13-mm), wide-necked aneurysm arising from the left MCA bifurcation. On further review, when the CTA is compared to the earlier CT, it is apparent that the associated hematoma has enlarged. This finding is consistent with additional bleeding from the aneurysm and emphasizes the need for urgent intervention to secure the aneurysm and evacuate the hematoma.

In general, intervention to secure a ruptured aneurysm should proceed as soon as possible to minimize the risks of rebleeding. Rebleeding is a major complication associated with an additional 50–60% risk of death and disability. For patients with untreated aneurysms, the risk of rebleeding is approximately 20% in the first 2 weeks and 50% at 6 months. The risk is highest during the first 24 hours (ranging from 4% to 6%). It then decreases and remains steady, at approximately 1.2% per day until day 14, before it gradually declines. Recent studies have suggested that the risk of rebleeding is higher in patients with larger aneurysms and in patients with large-volume SAH (modified Fisher grades 3 and 4).

The decision of whether to surgically clip or coil a ruptured aneurysm depends on its location, size, and findings on imaging studies. In patients with a large hematoma, such as the current case, the treatment of choice is craniotomy and clipping of the aneurysm, combined with the evacuation of the hematoma. However, when any delay in access to surgery is anticipated, coiling to secure the aneurysm, followed by craniotomy for hematoma evacuation, has been reported to be effective.

Questions

1. What is the significance of the hematoma for surgical management of this case?
2. What surgical approach would you use?
3. How would you manage the hematoma?

Surgical Procedure

The most common surgical approach for the management of ruptured MCA aneurysms is a pterional craniotomy. However, when rupture is associated with a large hematoma, surgical planning should include a larger exposure to allow bony decompression of the involved hemisphere, if necessary. Intraoperative placement of an EVD before craniotomy (if not already performed) may be useful in maximizing brain relaxation in patients with extensive aneurysmal SAH (modified Fisher grades 3 and 4).

After the craniotomy, the aneurysm should be exposed in the normal fashion, with initial steps taken to control the internal carotid artery and the proximal MCA. Once proximal control is obtained, subtotal evacuation of the hematoma can be performed to aid in brain relaxation. In the current case, the hematoma located in the anterior temporal lobe was evacuated and dissection was then carried out to widely open the sylvian fissure and expose the aneurysm neck for clipping. Temporary clipping of the distal M1 segment of the MCA before manipulation of the aneurysm dome should be considered to minimize the risk of intraoperative rupture, particularly in patients who have had a recent hemorrhage or a rebleeding episode. It is imperative to identify the proximal portions of the M2 branches of the MCA before clipping the aneurysm neck. A careful review of the preoperative angiogram aids the surgeon in this task.

Clipping of the aneurysm should be followed by intraoperative imaging. Intraoperative DSA and indocyanine green videoangiography are both reliable means of ensuring occlusion of the aneurysm and patency of the parent vessel and branches. Alternatively, microvascular Doppler ultrasonography can be used. The comparison of Doppler signals before and after clipping can identify changes in flow and the presence of clip-related stenosis. Puncture of the aneurysm dome with a tuberculin syringe (28-gauge needle) can be performed to confirm occlusion.

After clipping of the aneurysm, additional hematoma can be evacuated as indicated. It is important to recognize that much of the hematoma in the current patient appears to be expanding the sylvian fissure rather than dissecting into the surrounding brain. When the hematoma fills and expands the sylvian fissure, it makes substantial evacuation difficult to perform without causing injury to the MCA branches and perforating vessels. In such patients, a large decompressive craniotomy and duraplasty may reduce the risk of subsequent swelling and edema until the hematoma resolves. It may be preferable to leave the dura widely open and to place a layer of absorbable gelatin film (Gelfilm) both beneath and over the dura to prevent adhesions. Use of this technique greatly simplifies dissection for replacement of the bone flap. Placement of a drain between the layers of Gelfilm allows drainage of CSF through the sylvian fissure and may help clear blood from the SAH. (See the immediate postoperative CT and CTA images shown in Figure 6.3.)

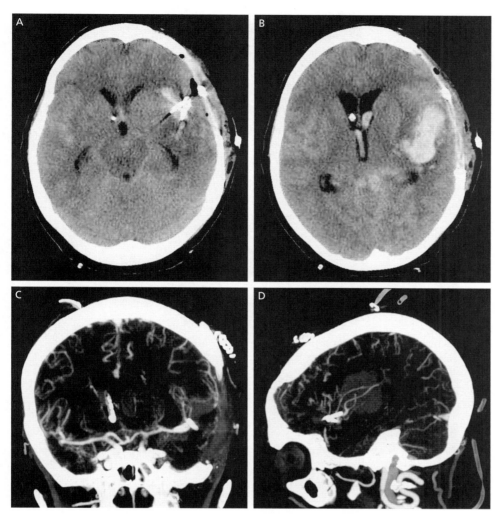

Figure 6.3 Immediate postoperative CT and CTA images. (A and B) Axial CT images demonstrate the decompressive craniotomy and the presence of two aneurysm clips in the region of the middle cerebral artery bifurcation. The hematoma has been cleared from the proximal sylvian fissure and the anterior temporal lobe. The residual hematoma in the distal sylvian fissure has been left in place (compare with Figures 6.3E and 6.3F). (C) Coronal and (D) sagittal CTA images demonstrate obliteration of the aneurysm and preservation of the parent vessel and branches (compare with Figures 6.3A and 6.3C).

Source: Used with permission from Barrow Neurological Institute, Phoenix, Arizona.

Oral Boards Review—Management Pearls

1. The goal of aneurysm treatment is complete, durable obliteration of the aneurysm. Although endovascular coiling may offer an advantage in early clinical outcome, it is associated with a clinically significant higher risk of aneurysm recurrence. The risk of aneurysm recurrence is related to aneurysm size, neck

morphology, and extent of occlusion. The overall risk of aneurysm recurrence that requires repeat endovascular treatment after coiling ranges from 10% to 20%, compared to 1% or 2% for clipping.

    a. The risk of recurrence after endovascular coiling is substantially higher in aneurysms with a maximum diameter >1 cm and in aneurysms with wide necks. A wide neck is defined as a neck diameter ≥4 mm or as an aneurysm dome diameter-to-neck width ratio <2. Stent-assisted coiling and flow diverters can reduce the risk of recurrence in this group, but they require initiation of dual antiplatelet therapy. For this reason, the use of these devices in patients with ruptured aneurysms is typically limited to rescue procedures such as management of vessel wall dissections or protruding coils.

2. Temporary proximal vessel occlusion can reduce the risk of intraoperative aneurysm rupture during dissection of the aneurysm dome, and it is typically well tolerated for 10–15 minutes. If the dome ruptures during dissection, temporary clips can also be applied to the M2 segment branches distal to the aneurysm dome for additional control.

    a. The risks of ischemic injury can be minimized by the induction of mild hypothermia, ranging from 34°C to 35°C, and by the initiation of electroencephalogram (EEG) burst suppression with barbiturates or propofol before temporary vessel occlusion. It is vital for blood pressure to be maintained in the normal range during periods of planned temporary vessel occlusion.

    b. Monitoring of EEG activity, somatosensory evoked potentials, and motor evoked potentials can identify patients in whom the elective use of temporary vessel occlusion is not well tolerated.

3. Visual inspection alone is not adequate to ensure complete occlusion of the aneurysm and vessel patency. Indocyanine green videoangiography avoids the drawbacks associated with intraoperative catheter angiography, and it has a reported diagnostic accuracy of approximately 90%, with the most commonly missed finding being small residual aneurysm neck remnants. At a minimum, flow in the parent vessel and all branches should be confirmed with a microvascular Doppler probe.

4. In patients with giant or complex aneurysms, preoperative surgical planning should include preparation for intraoperative DSA, including the use of a radiolucent head frame and surgical draping that allows appropriate vascular access.

Pivot Points

1. When patients present with an intracerebral hemorrhage from a ruptured aneurysm, the decision of whether to proceed with surgical clipping or endovascular coiling is influenced by the size of the hematoma. In patients with small hematomas, endovascular coiling can be used to secure the aneurysm and the hematoma can be closely monitored with CT imaging. For patients with large, life-threatening hematomas, surgery for evacuation of the hematoma should be combined with clipping of the aneurysm.

2. When patients present with a giant or complex aneurysm, it is important to consider options for revascularization, such as extracranial–intracranial and intracranial–intracranial bypass procedures. Preparation is important in such cases, and it may include preserving the superficial temporal artery during the craniotomy, draping the patient's neck for a possible bypass, and preparing an arm or leg for the potential harvesting of vascular grafts.

3. When intraoperative inspection reveals that one or more of the M2 branches arises from the aneurysm dome, bypass of the involved vessels should be performed before aneurysm occlusion or attempts at clip reconstruction.

Aftercare

The postoperative management of patients with ruptured aneurysms poses a number of unique issues that require prolonged monitoring in the ICU. Fluid and electrolyte abnormalities are common and necessitate careful monitoring, with the goal of maintaining normovolemia and avoiding hyponatremia. Typical ICU stays average 14–21 days.

The administration of oral nimodipine is strongly recommended for the prevention and limitation of vasospasm. Treatment should begin as soon as possible after hemorrhage and should be continued for 21 days or until the patient is discharged. Nimodipine is a calcium channel blocker that was originally developed for the treatment of high blood pressure; not surprisingly, hypotension is one of the side effects that may limit its use. The recommended dose is 60 mg every 4 hours, but when hypotension is an issue, 30 mg every 2 hours may be better tolerated, and further downward dose titration may be necessary for some patients.

Frequent neurological assessments are an essential aspect of treatment. They should be performed at least once per hour for the first 24 hours after surgery and then at 2- to 4-hour intervals. Any changes in neurological status must be rapidly evaluated. Typical causes of neurological deterioration include hydrocephalus, hyponatremia, infection, and vasospasm. For patients with aneurysmal hematoma, a mass effect from swelling and edema may necessitate emergency decompressive craniotomy, if it was not performed as part of the initial operative treatment.

As many as 50% of patients with SAH present with acute hydrocephalus and require emergency placement of an EVD. For patients who require long-term CSF drainage, attempts at EVD weaning are typically initiated 10–14 days after hemorrhage. Persistent hydrocephalus requires placement of a ventriculoperitoneal shunt in 20–30% of patients.

Most surgeons recommend immediate postoperative angiography to document aneurysm occlusion and patency of the parent vessels and branches. However, if DSA imaging is performed intraoperatively, early postoperative angiography may not be necessary.

Pharmacologic thromboprophylaxis for venous thromboembolism (VTE) is somewhat controversial in this group of patients. At a minimum, all patients should be treated with elastic compression hose and intermittent pneumatic compression devices. The use of elastic compression hose alone is not effective. Rates of VTE and pulmonary embolism in patients who have had neurosurgical procedures either with no VTE prophylaxis or with elastic compression hose alone are reported to range from 14% to 16%. Pharmacologic therapy with both unfractionated and low-molecular-weight heparin has been shown to significantly reduce the risk of VTE and pulmonary embolism.

Treatment with intermittent subcutaneous unfractionated heparin has the advantage of being readily reversible, and it should be initiated as soon as possible as determined by the surgeon—typically 24 hours after surgery or immediately after endovascular treatment.

If a decompressive craniectomy is performed, subsequent cranioplasty should be conducted as soon as possible upon resolution of swelling and edema. Early replacement of the bone flap minimizes the risks of postoperative complications associated with this procedure, avoids the symptoms of trephination, and allows for more aggressive rehabilitation therapy (Figure 6.4).

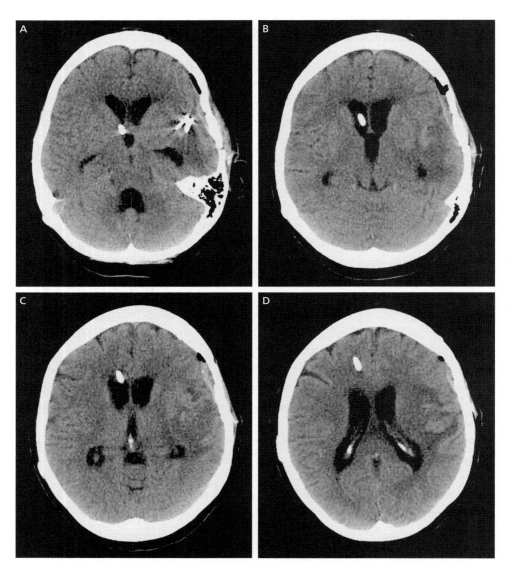

Figure 6.4 (A–D) Axial CT images obtained approximately 5½ weeks after decompressive craniotomy and clipping of the ruptured aneurysm and 10 days after cranioplasty with replacement of the bone flap. There are minimal postoperative changes underlying the craniotomy flap. The right frontal ventricular shunt catheter is in good position. Note the mild enlargement of the ventricles. The patient has a programmable shunt valve, which can be adjusted to minimize the risks of extra-axial fluid collection.

Source: Used with permission from Barrow Neurological Institute, Phoenix, Arizona.

Complications and Management

The delayed onset of ischemic deficits secondary to vasospasm is one of the major complications of SAH. Angiographic evidence of vasospasm, which is identified in 40–70% of patients on routine imaging, follows a time-dependent course after hemorrhage. It is seldom present before 3 days, reaches a peak 7–10 days after SAH, and then gradually resolves by 2 or 3 weeks after hemorrhage. Clinically, vasospasm refers to the ischemic complications associated with angiographic vasospasm that affects 20–30% of patients. Clinical vasospasm is typically characterized by the gradual onset of confusion or deterioration in the patient's level of consciousness, followed by the waxing and waning of focal neurological deficits. The course of clinical vasospasm follows the angiographic changes; onset is rare before day 5 or more than 2 weeks after a hemorrhage. Untreated clinical vasospasm can rapidly progress to stroke and death. Thus, early recognition of clinical vasospasm is critical. Initial treatment consists of quickly ruling out other causes of neurological deterioration and initiating normovolemic hypertensive therapy. At many centers, CTA is used to evaluate the severity of vasospasm, and patients with severe narrowing are referred for endovascular treatment such as balloon angioplasty or intra-arterial vasodilators.

One of the harbingers of vasospasm is hyponatremia, and daily monitoring of sodium levels should be considered for the first 2 weeks after hemorrhage. The infusion of 3% sodium chloride solution is reasonable in the acute management of hyponatremia and can be supplemented with oral sodium chloride tablets. Fludrocortisone has been reported to be effective in limiting the severity of hyponatremia, and demeclocycline may be useful in resistant cases.

EVD malfunction or displacement is a clinically significant risk in patients who present with acute hydrocephalus after aneurysmal SAH. Changes in neurological status should include a bedside assessment of EVD function, followed by CT when a malfunction is suspected. In patients with extensive intraventricular hemorrhage, repeated obstruction of the EVD catheter by blood can be limited by the intraventricular administration of recombinant tissue plasminogen activator after the aneurysm has been secured. Doses as small as 1 mg of tissue plasminogen activator once or twice per day have been reported to be effective in helping clear intraventricular hemorrhage. Daily CTs are used to monitor the need for continued thrombolytic treatment. Its use should be avoided in cases of significant hemorrhage along the EVD tract.

Bacterial ventriculitis is a clinically significant risk in patients who require prolonged extraventricular drainage. Multiple studies have demonstrated that the risks of CSF infection increase with the duration of EVD placement. Reported rates of infection range from 0% to 27% (mean = 9%). The risk of infection can be limited by careful attention to sterile technique during placement and by the use of antibiotic-impregnated catheters (Codman Bactiseal). There is no evidence to support the use of prophylactic antibiotics beyond the standard preprocedure dose, and prolonged antibiotics may increase the risk of nosocomial infection. The routine monitoring of CSF for cultures and laboratory studies is not supported by the medical literature and also may lead to an increased risk of infection. Unexplained changes in neurological status and fever of unknown origin should include evaluation of the CSF, including cell counts, Gram stain, glucose, protein, cultures, and antibiotic sensitivity testing. The most frequently identified organisms causing infection are normal skin flora (e.g., staphylococci, streptococci, and

Corynebacterium species), although *Pseudomonas* species and other opportunistic bacteria have been reported, particularly in patients receiving prolonged prophylactic antibiotic therapy. Initial treatment in suspected cases includes broad-spectrum antibiotics while awaiting the results of cultures. Daily treatment with intraventricular antibiotics (based on the CSF cultures) appears to speed the clearance of infection.

Oral Boards Review—Complications Pearls

1. Emergency surgical intervention is often necessary for the management of patients with large hematoma associated with ruptured MCA aneurysms. Despite the urgency of such cases, the surgeon must carefully consider the surgical options and make appropriate preparations. When the surgical plan includes management of the aneurysm, preparation should include electro-physiological monitoring and evaluation of the need for intraoperative imaging. When the case involves a complex or a giant aneurysm, it is important to consider the need for possible bypass procedures.
2. Preoperative planning should also include the potential for a large decompressive craniotomy or craniectomy because complete evacuation of the hematoma may not be possible, and delayed swelling and edema are common.
3. It is important to distinguish whether the hematoma associated with a ruptured MCA aneurysm is intraparenchymal or is expanding the sylvian fissure. Intraparenchymal hematoma is usually readily removed. In the case of sylvian hematoma, substantial evacuation of the hematoma beyond the proximal portion of the sylvian fissure is difficult to perform without injuring the MCA branches and perforating vessels.

Evidence and Outcomes

There are no randomized controlled trials addressing the management of the subgroup of patients who present with a hematoma secondary to a ruptured intracranial aneurysm. However, general recommendations can be made from the available published guidelines and from several prospective randomized controlled trials that have been published dealing with specific issues.

The most recent published guidelines for the management of SAH stress the importance of early intervention to secure the aneurysm and prevent rebleeding. Rebleeding is associated with a 50–60% risk of death and disability.

In general, MCA aneurysm rupture with concomitant large intraparenchymal or sylvian fissure hematoma formation carries a grave prognosis. Clinical grade on admission and hematoma volume are major predictors of outcome. In a recent retrospective review of 81 ruptured MCA aneurysms with an associated hematoma, only the clinical grade at the time of admission was found to correlate with outcome. A significant difference in favorable outcome (17% vs. 68%) was seen between patients with poor (Glasgow Coma Scale score <8) neurological condition and patients with good neurological condition at admission ($p < 0.01$). Patients with hematomas >50 mL had similar outcomes for coiling and clipping, and all underwent evacuation and decompressive craniotomy. Patients with hematomas <50 mL did not show differences in favorable outcome when comparing coiling and clipping groups, with or without evacuation and decompressive craniotomy.

Among the randomized controlled trials that have compared clipping and coiling for the obliteration of ruptured intracranial aneurysms, only the International Subarachnoid Aneurysm Trial (ISAT) demonstrated a clinically significant benefit for coiling over clipping in clinical outcome, but this study was limited to patients with small anterior circulation aneurysms who presented in good clinical condition. To avoid the selection bias of the ISAT, the investigators in the Barrow Ruptured Aneurysm Trial (BRAT) randomly assigned all patients with nontraumatic SAH to clipping or coiling regardless of clinical or imaging findings. The 6-year results of the BRAT demonstrated no difference in clinical outcome based on assignment to surgical clipping or endovascular coiling. However, rates of re-treatment and complete aneurysm obliteration at 6 years significantly favored patients who underwent clipping compared with those who underwent coiling. Aneurysm obliteration at 6 years was achieved in 96% of the clipping group and in 48% of the coiling group ($p < 0.001$), and overall re-treatment rates were 4.6% for clipping and 16.4% for coiling ($p < 0.001$).

Acknowledgment

I thank the staff of Neuroscience Publications at Barrow Neurological Institute for assistance with manuscript preparation.

Further Reading

Boogaarts HD, van Lieshout JH, van Amerongen MJ, et al. Aneurysm diameter as a risk factor for pretreatment rebleeding: A meta-analysis. *J Neurosurg.* 2015;122(4):921–928.

Roessler K, Krawagna M, Dorfler A, Buchfelder M, Ganslandt O. Essentials in intraoperative indocyanine green videoangiography assessment for intracranial aneurysm surgery: Conclusions from 295 consecutively clipped aneurysms and review of the literature. *Neurosurg Focus.* 2014;36(2):E7.

Salaud C, Hamel O, Riem T, Desal H, Buffenoir K. Management of aneurysmal subarachnoid haemorrhage with intracerebral hematoma: Is there an indication for coiling first? Study of 44 cases. *Interv Neuroradiol.* 2016;22(1):5–11.

Zabramski JM, Whiting D, Darouiche RO, et al. Efficacy of antimicrobial-impregnated external ventricular drain catheters: A prospective, randomized, controlled trial. *J Neurosurg.* 2003;98(4):725–730.

Zijlstra IA, van der Steen WE, Verbaan D, et al. Ruptured middle cerebral artery aneurysms with a concomitant intraparenchymal hematoma: The role of hematoma volume. *Neuroradiology.* 2018;60(3):335–342.

Unruptured Ophthalmic Artery Aneurysm Presenting with Vision Loss

Harry Van Loveren, Zeguang Ren, Pankaj Agarwalla, and Siviero Agazzi

7

Case Presentation

A 50-year-old female presented to an outside hospital with acute-onset headache and neck tenderness. Computed tomography angiography (CTA) showed a cerebral aneurysm, for which she was referred to a cerebrovascular neurosurgeon as an outpatient. Prior to a clinic visit, she presented to the emergency department with an episode of acute headache and new-onset right eye visual blurriness, which she described as "a film over my eye." Her family history was notable for ruptured intracranial aneurysms in her maternal aunt and cousin. On neurological examination, she had transient right monocular blurred vision.

Questions

1. Which aneurysm locations can cause blurred vision?
2. Does the ophthalmic artery arise intradurally or extradurally?
3. What is the most appropriate approach to determine whether a paraclinoid aneurysm is intradural or extradural?
4. What is the appropriate timing of the diagnostic workup?

Assessment and Planning

Due to the presentation of headache and intracranial aneurysm, rupture must first be ruled out. This patient had a head CT that was negative for subarachnoid hemorrhage (SAH) within the acute time window when CT scans are nearly 100% sensitive for detecting SAH. Her monocular visual difficulties indicated a likely paraclinoid region aneurysm with compression on the right pre-chiasmatic optic apparatus.

Based on her family history, neurological deficit, and known aneurysm, additional workup is warranted. Pretreatment neuro-ophthalmological assessment should be documented to serve as a baseline for future evaluation of treatment outcome. Prior to determining treatment choice, a diagnostic cerebral angiogram with three-dimensional (3D) reconstruction should be performed to assess the anatomy of the aneurysm. In addition, high-resolution CTA imaging is recommended to assess whether the aneurysm

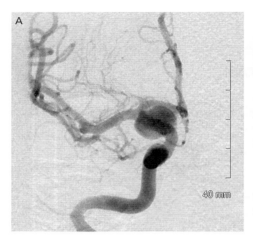
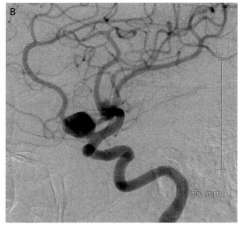

Figure 7.1 (A) Pretreatment anterior–posterior view of a right carotid injection angiogram demonstrating large superiorly pointing aneurysm. (B) Pretreatment lateral view of right carotid injection angiogram demonstrating a large paraclinoid region aneurysm projecting anteriorly and superiorly. Note the take-off of the ophthalmic artery immediately proximal and adjacent to the aneurysm.

is intradural or extradural, although even with the best imaging techniques, there can still be ambiguity.

The patient underwent a catheter-based diagnostic cerebral angiogram, which showed multiple intracranial aneurysms including (1) an 11-mm right paraclinoid aneurysm, (2) a 3-mm left supraclinoid internal carotid artery (ICA) aneurysm, and (3) a 2-mm basilar tip aneurysm. The paraclinoid aneurysm appeared to arise immediately distal to the take-off of the right ophthalmic artery pointing anterosuperiorly and medially (Figure 7.1). It measured 11 × 9 mm with a 4-mm neck. CTA suggested its intradural position based on its relationship with the optic strut and anterior clinoid, as discussed previously (Figure 7.2). There was also evidence of compression of the right anterior optic apparatus. In addition, the ophthalmic artery had delayed filling, and no significant tortuosity was noted on the right carotid.

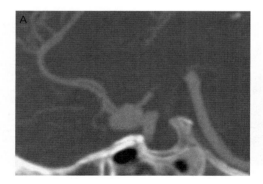
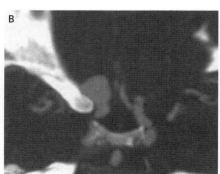
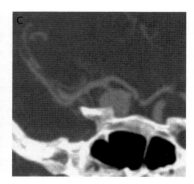

Figure 7.2 (A) Sagittal, (B) axial, and (C) coronal views of CTA of the head demonstrating a right paraclinoid aneurysm and its relationship to the anterior clinoid process.

Oral Boards Review—Diagnostic Pearls

1. For intracranial aneurysms, determination of rupture versus non-rupture is critical for decision-making. CT is most commonly used for diagnosis, although magnetic resonance imaging (MRI) is equally as sensitive as CT for acute SAH and has significant advantages over CT in the detection of subacute SAH. The most sensitive sequence is the gradient echo $T_2^\star$.

2. For suspicious cases with negative CT, particularly with a complaint of "worst headache of my life," lumbar puncture and assessment of cerebrospinal fluid xanthochromia is controversial.

3. Formal ophthalmological evaluation including visual fields and acuity are indicated to confirm optic nerve compression and to establish a baseline for assessment of outcome of treatment.

4. Intracranial aneurysms can be multiple, particularly with family history or genetic syndromes. With either of these, consider screening for all family members.

5. Smoking and hypertension remain the most important risk factors in the population for intracranial aneurysm, and these should be addressed with the patient and family members.

6. Conventional catheter-based cerebral angiogram with 3D reconstruction is the gold-standard test to assess aneurysm morphology, size, and treatment modality. For paraclinoid aneurysms, CTA is useful to assess intradural or extradural location.

In addition to understanding the vascular anatomy through angiography, other factors can play a role in decision-making. For example, aneurysm neck calcification, proximity to clinoid process or distal dural ring, and compression of critical neurovascular structures can influence decision-making. These factors can be verified on preoperative thin-section CT, CTA, and MRI. In this case, imaging confirmed the relationship to the optic strut, no intra-aneurysm thrombus, no calcification, and no ICA atherosclerosis. Based on the size and location of the aneurysm, the patient's age with subsequent lifetime risk of rupture, and her visual changes, a decision was made to treat her paraclinoid aneurysm electively.

The timing of treatment of an unruptured aneurysm associated with vision loss has not been clearly defined in the literature. For patients presenting with oculomotor palsy such as from a posterior communicating artery aneurysm, it is generally believed that earlier treatment affords improved outcomes. Interestingly, however, urgent treatment has not been demonstrated as critical for patients presenting with vision loss. Because this case was an unruptured aneurysm with only transient vision loss, the patient was treated within 2 weeks from initial presentation.

Questions

1. How do these clinical and radiological findings influence the decision to treat?

2. What is the most appropriate intervention in this patient based on these factors?
3. How do different treatment options affect risk of hemorrhage, time to obliteration, visual outcome, and treatment-associated morbidity?

Decision-Making

In the case of unruptured aneurysms, there is an extensive literature on the risk of hemorrhage and the decision to treat, and this is not reviewed in detail here. Because of the patient's age, multiple intracranial aneurysms, and visual deficit, the decision was made for treatment. In particular, her large paraclinoid artery aneurysm was treated because of the visual changes and also because of its size, knowing that the largest of multiple aneurysms (and certainly one that is symptomatic) is most likely to hemorrhage. Options include surgical clip obliteration, aneurysm trapping with surgical bypass, coil embolization with or without stent assistance, and flow diversion.

In the modern cerebrovascular era, decision-making for an unruptured paraclinoid aneurysm focuses on three important considerations: (1) treating the risk of hemorrhage; (2) improving neurological deficit, specifically vision in this case; and (3) minimizing morbidity. Here, we review different modalities and explain the rationale for use of flow diversion in this case.

Prior to the advent and spread of endovascular neurosurgery, surgical options for these aneurysms were clip obliteration, vessel occlusion, or aneurysm trapping and surgical bypass. In one study, of 17 patients with visual deficits and a paraclinoid aneurysm, 11 (65%) had improved visual outcomes after either direct clipping or indirect bypass. It was found that aneurysms with partial thrombosis or calcification tended to have worse visual outcomes, in part because of the challenge of decompressing the optic apparatus fully. Prior to the endovascular era, a number of classification schemata were proposed to assist in surgical decision-making. In general, aneurysms that project superiorly, are large, and have a wide neck have been traditionally treated with clipping or bypass. Additional studies have also reported visual outcomes from surgery for paraclinoid aneurysms, including simple clipping and complex bypass procedures. Unfortunately, the surgical series do emphasize a not insignificant risk of morbidity, including ischemic complications from high-flow bypass techniques.

In addition to open surgical management, coiling with or without stent-assistance first and flow diversion (FD) later have emerged as the primary treatment options for unruptured paraclinoid aneurysms, even with visual deficits. When comparing endovascular coiling with microsurgical clip obliteration, visual outcomes were similar. A recent meta-analysis showed that preoperative visual symptoms occurred in 38% of patients with paraclinoid aneurysms. Vision improved in 58% after clipping, 49% after coiling, and 71% after FD. Vision worsened in 11% of patients after clipping, 9% after coiling, and 5% after FD. New visual deficits were found in patients with intact baseline vision at a rate of 1% for clipping, 0% for coiling, and 0% for FD.

One of the concerns about both coiling and flow diversion is that the mass effect on the optic apparatus is not reduced, which can lead to worse visual outcomes. In particular, visual worsening can occur transiently after treatment because of aneurysm thrombosis resulting in an increase in aneurysm size and adjacent edema. This has been found to be a transient finding because aneurysm mass effect, size, and pulsation will improve in a delayed fashion. For FD, another concern is potential for ophthalmic artery occlusion. A case series of 95 patients reported that 7% of paraclinoid aneurysm patients treated with one type of flow diversion (Pipeline embolization device [PED]) showed occlusion of the ophthalmic artery, with only 1% of those reported to have symptomatic ophthalmic artery occlusion. To avoid this complication, it is necessary to minimize the number of devices covering the ophthalmic artery.

In the case presented here, due to the relatively wide neck, surgical clipping and flow diversion were considered the primary options. Because surgery would necessitate anterior clinoidectomy and neck exposure for proximal control, a potentially less morbid approach with FD was chosen (Figure 7.3).

Questions

1. What is the generally accepted mechanism for flow diversion in the treatment of aneurysms?
2. In the case presented in this chapter, what are the advantages and disadvantages of such an option?
3. How often does flow diversion result in new or worsened visual deficit?

Surgical Procedure

The surgical procedure of deployment of an FD device with intraoperative video has been published and is described briefly here. Prior to the procedure, the patient is started on aspirin 325 mg daily and clopidogrel 75 mg daily for 7–10 days. On the day of the procedure, antiplatelet function tests are generally performed to assess for response. If patients are not responders, then additional treatment should be given, including a

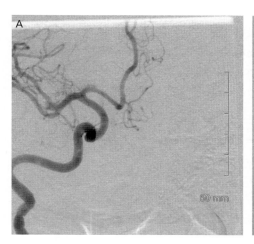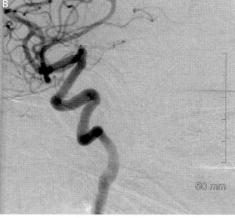

Figure 7.3 (A) Post-treatment anterior–posterior and (B) post-treatment lateral view demonstrating aneurysm obliteration, patency of ICA branches, and no stenosis/occlusion.

day-of-procedure loading dose. Commonly used alternative agents include ticagrelor and prasugrel.

Endovascular embolization of intracranial aneurysms is carried out under general anesthesia with a Foley catheter and an arterial catheter to monitor blood pressure. Paralysis is used to ensure absolutely no movement during the procedure. Vitals are monitored carefully as an indicator of any reaction or intraoperative rupture. Patients are positioned supine in standard fashion in the angiography suite. Both groin regions are prepared in case an additional vascular access point is needed.

Although there are some variations in the technical aspects, a standard triaxial system is used. A 6 Fr long sheath is advanced over a diagnostic catheter/glidewire under road map to the proximal common carotid artery. Then the guide catheter or other intermediate catheter is advanced into the petrosal ICA over a microcatheter. Finally, a microcatheter and microwire system is used to engage the location of the aneurysm and prepare for flow diverter deployment. In the United States, the most commonly used flow diverter is the PED.

Prior to embolization, a 3D angiogram is performed to identify the working views, which should clearly show the distal and proximal landing zones for the stent as well as the M1 segment of the middle cerebral artery for the guide wire past the landing zone. Next, the delivery microcatheter is advanced over a microwire past the deployment zone of the PED and into the M1 segment. After the microwire is removed and the PED delivery system is advanced into the microcatheter, the PED is ready for deployment. The PED is partially deployed to ensure that the distal end is opened fully and apposing the vessel wall. Using a combination of unsheathing and pushing simultaneously, the device is deployed and opened into the vessel.

Size selection is critical, including the diameter, which should fit the largest diameter of the target vessel, and the length, which should extend 5 mm both proximally and distally beyond the neck of the aneurysm. Once the PED is deployed, the push wire is recaptured with the microcatheter and removed. After PED deployment, contrast stagnation is expected, and a final diagnostic run is necessary to ensure no distal embolic events. The entire system is then withdrawn and the groin closed in standard fashion.

Occasionally, more than one device is necessary to ensure adequate flow diversion, which can increase the risk of in-stent thrombosis. Concurrent use of coils and an FD can reduce the number of diverters needed and can achieve rapid obliteration of aneurysms.

Oral Boards Review—Management Pearls

1. Pre-procedure dual antiplatelet therapy is critical to prevent flow diversion or stent thrombotic complications. Platelet function testing preoperatively is important to identify nonresponders and adjust regimen accordingly.
2. Heparin must be used intraoperatively to maintain therapeutic levels to prevent intraoperative thrombotic complications.
3. Accurate sizing of the parent vessel is necessary to select the appropriate FD size and hence obtain an optimal result.

Aftercare

If there are no immediate complications, patients are extubated and transferred to intensive care for overnight observation. Patients are generally discharged on postoperative day 1, and imaging is only obtained if there is a clinical indication. Most important, dual antiplatelet therapy of clopidogrel and aspirin must be continued for 3–6 months to prevent in-stent thrombosis followed by transition to aspirin only as long as patients are clinical responders. Follow-up angiography is performed within this time frame to assess for any stenosis, thrombosis, and aneurysm changes. In the current patient, follow-up angiogram demonstrated complete resolution of the aneurysm (Figure 7.3).

Complications and Management

The complication rate of FD for treatment of unruptured intracranial aneurysms is approximately 15%, which is significantly lower than that for ruptured aneurysms, perhaps due in part to the need for dual antiplatelet therapy. One of the complications of endovascular treatment, specifically whenever coils are used, is intraoperative aneurysm rupture. This can be particularly damaging when on antiplatelet or anticoagulant therapy. When this occurs, it is important to keep the microcatheter in place and advance more coils to occlude the rupture site if possible. One should not pull the catheter back because this could be blocking the perforation and it would make the complication worse. In-stent thrombosis or emboli can cause strokes both intraoperatively and postoperatively. If this occurs, embolectomy should be performed for any large vessel occlusion, and intra-arterial therapy using antiplatelet agents such as eptifibitide should be given for any intraluminal stenosis. This should be followed by postoperative administration of additional antiplatelet agents.

Technical complications can also occur. For example, it is possible that the device does not deploy completely or release from the deployment microwire. In the case of the newest iteration of the PED, the device is retrievable and can be repositioned and redeployed. Additional technical nuances are necessary for complex deployment challenges such as "wagging" the microcatheter or balloon angioplasty to assist in complete stent deployment. Finally, groin hematomas and pseudoaneurysms can occur at the entry site. Manual pressure often stops any hematoma, and pseudoaneurysms need to be followed, possibly in consultation with vascular surgeons.

Oral Boards Review—Complications Pearls

1. Prompt recognition of intraprocedural thrombus is essential to prevent thromboembolic complications. Additional heparin bolus in addition to intravenous or intra-arterial antiplatelet agents (abciximab or eptifibitide) should be administered, and repeat angiography should be performed. Should a thrombus persist, mechanical treatment (embolectomy and additional stent placement) may be necessary.
2. If the stent does not adequately deploy, it should be removed. If a portion of the stent is not well apposed to the vessel wall, balloon angioplasty can be performed.
3. In very large aneurysms treated with flow-diverting stents, some authors advocate for additional coiling of the aneurysm during stent placement to reduce the risk of delayed aneurysm rupture.

Evidence and Outcomes

The occlusion rate of aneurysms after FD treatment is as follows: complete occlusion in 89.1%, near-complete occlusion in 3%, and incomplete occlusion in 7.9%. Permanent morbidity occurs in 3.1%. Pooled analysis from a systematic review comparing clipping, coiling, and flow diversion for paraclinoid aneurysms demonstrated that 38% of patients had preoperative visual symptoms. FD treatment had the best therapeutic window with regard to visual symptoms, with 71% improvement in symptoms and only a 5% rate of worsening compared with worse outcomes for clipping and coiling. Furthermore, development of new visual deficit in patients without any preoperative symptoms occurred in 1% of clipping patients but 0% in the other two modalities. The combination of high obliteration rate and excellent visual outcomes with relatively low risk makes flow diversion treatment an excellent choice in the case presented here. In fact, the patient had complete obliteration of the aneurysm on 6-month follow-up angiogram (Figure 7.3). In addition, immediately after flow diversion treatment, she had persistent visual disturbance, but this too completely resolved at 6-month follow-up.

Further Reading

Chalouhi N, Daou B, Kung D, et al. Fate of the ophthalmic artery after treatment with the Pipeline embolization device. *Neurosurgery*. 2015;77(4):581–584.

Griessenauer CJ, Piske RL, Baccin CE, et al. Flow diverters for treatment of 160 ophthalmic segment aneurysms: Evaluation of safety and efficacy in a multicenter cohort. *Neurosurgery*. 2017;80(5):726–732.

Kim LJ, Tariq F, Levitt M, et al. Multimodality treatment of complex unruptured cavernous and paraclinoid aneurysms. *Neurosurgery*. 2014;74(1):51–61.

Matano F, Tanikawa R, Kamiyama H, et al. Surgical treatment of 127 paraclinoid aneurysms with multifarious strategy: Factors related with outcome. *World Neurosurg*. 2016;85:169–176.

Nossek E, Chalif DJ, Chakraborty S, Lombardo K, Black KS, Setton A. Concurrent use of the Pipeline embolization device and coils for intracranial aneurysms: Technique, safety, and efficacy. *J Neurosurg*. 2015;122(4):904–911.

Shimizu T, Naito I, Aihara M, et al. Visual outcomes of endovascular and microsurgical treatment for large or giant paraclinoid aneurysms. *Acta Neurochir (Wien)*. 2015;157(1):13–20.

Silva MA, See AP, Dasenbrock HH, Patel NJ, Aziz-Sultan MA. Vision outcomes in patients with paraclinoid aneurysms treated with clipping, coiling, or flow diversion: A systematic review and meta-analysis. *Neurosurg Focus*. 2017;42(6):E15.

Zhou G, Su M, Yin YL, Li MH. Complications associated with the use of flow-diverting devices for cerebral aneurysms: A systematic review and meta-analysis. *Neurosurg Focus*. 2017;42(6):E17.

Small Incidental Internal Carotid Artery Terminus Aneurysm

Tyler S. Cole, Dale Ding, Rami O. Almefty, Jacob F. Baranoski, Andrew F. Ducruet, and Felipe C. Albuquerque

8

Case Presentation

A 51-year-old male experienced acute onset of severe headache after bending over in the shower. He later developed nausea and vomiting and presented 1 day after onset of headache to the emergency department for evaluation. Computed tomography (CT) imaging demonstrated acute subarachnoid hemorrhage in the basilar cisterns, and based on the bleed pattern, he was determined to have a ruptured basilar tip aneurysm that was subsequently coiled. Imaging also demonstrated a 5-mm aneurysm at the bifurcation of the left internal carotid artery (ICA) and a 6-mm aneurysm at the left middle cerebral artery bifurcation (Figure 8.1). After securing the basilar aneurysm, the patient was recovering well. While still an inpatient, the patient and his family were concerned about the unruptured aneurysms and wished to pursue treatment.

Questions

1. What is the most appropriate imaging modality for further workup?
2. What aneurysmal features may be missed on CT angiography (CTA)?
3. What anatomical considerations of the aneurysm and parent vessels should be taken into account?

Assessment and Planning

Aneurysms at the ICA terminus are relatively uncommon, particularly considering the hemodynamic theory of aneurysm formation at major arterial branch points. The terminal segment of the ICA begins distal to the origin of the anterior choroidal artery, and it ends at its bifurcation into the middle and anterior cerebral arteries. Perforating branches into the anterior perforating substance, hypothalamus, mesial basal ganglia, and internal capsule may arise from the ICA terminal segment. These areas are collaterally perfused by the anterior choroidal artery. Given the extensive number of perforating branches from this area, open surgical treatment of ICA terminus aneurysms can be challenging. Specifically, superiorly projecting ICA terminus aneurysms can obscure visualization of the recurrent artery of Huebner, which courses posteriorly.

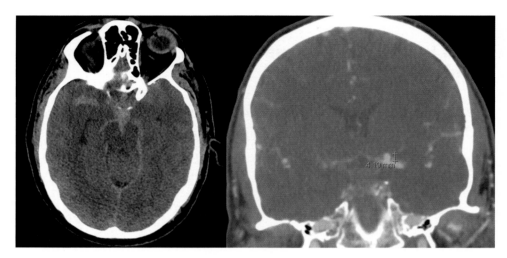

Figure 8.1 CT scan demonstrating acute subarachnoid hemorrhage in the basilar cisterns (left, axial view). Although the source was a ruptured basilar apex aneurysm, a small incidental left ICA terminus aneurysm was identified (right, coronal view).

Source: Used with permission from Barrow Neurological Institute, Phoenix, Arizona.

In this case, the patient's incidental aneurysm was found on a CTA workup after rupture of another aneurysm. CTA has excellent sensitivity and specificity compared to digital subtraction angiography (DSA). CTA is also very sensitive to calcified portions of the artery and aneurysm. To complete the assessment of ICA aneurysms, noninvasive imaging techniques may include magnetic resonance imaging (MRI) and magnetic resonance angiography (MRA) to assess for thrombotic portions of the aneurysm that may not be fully delineated on CTA. After completing any necessary noninvasive imaging, the next step is a DSA, which helps elucidate the flow dynamics at the ICA bifurcation complex (Figure 8.2). Rotational cerebral angiography, with three-dimensional (3D)

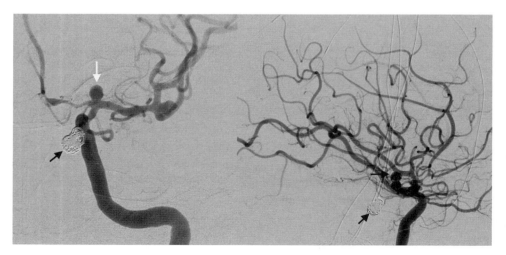

Figure 8.2 Anterior–posterior working angle view (left) and lateral view (right) during DSA demonstrate the aneurysm (white arrow). Note previously coiled basilar apex aneurysm (black arrow).

Source: Used with permission from Barrow Neurological Institute, Phoenix, Arizona.

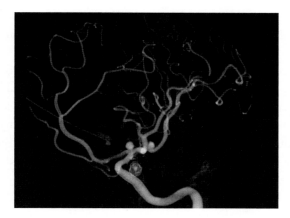

Figure 8.3 Three-dimensional rotational DSA of the aneurysm for treatment planning.

Source: Used with permission from Barrow Neurological Institute, Phoenix, Arizona.

reconstruction, can be helpful for defining the relationship between the aneurysm neck and branch arteries (Figure 8.3).

Questions

1. How do the radiographic findings influence treatment planning?
2. What patient characteristics may favor endovascular treatment?
3. What aneurysm characteristics may favor treatment over observation?

Oral Boards Review—Diagnostic Pearls

1. Use the bone window on CTA to get an accurate assessment of the extent and density of aneurysm or parent vessel calcification.
2. Mass effect near the aneurysm location should be examined and, if present, may indicate a non-opacifying thrombotic portion of the aneurysm.
3. A large, robust anterior choroidal artery may indicate a reciprocally lower contribution to perfusing deep anatomical locations directly from ICA perforators.
4. Multiple aneurysms are observed in approximately 40% of patients with ICA terminus aneurysms, so careful angiographic inspection of the entire cerebral vasculature is imperative.

Decision-Making

Factors to consider when deciding to treat an incidental aneurysm include the patient's age and medical comorbidities and the aneurysm's size, morphology, and orientation. Small aneurysms (diameter <5 mm) may be managed conservatively with serial imaging in most cases. Enlarging aneurysms or those with daughter sacs are more likely to rupture and should therefore be considered more strongly for treatment. Treatment should also be favored in patients with significant risk factors, including previously ruptured aneurysm (as in this case), history of smoking, hypertension, and family history of aneurysm rupture.

Treatment of unruptured aneurysms is generally elective, and for those located at the ICA terminus, there is relative equipoise between microsurgical and endovascular methods. Endovascular options have the advantage of a shorter hospital stay and avoidance of the surgical morbidity of a craniotomy. The main disadvantage of endovascular treatment is a higher recurrence rate than with microsurgical clipping, in most cases. Aneurysms with a higher dome-to-neck ratio are often considered better candidates for endovascular therapy with coiling alone, although balloon remodeling, dual microcatheters, and stent assistance are adjunctive endovascular techniques that have broadened the range of aneurysms treatable with endovascular techniques. Patients with a greater burden of medical comorbidities should be preferentially considered for endovascular treatment. Extensive aneurysm calcification is also a relative indication for endovascular treatment. An institutional interdisciplinary conference can help in decision-making for complex cases.

Questions

1. What pretreatment medication should be considered in these patients?
2. How does aneurysm morphology affect microcatheter tip choice?
3. For what treatment-related complications should equipment and pharmacotherapy be available?

Surgical Procedure

Preoperative medical clearance and laboratory workup should be obtained. If a stent is likely to be placed, the patient should be premedicated with dual antiplatelet therapy, which typically consists of aspirin (325 mg) and clopidogrel (75 mg) daily. Preoperative aspirin and P2Y12 reactivity assays can be performed to assess the patient's responsiveness to aspirin and clopidogrel, respectively, using point-of-care testing such as VerifyNow. Nonresponders should be switched to another antiplatelet agent. In general, central line placement is not necessary for unruptured aneurysm treatment. Normotension should be maintained throughout the procedure. General anesthesia is induced with a baseline activated clotting time obtained in preparation for an intravenous heparin bolus of 70–100 U/kg to reduce the risk of thromboembolic stroke during the procedure. Additional intravenous heparin should be administered to maintain an intraprocedural activated clotting time of at least 250 seconds. Somatosensory evoked potential electrophysiologic neuromonitoring may be considered. After the initial diagnostic angiogram is performed, including 3D rotational angiography to understand the morphology of the aneurysm in relation to the ICA, anterior cerebral artery, and middle cerebral artery, a suitable working angle is obtained for a clear view of the aneurysm neck and branch vessels.

For aneurysm coiling, a 6 Fr guide catheter is advanced to the distal cervical or petrous ICA, depending on the degree of proximal tortuosity; this provides microcatheter

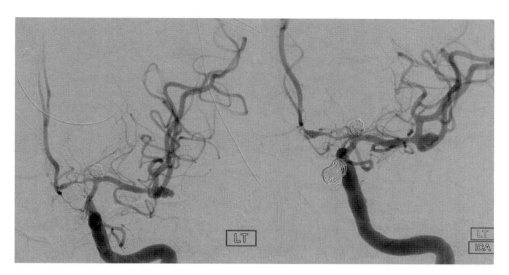

Figure 8.4 Post-coiling anterior–posterior standard view (left) and working-angle view (right) showing complete ICA terminus aneurysm obliteration. No thromboembolic complications were noted, clinically or radiographically.

Source: Used with permission from Barrow Neurological Institute, Phoenix, Arizona.

support. A microcatheter is then navigated over a micro guide wire under high magnification with road map visualization to selectively catheterize the aneurysm. The microcatheter is typically positioned one-half to two-thirds of the way into the aneurysm dome. In general, the optimal shape of the microcatheter should be guided by the direction of the aneurysm relative to the ICA bifurcation, and an S-shaped curve may be helpful.

A framing coil with a deployment diameter approximately equal to the aneurysm dome diameter creates a scaffold for the placement of additional coils, and it should outline the dome and neck of the aneurysm. Successive control angiograms are obtained through the guide catheter while deploying smaller coils to achieve sufficient packing density and aneurysm occlusion. A final working angle control angiogram or 3D rotational angiogram is used to assess the degree of aneurysm embolization, and a less-magnified post-embolization angiogram is used to confirm branch vessel patency (Figure 8.4). A closure device or manual compression is used to achieve hemostasis and prevent groin hematoma formation. Heparin reversal with protamine is not necessary after the procedure, but it can be performed if hemorrhagic complications (e.g., intraprocedural aneurysm rupture and retroperitoneal hematoma) are encountered.

Oral Boards Review—Management Pearls

1. Minimal coil herniation into the parent artery may be treated with antiplatelet agents, such as aspirin, to prevent embolic formation. Large areas of coil protrusion into the parent vessel that affect blood flow may require stent placement to pin the coil mass to the vessel wall and preserve parent vessel flow.

2. Intraoperative rupture should be followed by prompt reversal of anticoagulation (with protamine) and an expeditious completion of embolization. Balloon inflation across the aneurysm neck after intraoperative aneurysm rupture can mitigate additional hemorrhage while embolization is completed.

3. If the microcatheter position migrates from the aneurysm during coil placement, it can be advanced back into the aneurysm by pushing the microcatheter and withdrawing the coil at the same time.

4. Because of high aneurysm shear stress and constant arterial pulsation, aneurysms at T-shaped bifurcations have a high risk of recanalization.

Pivot Points

1. If the aneurysm has significant calcification, endovascular treatment should be strongly considered over surgical treatment.

2. Recurrence after endovascular treatment of an ICA bifurcation aneurysm may be more common than in aneurysms at other locations, so experienced microsurgical treatment might be preferred for ICA bifurcation aneurysms, especially for larger aneurysms.

3. Because stenting requires the use of antiplatelet agents, stenting in the setting of acute subarachnoid hemorrhage is associated with an increased risk of hemorrhagic complications.

Aftercare

The patient should be monitored overnight in an intensive care unit for hourly vital sign assessment and neurologic examination. Puncture site and flank pain should be monitored, and patients with a suspected retroperitoneal hematoma should undergo monitoring of serial serum hemoglobin/hematocrit levels. In severe cases of retroperitoneal hematomas, surgical evacuation may be required. Patients with distal pulse, extremity warmth, and subjective pain in the ipsilateral lower extremity should be monitored for possible arterial occlusion or thromboembolic events, and an immediate vascular surgery consult should be obtained if there is any concern for either of these complications. Post-procedural MRI can be used to detect intracranial thromboembolic complications, which are most readily apparent on diffusion-weighted imaging sequences. Any new neurological deficit should be assessed with immediate CTA and/or MRI/MRA to assess vessel patency and possible infarcts.

Follow-up angiographic assessment intervals vary by institution, but MRA and/or DSA are often recommended at 6 months, 1 year, and 2 years post-procedure, with modifications based on aneurysm occlusion status. CTA is not recommended for endovascular follow-up because artifact from the coils prevents adequate visualization of the aneurysm and branch vessels.

Complications and Management

The most feared intraprocedural complication during endovascular aneurysm treatment is rupture of the aneurysm. Intraprocedural rupture is evident on angiography as contrast extravasation into the subarachnoid space during the coiling process, but it can also be detected by a sudden increase in the patient's blood pressure, which should be continuously monitored through an arterial line during these cases. Rupture necessitates immediate heparin reversal with protamine and an urgent completion of the coil occlusion. In cases in which balloon assistance is used, inflation of the balloon can stem the hemorrhage. External ventricular drain placement should be performed after intraprocedural rupture in virtually all cases, except when the degree of subarachnoid hemorrhage is very minor and the patient awakes without a neurologic deficit.

Intraprocedural thromboembolic complications are treated as soon as they are identified, although their management depends on the severity. With large proximal occlusions of the ICA or proximal middle or anterior cerebral arteries, mechanical thrombectomy using an aspiration catheter or a stent retriever should be employed to rapidly recanalize the vessel. Smaller, more distal branch occlusions can be treated with superselective catheterization and direct intra-arterial infusion of a thrombolytic agent, such as abciximab or recombinant tissue plasminogen activator. If a stent is deployed without preoperative antiplatelet medication, the increased risk of stent thrombosis can be reduced with intra-arterial administration of abciximab or tirofiban (both glycoprotein IIb/IIIa receptor antagonists).

Upon guide catheter removal, brief contrast injections should be performed to assess for cervical ICA dissection and/or vasospasm. If a dissection is minor, it can be treated with antiplatelet medication and imaging follow-up. However, if the dissection is severe (related embolic events, active extravasation, associated pseudoaneurysm, or significant flow limitation with an obvious intimal flap), stent placement may be considered. Vasospasm, if moderate to severe, can be treated with intra-arterial infusion of calcium channel blockers, such as verapamil or nicardipine.

Patients should be consented regarding the possibility of renal injury due to contrast, delayed alopecia due to radiation exposure, and hematomas of the groin area or retroperitoneal space.

Oral Boards Review—Complications Pearls

1. Immediate attention to a cold, pulseless extremity with a lower extremity CTA and a vascular surgery consult can prevent significant morbidity from lower extremity thromboembolus.
2. Retroperitoneal hematoma can be deadly, and puncture of the femoral artery should always be below the inguinal ligament to reduce the hematoma risk. Ultrasound and prepuncture fluoroscopic localization of the femoral head should be used when obtaining vascular access.

Evidence and Outcomes

In a cohort of 37 ICA bifurcation aneurysms treated with endovascular methods, including 12 aneurysms ≤5 mm in size, a 2.7% procedural morbidity was reported. In the cohort, 28 of the aneurysms were unruptured, there were no intraoperative ruptures, and complete or near-complete occlusion was achieved in all cases. One patient had a thromboembolic event 10 days after the procedure. On longer term follow-up with a mean duration of 39.5 months, 23% of patients ($n = 7$) had incomplete aneurysm occlusion and 30% ($n = 9$) had near-complete occlusion, with a recurrence rate of 34% (12/35) and a mean time to recurrence of 13 months. In cases using flow diversion with PED, there were no complications. One patient with a known giant aneurysm recurrence died of rupture 30 months after coiling.

In the associated meta-analysis of endovascularly treated ICA bifurcation aneurysms comprising six studies and 158 patients with 163 aneurysms, the immediate post-embolization rate of complete or near-complete occlusion was 88%, which decreased to 82% on long-term follow-up. The rates of perioperative stroke, intraprocedural rupture, procedural morbidity, and procedural mortality were 3%, 3%, 4%, and 3%, respectively. The meta-analysis also showed a re-treatment rate of 14%, with good neurologic outcome in 93% of patients.

Another group published the results of its interdisciplinary treatment of ICA bifurcation aneurysms with either surgical ($n = 28$) or endovascular ($n = 30$) treatment, such that younger patients with larger aneurysms were generally favored to undergo surgery. All patients with combined factors or history of subarachnoid hemorrhage, superiorly projecting aneurysms, and aneurysms originating from the ICA bifurcation were assigned to coiling ($n = 10$). Complete or near-complete occlusion was achieved in 96% of coiled versus 100% of clipped aneurysms at a mean follow-up of 30 months. Minor recanalization of the neck was found in 42% of the endovascular group, although only 1 patient (4%) had a major recanalization and subsequently underwent surgical treatment. Analysis showed a lower recurrence rate when the A1/M1 segments were involved (10%) versus a higher recurrence rate for the bifurcation-only aneurysms (69%), with a trend toward a greater likelihood of recurrence for superiorly projecting aneurysms. There were no differences in procedural morbidity between the treatment groups, and there were no instances of post-procedural hemorrhage. Although the favorable results of both treatment methods are biased by the treatment allocation preferences of a single institution, the authors noted that selection biases arise frequently with interdisciplinary consensus and therefore are reflective of real-world situations.

A study of 65 patients with ICA bifurcation aneurysms (82% unruptured, 41 patients, and <5-mm aneurysm diameter), who were not included in the aforementioned meta-analysis, reported that all patients were able to achieve immediate aneurysm occlusion, with 88.7% stable occlusion, 7.5% minor recanalization, and 3.8% major recanalization rates at a mean follow-up of 27 months. A single microcatheter technique was used in more than half of the patients; however, 14 (21.2%) required balloon remodeling, 10 (15.1%) required multiple microcatheters, and 5 (7.6%) required stent assistance. A procedural complication occurred in 7 patients, with six instances of subclinical thrombosis (resolved with intra-arterial tirofiban infusion) and one instance of hemorrhage. The authors reported no cases of clinical morbidity or mortality. There were no instances of delayed cerebral infarction or hemorrhage, although 3.8% ($n = 2$) of patients with major recanalization underwent repeat treatment.

Acknowledgment

We thank the staff of Neuroscience Publications at Barrow Neurological Institute for assistance with manuscript preparation.

Further Reading

Backes D, Rinkel GJE, Greving JP, et al. ELAPSS score for prediction of risk of growth of unruptured intracranial aneurysms. *Neurology* 2017;88:1600–1606.

Cekirge SH, Yavuz K, Geyik S, et al. HyperForm balloon-assisted endovascular neck bypass technique to perform balloon or stent-assisted treatment of cerebral aneurysms. *AJNR Am J Neuroradiol*. 2007;28:1388–1390.

Ding D, Etminan N. A model for predicting the growth of unruptured intracranial aneurysms: Beyond fortune telling. *Neurology* 2017;88:1594–1595.

Ingebrigtsen T, Morgan MK, Faulder K, et al. Bifurcation geometry and the presence of cerebral artery aneurysms. *J Neurosurg*. 2004;101:108–113.

Konczalla J, Platz J, Brawanski N, et al. Endovascular and surgical treatment of internal carotid bifurcation aneurysms: Comparison of results, outcome, and mid-term follow-up. *Neurosurgery*. 2015;76:540–550.

Lee WJ, Cho YD, Kang HS, et al. Endovascular coil embolization in internal carotid artery bifurcation aneurysms. *Clin Radiol*. 2014;69:e273–e279.

Lehecka M, Dashti R, Romani R, et al. Microneurosurgical management of internal carotid artery bifurcation aneurysms. *Surg Neurol*. 2009;71:649–667.

Morales-Valero SF, Brinjikji W, Murad MH, et al. Endovascular treatment of internal carotid artery bifurcation aneurysms: A single-center experience and a systematic review and meta-analysis. *AJNR Am J Neuroradiol*. 2014;35:1948–1953.

Park MS, Stiefel MF, Albuquerque FC, et al. Endovascular treatment of cerebral aneurysms. In: Nader R, Gragnaniello C, Berta SC, et al., eds. *Neurosurgery Tricks of the Trade: Cranial*. New York: Thieme; 2013; 429–431.

Patel BM, Ahmed A, Niemann D. Endovascular treatment of supraclinoid internal carotid artery aneurysms. *Neurosurg Clin North Am*. 2014;25:425–435.

Pritz MB. Perforator and secondary branch origin in relation to the neck of saccular, cerebral bifurcation aneurysms. *World Neurosurg*. 2014;82:726–732.

Starke RM, Durst CR, Evans A, et al. Endovascular treatment of unruptured wide-necked intracranial aneurysms: Comparison of dual microcatheter technique and stent-assisted coil embolization. *J Neurointerv Surg*. 2015;7:256–261.

Villablanca JP, Duckwiler GR, Jahan R, et al. Natural history of asymptomatic unruptured cerebral aneurysms evaluated at CT angiography: Growth and rupture incidence and correlation with epidemiologic risk factors. *Radiology* 2013;269:258–265.

Medium-Sized Incidental Anterior Choroidal Artery Aneurysm

Jan-Karl Burkhardt and Michael T. Lawton

9

Case Presentation

A 38-year-old female presented with worsening headaches. She has had chronic headaches for the past 10 years. She was evaluated with brain imaging including computed tomography (CT) angiogram, magnetic resonance imaging (MRI), and magnetic resonance angiography (MRA). A small vessel abnormality was noted at the left internal carotid artery (ICA) near the origin of the posterior communicating artery (PCoA). No hemorrhage or other abnormalities were seen. The patient was neurologically intact without any focal neurological deficits. Her past medical history was unremarkable except for hypertension. The patient is married and has two healthy children, but her father died from a ruptured intracranial aneurysm 5 years ago.

Questions

1. What is the likely diagnosis?
2. What is the most appropriate imaging modality in this situation?
3. What are the most likely vessel locations of this lesion based on cross-sectional imaging?
4. What is the appropriate timing of the diagnostic workup?
5. What are risk factors for this disease?

Assessment and Planning

An unruptured incidental intracranial supraclinoid aneurysm is suspected, associated with either the posterior communicating or the anterior choroidal artery. Other possible diagnoses in the differential are rare and might include vascular tumors or vascular malformations. To confirm the diagnosis, catheter angiography is the next diagnostic step of choice. Because this patient's presenting symptoms include chronic headache, without a thunderclap component or a new neurological deficit, outpatient testing is appropriate for this unruptured intracranial aneurysm (UIA).

The catheter angiogram shows a 3-mm aneurysm arising off of the left anterior choroidal artery (AChA) with a 2-mm aneurysm neck (Figure 9.1). In addition, a 1.5-mm sessile aneurysm is seen within the cavernous segment of the left ICA. No other aneurysms, arteriovenous malformations, stenosis, or other vessel abnormalities are seen.

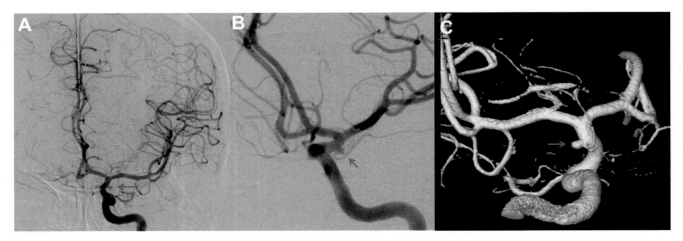

Figure 9.1 Preoperative catheter angiography with anterior–posterior (A), oblique (B), and three-dimensional (C) views demonstrates the left AChA aneurysm (arrows).

Risk factors for aneurysm rupture include a positive family history and hypertension. In general, other risk factors include patient age; previous subarachnoid hemorrhage (SAH) from another aneurysm; aneurysm characteristics such as size, location, shape, and multiplicity; connective tissue disease; and smoking history.

Questions

1. What are the management options for this diagnosis?
2. What scales or scores help the patient/physician during the decision-making process?
3. What is the most appropriate timing for intervention in this patient?

Oral Boards Review—Diagnostic Pearls

1. Catheter angiography is the gold standard to diagnose intracranial aneurysms. Especially with small aneurysms located in the posterior circulation or close to the skull base (as with this AChA aneurysm), catheter angiography can more accurately display the parent vessel and aneurysm with its possible branching vessels and aneurysm characteristics such as daughter sacs.
2. The quality of CTA and MRA has improved during the past several years, and these might be used as an alternative in cases in which catheter angiography is contraindicated, or in elderly patients, to avoid potential complications from catheter angiography.
3. Catheter angiography is an invasive test with a small risk of potential complications, including a permanent neurological complication rate of 0–5.4%.

Decision-Making

Patients presenting with ruptured aneurysms need to be treated within 24 hours due to the high risk for re-rupture within the first days after SAH. The management of patients with UIAs requires a fine judgment balancing the risk of aneurysm rupture with a decision to observe versus the risk of complications from treatment with a decision to intervene. Rupture risk ranges between 0.1% and 4% per year and depends on different patient or aneurysm risk factors, such as aneurysm size and location and patient age. The International Study of Unruptured Intracranial Aneurysms trial and the Unruptured Cerebral Aneurysm Study stratified the risk of rupture for UIAs according to aneurysm size, which showed a very small annual rupture risk for UIAs <7 mm. A useful score to calculate the patient individual aneurysm rupture risk is the UIA treatment score. The UIA treatment score can be used to compare individualized aneurysm rupture risk during observation versus complication rate during aneurysm treatment. All scores and scales take into account demographic and aneurysm characteristics, are compared to published rates of rupture, and provide suggested annualized risks of rupture to aid in treatment decision-making, although no scale is perfect.

If the decision for treatment is made, both microsurgical clipping and endovascular embolization are treatment options. Microsurgical clipping for small UIAs is effective and advantageous in young patients with a long life expectancy because of its durability and lower recurrence rate and re-treatment rate compared to endovascular coiling. Aneurysms with small dome size and wide necks are more favorable for surgical clipping than endovascular coiling, although the advent of stent-assisted coiling and flow-diverting stents permits safe endovascular treatment of wide-necked aneurysms. For older patients or those with surgical comorbidities, endovascular treatment is preferable. Surgical clipping is more favorable for aneurysms in particular locations, such as the AChA (because aneurysm coils may occlude the origin on the AChA).

Questions

1. What are the risks of microsurgical clipping in this patient?
2. Which surgical approach would you choose and what intraoperative adjuvants are helpful to treat this aneurysm?

Surgical Procedure

Microsurgical clipping of an aneurysm is a major procedure carried out under general anesthetic with a Foley catheter and duplicate intravenous access in place. Intraoperative neuromonitoring including somatosensory evoked potentials (SEPs) and motor evoked potentials (MEPs) can alert the surgeon to ischemia during and after clipping and can measure the degree of burst suppression in the case of temporary clipping.

AChA aneurysms are treated through a pterional or mini-pterional approach. The patient is positioned supine in the Mayfield holder with the head rotated 15–20 degrees away from the side of the aneurysm and extended 20 degrees, allowing gravity to retract the frontal lobe away from the anterior fossa; the malar eminence is the highest point. A curvilinear skin incision begins at the zygomatic arch, 1 cm anterior to the tragus, and either arcs to the midline behind the hairline (pterional approach) or stops halfway behind the hairline (mini-pterional approach). After skin incision, the scalp and temporalis muscle are mobilized forward, and a pterional or mini-pterional craniotomy flap is turned. The dura is tacked up circumferentially, and the lateral aspects of the sphenoid wing are drilled until flat. The dura is then opened circumferentially based on the pterion.

The microscope is brought into the field, and the sylvian fissure is widely split, separating the frontal and temporal lobes. The middle cerebral branch arteries are followed down into the sylvian fissure and down to the ICA and its bifurcation. The anterior choroidal artery aneurysm comes into view, and the ICA is dissected for temporary clip placement (Figure 9.2). Then the aneurysm is dissected carefully to fully visualize the aneurysm neck, AChA, and PCoA. This aneurysm can be clipped with a straight 5-mm titanium clip, which occludes the aneurysm dome while preserving the AChA. An indocyanine green (ICG) videoangiogram helps confirm the complete

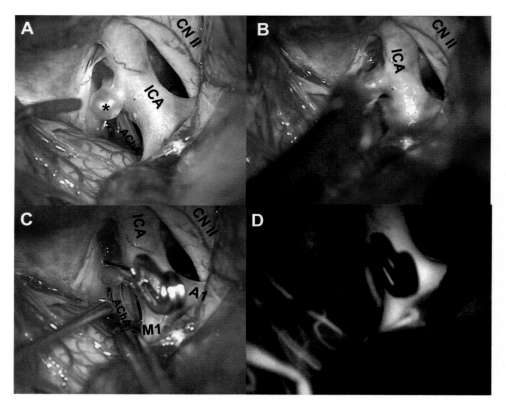

Figure 9.2 Intraoperative images demonstrate the AChA aneurysm (asterisk) before clipping (A), during clipping with a straight 5-mm clip (B), and after clipping (C). ICG angiography confirms complete aneurysm occlusion and patency of the AChA (D). A1, A1 segment anterior cerebral artery; AChA, anterior choroidal artery; CNII, optic nerve; ICA, internal carotid artery; M1, M1 segment middle cerebral artery.

clipping of the aneurysm with no compromise of the AChA. The aneurysm sac can be punctured to confirm complete occlusion. Both MEPs and SEPs are monitored throughout the surgery. In case of changes after clipping, immediate adjustment of the clip is important to prevent AChA stroke. Cisternal irrigation with vasodilators (e.g., nicardipine and papaverine) can reverse or prevent vasospasm associated with surgical manipulation, preventing ischemia in small vessels.

After irrigation, the dura is closed with running 4–0 sutures and the bone flap is replaced with titanium plates and screws. Temporalis muscle and galea are re-approximated with interrupted 2–0 sutures. The skin is closed with staples or suture.

Questions

1. How many days will the patient be admitted perioperatively?
2. When should the patient be followed up after surgery?

Oral Boards Review—Management Pearls

1. Complete aneurysm occlusion is necessary to prevent aneurysm recurrence and eliminate the risk of aneurysm rupture.
2. In approximately 5% of cases, a duplication of the AChA is present and needs to be taken into consideration during clipping.
3. Before clipping, it is important to expose both the PCoA and the AChA in the carotid–oculomotor triangle to prevent unintentional clipping of these two important arteries.
4. A wide sylvian fissure dissection is needed to expose the terminal ICA and AChA to have enough exposure for clipping.

Pivot Points

1. If intraoperative MEP/SEP waves change after clipping, immediately readjust clips to prevent AChA infarct.
2. Aneurysm recurrence after clipping is rare and significantly lower compared to that after coiling. A 3- to 5-year follow-up catheter angiography is recommended to check for recurrence and de novo aneurysms.

Aftercare

Patients with UIAs are usually admitted in the morning on the day of surgery. After surgery, the patient stays for 1 night in the intensive care unit followed by 1 or 2 nights on a step-down ward. The patient can be discharged when there are no complications, the surgical wound looks intact, and an angiogram or CTA confirms complete aneurysm occlusion (Figure 9.3). Staples/sutures can be removed 10 days after surgery, and a first clinical

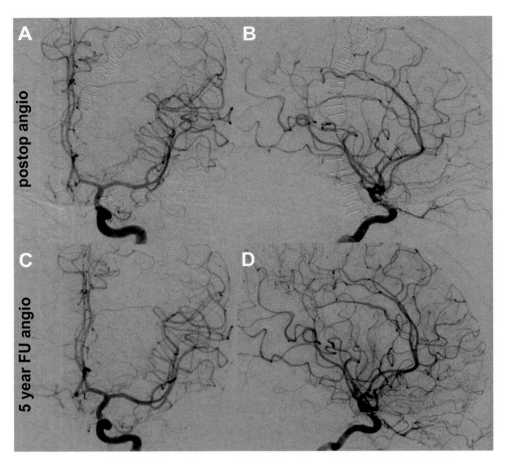

Figure 9.3 Direct postoperative catheter angiography (A and B) and 5-year follow-up (FU) catheter angiography (C and D) in anterior–posterior (A and C) and lateral (B and D) views. Complete aneurysm occlusion was confirmed with patency of parent vessels. Five-year follow-up catheter angiography showed stable condition without aneurysm regrowth or any de novo aneurysms.

outpatient follow-up visit is scheduled 6 weeks after surgery. A long-term follow-up catheter angiogram is scheduled 3–5 years after surgery to rule out the rare event of aneurysm recurrence or de novo aneurysm formation at another location (see Figure 9.3).

Questions

1. Which symptoms will the patient have if the AChA is occluded during clipping?
2. How can you avoid complications during surgery?

Complications and Management

In addition to general surgical complications such as infection and postoperative hemorrhage, the complication risk during aneurysm clipping may include intraoperative aneurysm rupture, stroke due to unintended injury/occlusion of intracerebral arteries or veins, and incomplete aneurysm occlusion.

The AChA aneurysm location is especially delicate because occlusion or injury of the parent AChA artery may lead to an anterior choroidal infarct with devastating consequences, including contralateral hemiplegia; contralateral hemi-hypoesthesia; and homonymous hemianopsia due to partial damage of the posterior limb of the internal capsule, thalamus, and lateral geniculate body. If the infarct is in the dominant hemisphere, an AChA infarct may also lead to aphasia. Indocyanine green videoangiography and MEP/SEP monitoring are important surgical adjuncts in detecting a possible AChA occlusion early during surgery, when corrective action such as clip adjustment or vasodilator irrigation can be taken. Postoperative detection of neurological deficits related to AChA occlusion should prompt immediate surgical re-exploration and clip adjustment. Symptoms of AChA infarcts may improve over time because the posterior limb of the internal capsule also receives lenticulostriate artery supply from the middle cerebral artery. However, the recovery time can take weeks or months.

Questions

1. Is there a difference in aneurysm recurrence rates for clipped versus coiled aneurysms?
2. Is the AChA aneurysm location a common or rare aneurysm location?

Oral Boards Review—Complications Pearls

1. Careful perioperative assessment of the AChA using intraoperative monitoring (MEP and SEP) and ICG videoangiography helps prevent an AChA infarct.
2. Incomplete aneurysm occlusion may need re-surgery. Therefore, postoperative angiography is important during the hospitalization to rule out any aneurysm residual.

Evidence and Outcomes

Both microsurgical clipping and endovascular coiling of AChA aneurysms are effective. However, the aneurysm recurrence rate is lower for clipped aneurysm compared to coiling, and endovascular treatment may put the AChA at risk of occlusion if the aneurysm incorporates the AChA.

Further Reading

André A, Boch AL, Di Maria F, et al. Complication risk factors in anterior choroidal artery aneurysm treatment. *Clin Neuroradiol.* 2018;28(3):345–356. doi:10.1007/s00062-017-0575-y.

Bekelis K, Gottlieb DJ, Su Y, et al. Comparison of clipping and coiling in elderly patients with unruptured cerebral aneurysms. *J Neurosurg.* 2017;126(3):811–818.

Chalouhi N, Bovenzi CD, Thakkar V, et al. Long-term catheter angiography after aneurysm coil therapy: Results of 209 patients and predictors of delayed recurrence and retreatment. *J Neurosurg.* 2014;121:1102–1106.

Davies JM, Lawton MT. Advances in open microsurgery for cerebral aneurysms. *Neurosurgery.* 2014;74(Suppl 1):S7–S16.

Jang CK, Park KY, Lee JW, et al. Microsurgical treatment of unruptured anterior choroidal artery aneurysms: Incidence of and risk factors for procedure-related complications. *World Neurosurg.* 2018;119:e679–e685. doi:10.1016/j.wneu.2018.07.241.

Srinivasan VM, Ghali MGZ, Cherian J, et al. Flow diversion for anterior choroidal artery (AChA) aneurysms: A multi-institutional experience. *J Neurointerv Surg.* 2018;10(7):634–637. doi:10.1136/neurintsurg-2017-013466.

Giant Aneurysm of the Middle Cerebral Artery Presenting with Headache

Robert T. Wicks and Robert F. Spetzler

10

Case Presentation

A 32-year-old female presents to the emergency department with a severe headache that has waxed and waned during the past week. She reports that it started 1 week ago when she experienced the worst headache of her life. She did not seek medical care at that time. She denies nausea, vomiting, and photophobia. Her only prior medical history consists of panic attacks. She denies any family history of vascular disorders. She is awake and notably anxious but is otherwise neurologically intact without any focal deficits or nuchal rigidity.

A head computed tomography (CT) scan without contrast was obtained and was negative for acute hemorrhage. A lumbar puncture was then performed, which revealed xanthochromia documenting a prior subarachnoid hemorrhage. A CT angiogram (CTA) was performed that revealed a giant fusiform aneurysm of the right middle cerebral artery (MCA) (Figure 10.1).

Questions

1. What additional information should be gathered from the CTA? When should a six-vessel diagnostic angiogram be performed?
2. What are the three morphological subtypes of giant MCA aneurysms? How does the morphology affect the management strategy?
3. What management options are available, both endovascular and microsurgical, for giant MCA aneurysms?

Assessment and Planning

A comprehensive history should be obtained, and a thorough physical examination should be performed to establish the patient's appropriateness for surgical intervention. The CTA should be of adequate quality to visualize the aneurysm morphology along with the branching vasculature. Both internal and external carotid vasculature of the head and neck should be visualized to evaluate potential bypass options. If CTA adequately provides this information, then a digitally subtracted angiogram is not necessary.

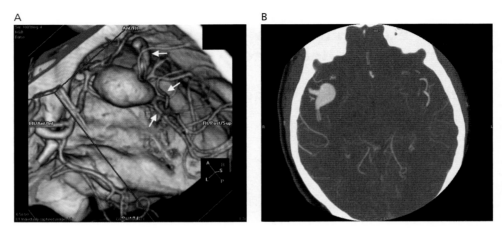

Figure 10.1 (A) CTA revealing a giant MCA fusiform aneurysm with fusiform branch segment and two distal branching arteries (white arrows). (B) Axial CTA revealing the distal portion of the fusiform aneurysm with filling of the dilated MCA segment and one major and two smaller distal branches.

Oral Boards Review—Diagnostic Pearls

1. Detailed preoperative planning is necessary. Determine whether any branching arteries are involved in the giant MCA aneurysm and which, if any, will remain patent with clip reconstruction. Assess what potential bypass procedures may be necessary.
2. Analyze the anatomy of the STA and predict whether the STA is of adequate size to allow for a bypass to be performed and whether both the frontal and parietal divisions of the STA are of sufficient size to perform a double-barrel bypass if this is required.
3. When pursuing microsurgical management of a giant aneurysm, always consider what high-flow bypass options may be available. If a radial artery graft is feasible, plan to prepare the forearm and position the patient accordingly to ensure access.
4. Referral to a high-volume center for the management of complex giant aneurysms should always be considered depending on the level of open cerebrovascular surgical experience.

Questions

1. Is the superficial temporal artery (STA) of adequate size to allow for a bypass if one were to become necessary? Are both frontal and temporal branches of the STA present and of adequate size in the event that a double-barrel bypass procedure is necessary?
2. What steps should be taken during preparation for microsurgical intervention? What additional precautions should be taken in regard to positioning?

3. Will the mass effect of the aneurysm be fully reduced once the vascular inflow is occluded or the parent vessel is reconstructed? Or, is there a significant thrombosed portion to the aneurysm that will require internal debulking with an ultrasonic aspirator?

Decision-Making

Giant aneurysms, defined as larger than 2.5 cm in size, represented 4.7% of aneurysms in the International Study of Unruptured Intracranial Aneurysms (ISUIA) study. In larger series of MCA aneurysms alone, giant MCA aneurysms represent approximately 3–5%. Although rare, the prognosis for untreated giant intracranial aneurysms is poor. One study reported mortality rates of 68% at 2 years and 85% at 5 years. In the subset of unruptured giant aneurysms of the anterior circulation that were monitored in the ISUIA trial, a 5-year cumulative rupture rate of 40% was described.

Giant aneurysms of the MCA can take on one of three forms: saccular, fusiform, and serpentine. The first, most common, form is saccular, which develops through the gradual enlargement of a smaller saccular aneurysm typically at the MCA bifurcation. As the artery enlarges, the neck will often envelop the branching arteries, making bypass procedures necessary. Fusiform aneurysms, in contrast, develop through progressive atherosclerotic change over a long segment of the parent vessel. These aneurysms by definition do not have a true neck. They will often eventually envelop major branching arteries, making complex reconstructive and bypass procedures necessary. Giant serpentine aneurysms are a group of partially thrombosed aneurysms with a small persistent "serpentine" vascular channel. These aneurysms have a large surrounding avascular, thrombosed portion that will cause mass effect and can be associated with surrounding edema. Serpentine giant aneurysms are rarely associated with hemorrhage or rupture. Internal debulking of the aneurysm, however, is often necessary to decrease its mass effect.

Two treatment strategies exist in regard to giant MCA aneurysms: open microsurgical and neuroendovascular. Surgical management of giant aneurysms was historically limited to Hunterian ligation—a procedure named for the Scottish surgeon John Hunter, who first described the surgical occlusion of the parent artery for treatment of a popliteal artery aneurysm in 1793. The cooperative aneurysm study revealed a 59% rate of ischemic complications with acute ligation of the internal carotid artery and a 32% rate of complications with ligation of the common carotid artery; complication rates with graduated occlusion were slightly lower. With the development of microneurosurgery and the field of neuroanesthesia within the latter half of the 20th century, successful techniques for clip reconstruction and extracranial–intracranial bypass were developed. Initial treatment series with microsurgical management revealed significant improvement in outcomes with surgical mortality rates between 5% and 22%, with good or excellent outcomes seen in 61–87% of patients. One study revealed surgical outcomes to be excellent in 74% of patients, with a morbidity rate of 12% and mortality rate of 9%. A more recent series of ruptured and unruptured giant aneurysms revealed similar rates, with a neurologic morbidity related to surgery of 9% and mortality rate of 13%. In a separate series reviewing the surgical management of large or giant fusiform MCA aneurysms, no mortalities were noted and a modified Rankin Scale score of ≤2 was achieved in 90% of patients. Given the poor natural history of giant cerebral aneurysms with relatively favorable surgical outcomes, aggressive surgical management of these complex lesions has been advocated.

Due to both the distal location and the frequent involvement of branching arteries within the aneurysm neck, endovascular options are often suboptimal when evaluating giant MCA aneurysms. The largest early series of giant intracranial aneurysms treated with endovascular techniques revealed a 26% morbidity rate and 29% mortality rate at last follow-up, with a 95% occlusion rate in 64% of aneurysms and 100% occlusion rate in 36% of aneurysms. A review of the literature through 2007 revealed that coiling and balloon-assisted stent coiling of all giant aneurysms have been noted to provide occlusion rates of approximately 57%, a mean mortality rate of 7.7%, and a major morbidity rate of 17.2%. Giant MCA aneurysms present a greater challenge. Liquid embolization with materials such as Onyx is not feasible given the multiple branching arteries. With the advent of the Pipeline embolization device (PED), which was initially applied to distal giant aneurysms but in one case involved an M1 division giant MCA, combined PED with coiling resulted in the unfortunate collapse of the stent due to the size of coil mass required to embolize the aneurysm. Although dense coil packing is not necessary with PED, additional difficulty is found in that the proximal MCA territory involves the many branching lateral lenticulostriate arteries, which are at risk of thrombosis due to the flow-diverting stent, and the distal MCA has multiple large branching arterial divisions. Notwithstanding, a study described 10 patients with complex MCA aneurysms, five of which were large MCA aneurysms and three were giant, who were treated with PED. One morbidity and no mortalities were noted. Outcomes for the giant MCA aneurysms alone are not clearly presented in isolation, although all giant aneurysms described in the series were fusiform in nature. Overall, three of five patients with MCA M1 division aneurysms were successfully occluded and one of three MCA bifurcation aneurysms were occluded at last follow-up between 7 and 12 months. Delayed aneurysm rupture can remain a persistent problem in large or giant aneurysms treated with PED.

Questions

1. What endovascular options are feasible and under what circumstance should they be applied?
2. What surgical approach and preparations should be made in this patient?
3. What particular steps should be considered if the parent artery must be occluded and none of the branching vessels can be preserved?

Surgical Procedure

Microsurgical clip reconstruction with STA–MCA bypass was planned. The patient was positioned supine, and the patient's head was placed into a radiolucent three-point head clamp in the event that intraoperative neuroangiography became necessary. The head was turned approximately 45 degrees and slightly extended. The patient's right neck was prepared, in addition to the right forearm in preparation for a potential radial artery graft, and the right groin was prepared for potential intraoperative angiogram. A Doppler probe was used to identify the STA parietal branch. Dissection of the frontal branch of the STA was not believed to be necessary. The skin incision was planned behind the hairline approximating the path of the STA.

The approach chosen was a modified two-piece orbito-zygomatic craniotomy. The STA was dissected free for a length of approximately 7 cm. The artery was kept in continuity. The temporalis muscle was incised, and the myocutaneous flap was dissected free from the bone and brought forward. The roof of the orbit was dissected free of the periorbita. A pterional craniotomy flap was turned in the usual fashion. A sagittal cutting saw was then used to make the following cuts: (1) along the medial aspect of the orbit through the roof of the orbit immediately lateral to the supraorbital nerve, (2) lateral to the fronto-zygomatic suture, and (3) across the roof of the orbit connecting to the McCarty keyhole. An osteotome was used to free the modified orbito-zygomatic bone flap.

After smoothing of the pterional ridge with a high-speed drill, the dura was opened in a curvilinear fashion and tacked forward. The proximal sylvian fissure was then opened. The proximal M2 artery was identified, and with it, the aneurysm. The M1 branch was then identified, and a site for proximal control was exposed. The aneurysm was then dissected free of the surrounding vessels and brain. It consisted of a large bulbous portion and large outflow branch. Distal on the aneurysm, two additional small outflow branches were identified. Intraoperative indocyanine green (ICG) study was then performed to confirm which were the inflow and outflow branches of the aneurysm (Figure 10.2).

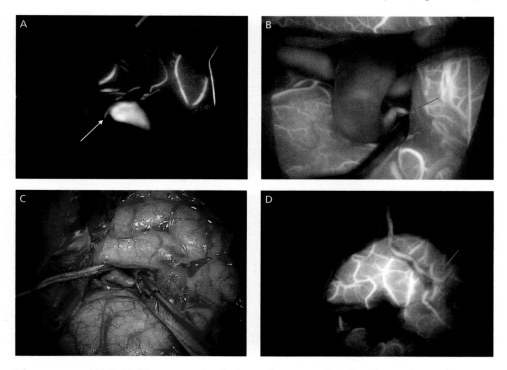

Figure 10.2 (A) Initial intraoperative indocyanine green (ICG) videoangiography revealing the proximal MCA inflow (white arrow) and major proximal outflow (red arrow) of the giant fusiform MCA aneurysm. (B) Initial intraoperative ICG videoangiography revealing the distal outflow (red arrow) of the giant fusiform MCA aneurysm into two immediately adjacent branching arteries. (C) Intraoperative photograph of the proximal clip ligation of the giant MCA fusiform aneurysm while maintaining perfusion of the proximal major MCA branch. (D) Final intraoperative ICG videoangiography revealing patency of the STA to M3 division bypass (red arrow).

It was clear from the ICG study that one of the outflow branches from the aneurysm could be maintained with clip reconstruction of the proximal part of the aneurysm. The temporal lobe was supplied by MCA feeders from the proximal aneurysm. The decision was made that a STA bypass to a frontal M3 artery would be necessary. The STA was then prepared by placing a temporary clip at the distal end and disconnecting the artery at its distal end. All soft tissue was cleared from the end, and the STA was then anastomosed to the M3 branch using two running 10–0 Prolene sutures. A straight clip was placed proximally on the aneurysm to reconstruct the deep inflow and one outflow branch. A final ICG was then run that revealed good filling of the outflow branch with clip reconstruction and no filling of the aneurysm. Good flow was noted through the STA–MCA bypass and the entirety of the cortical surface.

Oral Boards Review—Management Pearls

1. Endovascular approaches often do not provide adequate management options to effectively treat giant MCA aneurysms.
2. Be prepared to perform a high-flow bypass. Consider preparing a forearm in the event that a radial artery donor graft is required. If a radial artery graft is planned, assess the radial artery with an ultrasound to confirm patency prior to planning the dissection.
3. Total intravenous anesthesia should be considered early on during the surgical procedure in situations in which significant cerebral edema or prior preoperative hemorrhage is a concern.
4. Neuromonitoring with electroencephalogram (EEG), somatosensory evoked potentials (SSEPs), and motor evoked potentials is recommended. EEG is useful in confirming anesthetic burst suppression during periods of temporary occlusion.
5. Place cardioversion pads on the chest in the event that intraoperative adenosine is necessary for temporary cardiac arrest if premature aneurysm rupture occurs.
6. Prior to performing the craniotomy, take additional time to ensure the STA is preserved. Then, dissect out the STA in preparation for bypass prior to proceeding with the craniotomy. It is best to keep the STA in continuity until the required time to perform the bypass. Consider whether a double-barrel bypass may be necessary to fully restore flow to the arterial branches whose parent artery will be sacrificed. If so, prepare to dissect both parietal and frontal branches of the STA a sufficient length to use in bypass, generally approximately 7 cm.
7. Have wrapping material such as cotton available in the event that a complete clipping while maintaining all branching vasculature is not possible.

Pivot Points

1. If the giant MCA aneurysm involves the proximal M1 segment and is not located at the bifurcation, a high-flow bypass to the MCA segment distal to the aneurysm will likely be necessary.

2. If the aneurysm is located at the MCA division point and two major branching vessels are to be sacrificed in the reconstruction, a double-barrel STA bypass may need to be considered.

3. If there is a significant thrombosed portion to the aneurysm causing symptomatic mass effect or surrounding edema, the aneurysm may need to be opened and decompressed (frequently using an ultrasonic aspirator) prior to completing the definitive clip reconstruction.

Aftercare

The initial postoperative period is critical in situations of giant MCA aneurysm management, especially when a bypass procedure is performed. Systolic blood pressure should generally be maintained within the range of 100–140 mmHg to maintain perfusion through the bypass while preventing hemorrhage during the postoperative period. If a bypass is performed, aspirin 325 mg daily should be initiated immediately postoperatively. Immediate postoperative angiography should be performed (Figure 10.3), with repeat angiography with a diagnostic cerebral angiogram is recommended at 6 months and 2 years following treatment. If aneurysm residual is observed, it can be monitored or subsequently treated with repeat surgery or endovascular methods, as in this case (Figure 10.4).

Complications and Management

Many of the most dreaded complications of giant MCA aneurysm surgery can be prevented through detailed microsurgical technique and careful consideration of

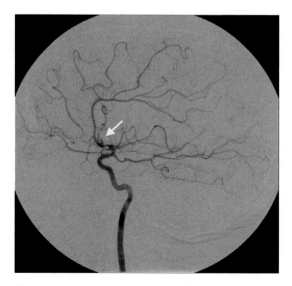

Figure 10.3 Immediate postoperative angiogram showing a right internal carotid artery injection, lateral projection. There is small residual filling of the giant fusiform MCA aneurysm proximal to the aneurysm clip (arrow). This residual portion was necessary in order to maintain patency of the first major branching artery.

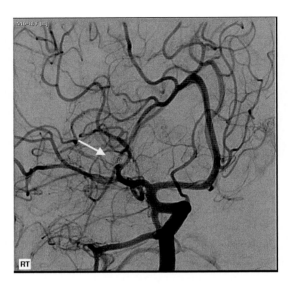

Figure 10.4 The residual portion of the aneurysm was monitored over time. Definitive coiling of the residual aneurysm component was performed in a delayed fashion at 2 years. Right carotid artery injection, oblique projection. Definite coiling is seen (arrow) with patency of all branching arteries.

contingency plans for management of the most common complications—that is, premature aneurysm rupture, occlusion of branching arteries, incomplete aneurysm obliteration, prolonged temporary occlusion with resulting ischemia, and occlusion of bypass. To be prepared for premature aneurysm rupture, intraoperative monitoring with SSEPs and EEG should be performed in the event temporal arterial occlusion is necessary. Cardioversion pads should be placed in the event that adenosine is necessary for temporary cardiac flow arrest. Temporary clipping should be used judiciously and the occlusion time minimized to absolute necessity to avoid ischemic complications. If, based on preoperative imaging, there is a high likelihood that permanent proximal MCA artery occlusion may be necessary, preoperative preparations for high-flow bypass should be made. The radial artery should be assessed preoperatively with ultrasound to confirm its patency. Patients with frequent or prolonged prior hospitalizations may occlude their radial arteries secondary to multiple arterial line placements. An alternative saphenous vein graft can also be considered. If the giant MCA aneurysm is located at a more distal MCA division point, an STA–MCA bypass may suffice. In our series of unclippable giant MCA aneurysms that required extracranial–intracranial bypass procedures, 75% of aneurysms (12 of 16 cases) were occluded successfully. A small residual was noted in the other cases that were later re-treated. The management strategy was associated with three infarctions but no perioperative deaths. In another series of surgically treated giant aneurysms, a rebleeding rate of 3% and re-treatment rate of 1% were reported. If proper steps are taken throughout these complex surgical procedures, complications can be reduced and successful treatment outcomes can be achieved.

Oral Boards Review—Complications Pearls

1. Intraoperative monitoring with EEG and SSEPs is helpful in establishing burst suppression and preventing ischemic injury during temporary arterial occlusion. Limit temporary clipping time to no more than 8–10 minutes to help lower the risk of permanent ischemic injury.
2. Be prepared that if the M1 must be sacrificed, high-flow bypass or double-barrel STA bypass options will likely be required.
3. Remember to initiate antiplatelet therapy postoperatively if a bypass procedure is performed.
4. During the postoperative period, close monitoring of blood pressure is critical to preventing postoperative hemorrhage.

Evidence and Outcomes

Some series show similar outcomes with giant MCA aneurysm treatment as with other MCA aneurysm management when unruptured. In a series of 750 unruptured MCA aneurysms, 26 were considered giant. There were no reported mortalities throughout the series, and only 1 giant aneurysm experienced a treatment-related complication of a deep vein thrombosis. In the series of ruptured and unruptured large or giant fusiform aneurysms of the MCA, complete obliteration was found in 19 out of 20 total aneurysms (95%), and a good outcome (modified Ranking Scale score ≤2) was seen in 18 patients (90%), only 1 of which had worsened after the operation.

Further Reading

Eller JL, Dumont TM, Sorkin GC, et al. Endovascular therapies for middle cerebral artery aneurysms. In: Spetzler RF, Kalani MYS, Nakaji P, eds. *Neurovascular Surgery*. 2nd ed. New York: Thieme; 2015:569–583.

Jahromi BS, Mocco J, Bang JA, et al. Clinical and angiographic outcome after endovascular management of giant intracranial aneurysms. *Neurosurgery*. 2008;63(4):662–674.

Kalani MY, Zabramski JM, Hu YC, Spetzler RF. Extracranial–intracranial bypass and vessel occlusion for the treatment of unclippable giant middle cerebral artery aneurysms. *Neurosurgery*. 2013;72(3):428–435.

Lawton MT, Spetzler RF. Surgical management of giant intracranial aneurysms: Experience with 171 patients. *Clin Neurosurg*. 1995;42:245–266.

Mizoi K, Yoshimoto T. Permissible temporary occlusion time in aneurysm surgery as evaluated by evoked potential monitoring. *Neurosurgery*. 1993;33(3):434–440.

Morley TP, Barr HW. Giant intracranial aneurysms: Diagnosis, course, and management. *Clin Neurosurg*. 1969;16:73–94.

Nussbaum ES, Madison MT, Goddard JK, Lassig JP, Kallmes KM, Nussbaum LA. Microsurgical treatment of unruptured middle cerebral artery aneurysms: A large, contemporary experience. *J Neurosurg*. 2018 June 22.

Peerless S, Wallace M, Drake C. Giant intracranial aneurysms. In: Youmans J, ed. *Neurological Surgery: A Comprehensive Reference Guide to the Diagnosis and Management of Neurological Problems*. Philadelphia: Saunders; 1990:1742–1763.

Reynolds MR, Osbun JW, Cawley CM, Barrow DL. Giant aneurysms of the anterior circulation. In: Rangel-Castilla L, Nakaji P, Siddiqui AH, Spetzler RF, Levy E, eds. *Decision Making in Neurovascular Disease*. New York: Thieme; 2018:203–211.

Sharma BS, Gupta A, Ahmad FU, Suri A, Mehta VS. Surgical management of giant intracranial aneurysms. *Clin Neurol Neurosurg*. 2008;110(7):674–681.

Siddiqui AH, Kan P, Abla AA, Hopkins LN, Levy EI. Complications after treatment with pipeline embolization for giant distal intracranial aneurysms with or without coil embolization. *Neurosurgery*. 2012;71(2):E509–E513.

Spetzler RF, Carter LP. Revascularization and aneurysm surgery: Current status. *Neurosurgery*. 1985;16(1):111–116.

Sughrue ME, Saloner D, Rayz VL, Lawton MT. Giant intracranial aneurysms: Evolution of management in a contemporary surgical series. *Neurosurgery*. 2011;69(6):1261–1270.

Wiebers DO, Whisnant JP, Huston J, 3rd, et al. Unruptured intracranial aneurysms: Natural history, clinical outcome, and risks of surgical and endovascular treatment. *Lancet*. 2003;362(9378):103–110.

Xu F, Xu B, Huang L, Xiong J, Gu Y, Lawton MT. Surgical treatment of large or giant fusiform middle cerebral artery aneurysms: A case series. *World Neurosurg*. 2018;115:e252–e262.

Ruptured Pericallosal Artery Aneurysm

Kristine Ravina, Jonathan J. Russin, and Steven L. Giannotta

11

Case Presentation

A 41-year-old female is admitted with a 4-day history of gradual-onset neck pain, lower back pain, and headache that had worsened after an unsuccessful chiropractic treatment. The patient has no significant past medical history and denies any head injuries. Detailed neurological examination reveals nuchal rigidity and lethargy. The patient is fully oriented and displays no ocular movement restriction, no visual impairment, and no other cranial nerve deficits. She has symmetric muscle strength, tone, and reflexes. Head computed tomography (CT) imaging without contrast reveals subarachnoid hemorrhage (SAH) within the cingulate, callosal, and frontal sulci and communicating hydrocephalus (Figure 11.1).

Questions

1. What is the differential diagnosis?
2. What additional imaging is necessary for surgical planning?
3. Which features in the initial imaging indicate location of the lesion?

Assessment and Planning

Suspecting a vascular lesion, a CT angiogram (CTA) is performed, which reveals a saccular (2.8 × 2.6 mm), bilobed anterior cerebral artery (ACA) A3 or pericallosal segment aneurysm. The aneurysm can be seen arising immediately proximal to the origin of the callosomarginal artery on the left (Figures 11.2 and 11.3A). Based on traditional ACA anatomic classification, the A2 segment begins at the anterior communicating artery (ACoA) and transitions to be the A3 segment at the junction of the rostrum and genu of the corpus callosum. The A3 segment then continues around the genu and terminates where the artery turns sharply posterior above the genu. The A4 and A5 segments then run along the superior surface of the corpus callosum and are typically divided by the coronal suture. In 85% of cases, distal ACA aneurysms originate from the A3 segment. Distal ACA aneurysm rupture typically causes SAH over the genu and body of corpus callosum, which can further extend into the adjacent sulci, as seen in Figure 11.1.

ACoA or proximal ACA aneurysms are included in the differential diagnosis, although they would typically present with an interhemispheric and/or perimesencephalic SAH pattern. Although unlikely in the presented case, differential diagnoses can also include other vascular lesions, such as a ruptured frontal arteriovenous malformation or traumatic

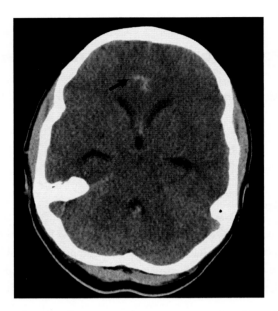

Figure II.I Presented patient's preoperative noncontrast head CT image showing communicating hydrocephalus and SAH (arrow).

pseudoaneurysm, as well as non-aneurysmal SAH or reversible cerebral vasoconstriction syndrome. ACA aneurysmal hemorrhage commonly has an intraparenchymal and/or intraventricular extension and can be associated with hydrocephalus as in the presented case. Distal ACA aneurysms are not typically associated with cranial nerve deficits, such as visual disturbances that can be seen with mass effect from large ACoA aneurysms. In the absence of a typical sudden, severe "thunderclap" headache with the presence of nuchal rigidity and back pain, the diagnosis of meningitis should also be considered when initial imaging is not conclusive for SAH.

A noncontrast head CT is very sensitive for SAH and is helpful during the initial workup to diagnose subarachnoid, intraparenchymal, and/or intraventricular

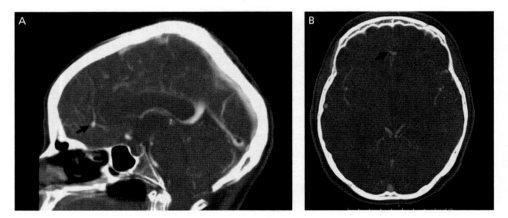

Figure II.2 Presented patient's re-operative CTA showing the left anterior cerebral artery A3 segment aneurysm (arrow) arising immediately proximal to the origin of the callosomarginal artery in sagittal (A) and axial (B) planes.

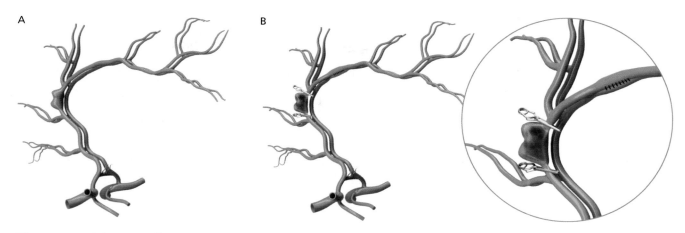

Figure 11.3 Schematic illustration of the presented case showing left anterior cerebral artery A3 segment aneurysm (A) and microsurgical management with clip-trapping and side-to-side microvascular bypass (B).

hemorrhage as well as the presence of hydrocephalus. A CTA is a rapid, noninvasive, and relatively safe secondary imaging modality and should be utilized whenever there is concern for vascular pathology based on clinical presentation and the initial noncontrast CT. The CTA also allows for three-dimensional (3D) image reconstruction, which can help with spatial examination of the vascular lesion and its relationship to the surrounding structures.

The gold standard for vascular imaging is a digital subtraction angiogram of all cerebral vessels in at least two projections (anteroposterior and lateral), as well as 3D reconstructions when indicated. Catheter angiography provides detailed, high-resolution information on aneurysm morphology, filling dynamics, and collateral circulation, and it can rule out any other vascular pathology. It can also evaluate the extracranial circulation when a revascularization procedure may be required.

Oral Boards Review—Diagnostic Pearls

1. Pseudoaneurysms of the ACA
   a. Traumatic pseudoaneurysms: The distal ACA segments' proximity to the falx cerebri renders it sensitive to traumatic pseudoaneurysm formation that can occur even with mild closed head injury, more commonly in children. Typical for motor vehicle accidents, acceleration–deceleration-induced brain movement against the falx cerebri can cause arterial wall injury resulting in pseudoaneurysm formation. Arterial injury can also be caused by penetrating head injuries and skull fractures.
   b. Iatrogenic pseudoaneurysms: Surgical procedures such as frontal lobe and skull base tumor resection, especially via the endoscopic, trans-sphenoidal route, can be complicated by iatrogenic arterial injury. Certain tumors, particularly craniopharyngiomas, tend to have capsules that can adhere to adjacent blood vessels and result in pseudoaneurysm formation during

resection. In these cases, arterial injury typically occurs on more proximal ACA or distal internal carotid artery segments.

c. Diagnosing pseudoaneurysms: The natural history of pseudoaneurysms is associated with a very high mortality rate due to recurrent hemorrhages. These vascular lesions can be easily overlooked in cases of traumatic brain injury in which there are hemorrhages in multiple intracranial locations. Pseudoaneurysms typically lack a defined neck or walls; are not necessarily located at arterial branch points; and can present with delayed, recurrent hemorrhages weeks or even years after the initial injury. It is important to obtain and carefully review a CTA in cases of head trauma in which there is any concern for a traumatic pseudoaneurysm. When the clinical suspicion for a traumatic pseudoaneurysm is high, a negative CTA should be supplemented with a catheter angiogram. In addition, follow-up CTA or catheter angiograms should be obtained at approximately 7 days and 3 months post injury if initial studies are negative. Regardless of the pathogenesis, a pseudoaneurysm should be treated as soon as possible to prevent life-threatening recurrent hemorrhage.

2. False-negative imaging
   a. After excluding an intracranial mass lesion and SAH on initial CT imaging, a lumbar puncture or brain magnetic resonance imaging can be performed when the clinical history suggests a ruptured aneurysm. When a lumbar puncture is required, blood-tinged or xanthochromic cerebrospinal fluid (CSF) requires further angiographic evaluation.
   b. A false-negative angiogram in the presence of SAH on CT is more characteristic of communicating ACA segment aneurysms. In cases of angio-negative SAH, a repeat angiogram, including all six vessels but specifically focused on the suspicious vascular segment, should be obtained approximately 1 week after presentation. If the 1-week angiographic follow-up is negative, a 3-month follow-up angiogram is typically recommended.

Questions

1. How do these radiological findings influence surgical planning?
2. Is revascularization a consideration in this case?
3. What are the key points in surgical approach planning?

Decision-Making

Distal ACA aneurysms tend to rupture at a smaller size (<7 mm) compared to other circle of Willis aneurysms. For this reason, treatment of a small, unruptured distal ACA aneurysm in an otherwise healthy patient should be considered when such a lesion would likely be recommended for observation in other anatomic locations. Endovascular treatment of distal ACA aneurysms is possible in certain circumstances, but it is generally not favored due to the relatively small diameter of the parent artery and the typical wide-necked morphology of these aneurysms.

In cases in which the aneurysm morphology is such that the parent artery will be at risk with attempted clip reconstruction or when trapping of the aneurysmal segment is being planned, revascularization should be considered (Figure 11.3B). The distal A3/A4 segments coursing along the corpus callosum are ideal candidates for a side-to-side in situ bypass to revascularize the distal ACA segments. In the current case, an A3–A3 bypass was performed after exploring the aneurysm and deciding that clip reconstruction would place the parent artery at risk or a significant aneurysmal remnant would remain.

Distal ACA aneurysms are typically approached using a frontal interhemispheric craniotomy. Utilizing this approach, both A3 segments can be accessed under the inferior edge of the falx cerebri. The exact location of the aneurysm along the course of ACA determines the location of the bone flap. The more proximal the aneurysm is located, the more anterior the craniotomy should be. The correct approach angle will prevent the genu of the corpus callosum from obstructing the surgeon's view of the ACA segment proximal to the aneurysm. If a side-to-side bypass is planned, the craniotomy needs to be large enough to allow sufficient room for the anastomosis to be performed distal to the aneurysm.

Questions

1. What surgical approach is the most optimal for A3 segment aneurysms and why?
2. What are the technical pitfalls associated with the interhemispheric approach and how do you avoid them?
3. Which imaging and intraoperative findings would indicate the need for revascularization and what are the benefits and disadvantages of different kinds of bypasses in this location?

Surgical Procedure

As per routine protocol, patients receive antibiotics, diuresis, and antiepileptics following the induction of general anesthesia. Intraoperative monitoring of somatosensory and motor evoked potentials, as well as electroencephalography, is recommended. CSF diversion should be considered in all cases of distal ACA aneurysms. This can help reduce the need for retraction when dissecting the interhemispheric fissure. Patient positioning is dependent on the anticipated need for revascularization. In the case of anticipated clip ligation, the patient is supine, and the head is maintained neutral or with slight flexion. When an A3–A3 bypass is being considered, the patient is placed supine with a unilateral shoulder roll. The head is turned so the aneurysmal ACA is dependent. The falx cerebri is positioned almost parallel with the floor. A slight tilt is maintained to facilitate the runoff of irrigation during the microvascular anastomosis. The vertex is slightly flexed as the final positioning maneuver. Head positioning approximately 20 cm above the level of the heart is recommended to reduce venous bleeding into the operative field and is achieved by elevating the back of the table after securing the skull clamp. In the presented case, the patient was not planned for bypass and was positioned supine with the head in neutral position and slightly flexed.

Patient positioning and operative planning can be facilitated by neuronavigation from the preoperative CTA. A "partial" Souttar incision was planned, starting approximately 1 cm in front of the left tragus and extending across the midline up to the contralateral anteriormost point of the hairline. Alternatively, a "true" Souttar or bicoronal incision can be used, although sufficient exposure can typically be acquired with a smaller incision and scalp retraction, as illustrated by the current case. The scalp flap is reflected down to approximately the orbital rim, and the temporalis fascia and muscle are not dissected. Burr holes are then placed on either side of the midline with the bone flap planned out to be one-third posterior and two-thirds anterior to the coronal suture. The bone flap must be large enough to allow for both distal A3 segment access for side-to-side bypass and proximal A3 segment access for aneurysm trapping. A C-shaped dural incision is made with its base against the superior sagittal sinus and reflected with sutures. During the dural opening, care should be taken not to sacrifice any bridging veins. The operative microscope is then used to enter the interhemispheric fissure.

The dissection is performed along the falx cerebri down onto the corpus callosum and the ACAs (Figure 11.4A). Care is taken to avoid excessive retraction to prevent infarcts and intraoperative aneurysm rupture. As an alternative, rolled cottonoids can be placed in the fissure to assist with hemisphere separation. After the dural opening, 10–15 mL of CSF can be drained at a time for up to a total of 30–50 mL to facilitate brain relaxation.

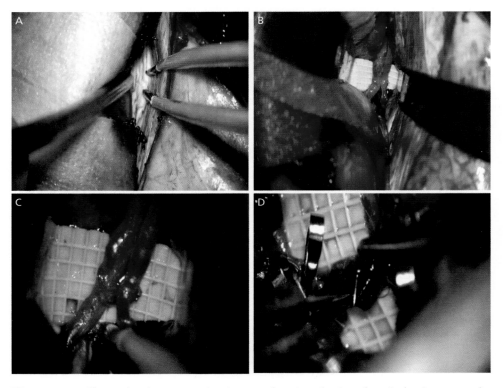

Figure 11.4 Illustrative intraoperative images showing the interhemispheric approach (A), isolation of bilateral A3 segments (B), and microvascular side-to-side bypass (C and D).

At the inferior edge of the falx, the dissection plane runs in between the cingulate gyri, which are typically adherent. Care should be taken to avoid damage or retraction of the cingulate gyri to prevent postoperative akinetic mutism. Although pericallosal ACAs can sometimes be found in the cingulate sulcus, they are typically located deeper, directly over the corpus callosum. The corpus callosum can be identified by its whitish color and transverse fibers. Once the bilateral A3 segments are identified (Figure 11.4B), they are followed proximally along the body and genu of the corpus callosum to localize the aneurysm. Important landmarks here are the callosomarginal artery, the genu of the corpus callosum, and any other specific anatomic characteristics identified in preoperative imaging. The initial goal is to ensure access for proximal temporary clip control of the parent A3 segment. Partial hematoma evacuation can aid in brain relaxation when diuresis and CSF diversion do not suffice.

In the presented case, the aneurysmal A3 segment was found to be circumferentially dilated and dysplastic, which would render simple aneurysm neck clipping insufficient. Clip reconstruction was considered but would require that a significant amount of aneurysm remain in order to reconstruct the parent artery. A decision was made to trap the aneurysmal segment after a side-to-side A3–A3 bypass was performed beyond the aneurysm.

The bilateral A3 segments are followed distally over the corpus callosum and circumferentially dissected for approximately 1.5 cm to allow enough room for side-to-side bypass. At this point, electroencephalographic burst suppression is induced for neuroprotection using titrated doses of anesthetics. A microgrid background is placed underneath the dissected segments to facilitate visualization of the anastomosis (Figure 11.4C). A continuous microsurgical suction is then placed deep in the interhemispheric fissure, and temporary clips are applied proximally and distally to the anastomosis site on both A3 segments. Arteriotomies are made, which are typically three times the diameter of the vessels. A running side-to-side anastomosis is performed using a 10–0 nylon suture. The posterior wall suturing is done from inside the lumen while the anterior wall is sutured from outside of the lumen in a continuous fashion (Figure 11.4D). After completion of the anastomosis (Figure 11.5A), the temporary clips are removed, and

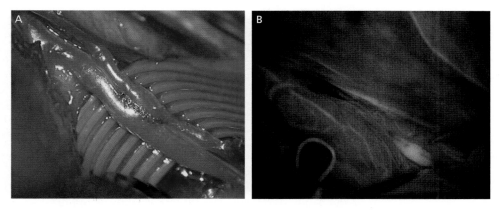

Figure 11.5 Illustrative intraoperative images showing a completed A3–A3 bypass (A) with its patency confirmed using intraoperative indocyanine green angiography (B).

bypass patency is evaluated using intraoperative indocyanine green angiography (Figure 11.5B) and micro-Doppler. Once the bypass is completed and patency confirmed, the aneurysmal segment is again inspected and then trapped using permanent clips placed proximal and distal to the aneurysm.

In cases in which direct aneurysm clipping is possible, proximal temporary clip control is recommended while performing the final aneurysm dissection. Distal-only clipping after bypass typically results in spontaneous aneurysm thrombosis and can be considered in cases of large, dysplastic, fusiform aneurysms in which proximal access is not feasible through the same exposure.

Following aneurysm trapping, electroencephalographic burst suppression is discontinued, and somatosensory and motor evoked potential responses are checked. Meticulous hemostasis of the operative field is achieved, and a watertight dural closure is performed followed by replacement of the bone flap using cranial plates.

Oral Boards Review—Management Pearls

1. Careful preoperative approach trajectory planning and vascular anatomy analysis are crucial for surgical success in the narrow and deep surgical corridor of the interhemispheric fissure, especially if a ruptured aneurysm is associated with a large hematoma and extensive cerebral swelling.
2. Care should be taken to avoid bridging vein injury during dural opening and entry into the interhemispheric fissure.
3. Extensive retractor use should be avoided to prevent ischemic complications and intraoperative aneurysm rupture. A proper use of bipolar forceps, suction, microscissors, and cottonoids can be aided with gentle cotton roll placement at the opposite ends of the working segment of interhemispheric fissure.
4. When significant compromise or complete occlusion of the parent artery is unavoidable while securing the aneurysm, revascularization of distal arterial segments is necessary. Although technically challenging, an A3–A3 anastomosis is a convenient option that avoids the limitations of an extracranial-to-intracranial end-to-side bypass.

Pivot Points

1. Preoperative imaging should be carefully inspected for sclerotic changes in the aneurysm and parent artery as well as the proximity of branching arteries, which can significantly complicate temporary and/or permanent clip placement. Alternative strategies such as distal-only clipping or trapping of the aneurysm with distal revascularization can then be considered and planned accordingly.
2. CSF diversion should be established via external ventricular or lumbar drain along with diuretic and mannitol treatment to aid intraoperative brain relaxation, which is especially important for the management of ruptured aneurysms.

3. Intraoperative somatosensory, motor evoked potential, and electroencephalogram monitoring should be used, and responses should be checked at multiple points throughout the procedure, especially if a revascularization is planned.

Aftercare

In the presented case, postoperative CT and CTA were ordered to evaluate the patency of the bypass and to ensure occlusion of the aneurysm (Figure 11.6A). Although CTA is adequate, a catheter angiogram is preferred after complex revascularization procedures.

Aneurysmal SAH patients remain in the intensive care unit for vasospasm monitoring for approximately 14 days post-presentation. Vasospasm monitoring includes serial neurological exams, careful monitoring of serum sodium levels, and daily transcranial Doppler ultrasonography. All patients with SAH also receive oral nimodipine at a dose of 60 mg every 4 hours for 21 days after presentation. Standard prophylactic antibiotics such as cefazolin are continued for 24 hours postoperatively. Therapeutic antiepileptic medication levels may be maintained for up to 2 or 3 months postoperatively.

Complications and Management

Compared to more proximal lesions, there are unique technical complications related to the interhemispheric approach and distal ACA dissection. Retraction injury and damage to bridging veins may result in postoperative cortical venous infarcts. Small ACA branch or perforator injury may lead to ACA distribution frontal lobe infarcts. Retraction or other ischemic insult to the cingulate gyri can cause postoperative akinetic mutism, which is typically transient. Other deficits can include bilateral leg weakness and behavioral and cognitive impairment that can be related to bilateral ischemic or mass effect injury to the supplementary motor area and limbic structures. Meticulous surgical

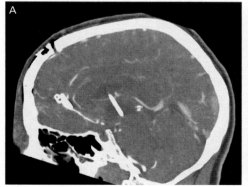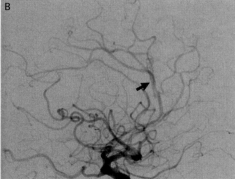

Figure 11.6 Presented patient's postoperative CTA (A) showing trapped left A3 segment aneurysm and a catheter angiogram (B) with right carotid injection showing contralateral distal anterior cerebral artery filling through the A3–A3 bypass (arrow). No evidence of vasospasm can be identified.

technique, thorough preoperative planning, and the correct approach can help minimize the risks.

In the case of intraoperative bypass failure, an extracranial-to-intracranial bypass from the ipsilateral superficial temporal artery stump with a radial artery graft can be considered. In cases of postoperative bypass failure, an additional extracranial-to-intracranial bypass should only be considered when the patient is symptomatic with radiographic evidence of a perfusion deficit that has not yet resulted in a completed infarct.

If a clinical deterioration on exam or an increase in transcranial Doppler velocities is noted, an urgent head CT should be obtained to rule out acute conditions such as hydrocephalus or intracranial hemorrhage. A CTA or catheter angiogram should follow to evaluate for radiographic vasospasm. Upon suspicion of a vasospasm, the patient should be treated with vasopressors, or if necessary, a catheter angiogram can be performed to deliver intra-arterial vasodilators or to perform angioplasty.

The presented patient developed new neurologic symptoms on postoperative day 1 without evidence of vasospasm on catheter angiogram (Figure 11.6B). Magnetic resonance imaging revealed areas of diffusion restriction along the posterior body of corpus callosum and bilateral anterior cingulate gyri likely related to retractor use (Figure 11.7). The patient's neurologic status improved during the remainder of the postoperative course, and she regained full strength in all extremities on postoperative day 5. A noncontrast CT performed on postoperative day 9 showed no new infarction and complete resolution of the SAH. The patient was discharged neurologically intact on postoperative day 10. At 1-month follow-up, the patient was living independently without neurological deficit.

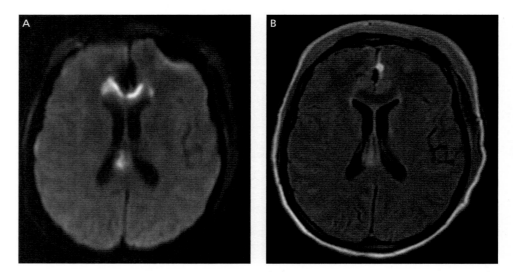

Figure 11.7 Presented patient's postoperative magnetic resonance diffusion-weighted (A) and T$_2$ sequence (B) imaging showing intraoperative retraction-related ischemic changes.

Oral Boards Review—Complications Pearls

1. Technical complications can be minimized with preoperative imaging and planning as well as meticulous surgical technique.
2. Ruptured aneurysm patients should remain in the intensive care unit postoperatively for vasospasm monitoring. Serial neurological exams and transcranial Doppler ultrasonography are useful tools for early vasospasm detection. Hypertensive therapy is the first-line treatment, whereas intra-arterial vasodilators and angioplasty are secondary means in resistant or severe vasospasm cases.

Evidence and Outcomes

Distal ACA aneurysms comprise 2–9% of all intracranial aneurysms and are more often associated with intracerebral hemorrhage and multiple aneurysms. Good outcomes have been reported for the microsurgical management of ruptured distal ACA aneurysms. A lower mortality risk than that of ruptured aneurysms in other locations has also been shown. Independent risk factors associated with unfavorable outcomes are advanced age, poor Hunt and Hess grade, rehemorrhage before treatment, intracerebral hemorrhage, intraventricular hemorrhage, and severe preoperative hydrocephalus.

There are no prospective, controlled trials comparing endovascular and microsurgical treatment for distal ACA aneurysms. Microsurgical management is still a treatment option for these aneurysms, although individual treatment should be evaluated on a case-by-case basis, ideally within a multidisciplinary team. The rapid advancement of endovascular access and treatment devices will likely impact the management of these lesions in the near future.

Further Reading

Lee JW, Lee KC, Kim YB, Huh SK. Surgery for distal anterior cerebral artery aneurysms. *Surg Neurol*. 2008;70(2):153–159.

Lee SH, Jung Y, Ryu JW, Choi SK, Kwun BD. Surgical revascularization for the treatment of complex anterior cerebral artery aneurysms: Experience and illustrative review. *World Neurosurg*. 2018;111:e507–e518.

Lehecka M, Dashti R, Hernesniemi J, et al. Microneurosurgical management of aneurysms at A3 segment of anterior cerebral artery. *Surg Neurol*. 2008;70(2):135–152.

Lehecka M, Lehto H, Niemela M, et al. Distal anterior cerebral artery aneurysms: Treatment and outcome analysis of 501 patients. *Neurosurgery*. 2008;62(3):590–601.

Lehecka M, Porras M, Dashti R, Niemela M, Hernesniemi JA. Anatomic features of distal anterior cerebral artery aneurysms: A detailed angiographic analysis of 101 patients. *Neurosurgery*. 2008;63(2):219–228.

Incidental Medium-Sized Basilar Tip Aneurysm

Ethan A. Winkler, W. Caleb Rutledge, Alex Lu, and Adib A. Abla

12

Case Presentation

A 47-year-old female presented to the neurosurgery clinic complaining of headaches. A magnetic resonance angiogram (MRA) and, later, a computed tomography angiogram (CTA) demonstrated a 2-mm basilar tip aneurysm. She is a current smoker, and her family history is remarkable for two grandparents who died from ruptured cerebral aneurysms and subarachnoid hemorrhage (SAH). A detailed neurologic examination was unremarkable. After a detailed discussion of the natural history of this aneurysm, she was advised to stop smoking and to follow the aneurysm with serial imaging. However, she continued to have headaches and returned to the clinic 4 months later. A repeat CTA demonstrated interval growth of the aneurysm. The aneurysm now measured 5 mm in diameter and had approximately tripled in volume (Figure 12.1). She had had no episodes of sudden severe headache concerning for either a sentinel bleed or SAH. Her neurologic exam showed no deficit.

Questions

1. What is the appropriate interval follow-up and preferred image modality to follow incidental unruptured aneurysms?
2. When should treatment be considered for incidental unruptured aneurysms of the basilar apex?
3. What treatment modalities are available and how is the optimal treatment strategy determined?

Assessment and Planning

Assessment of unruptured cerebral aneurysms involves careful review of cerebrovascular imaging modalities, including CTA, MRA, and conventional catheter-based digital subtraction angiography. Although the gold standard remains conventional angiography, technological improvements with CTA and MRA have resulted in sensitivities of >90% that vary with aneurysm size and location. If there are clinical signs or symptoms suggestive of rupture, such as worst headache of life, depressed mental status, and/or focal neurologic deficits, a noncontrast CT scan and, if negative, subsequent lumbar puncture are warranted to evaluate for potential SAH. Evaluation of noncontrast studies also provides additional information regarding partial thrombosis of the aneurysm and/or calcification of parent arteries that may influence treatment decisions.

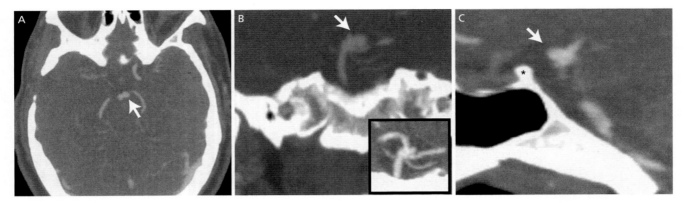

Figure 12.1 Preoperative imaging of unruptured basilar tip artery aneurysm. (A) Axial, (B) coronal, and (C) sagittal images of preoperative CTA of unruptured basilar tip aneurysm. Inset, higher magnification view of aneurysm in coronal plane; arrows, basilar tip aneurysm; asterisk, dorsum sellae. Note that when selecting the surgical approach, it is important to appreciate the relative position of the aneurysm with the dorsum sellae.

The decision to treat or observe an unruptured aneurysm must balance the risks of rupture or neurologic deficit with the potential morbidity of treatment. To estimate risks of rupture, a detailed patient history and careful review of aneurysm size, location, and morphology are required. In the International Study of Unruptured Intracranial Aneurysms (ISUIA), the cumulative 5-year rupture rates for posterior circulation aneurysms—including basilar tip aneurysms—were 14.5%, 18.4%, and 50% for aneurysms 7–12, 13–24, and ≥25 mm, respectively. For aneurysms ≤7 mm, rupture rates varied based on whether the patient had prior SAH (no SAH, 2.5%; prior SAH, 3.4%). These statistics reflected pooled data of aneurysms from multiple sites in the posterior circulation, and aneurysms of the basilar tip are associated with greater odds of rupture. Despite this predictive modeling, small aneurysms (<10 mm) account for the majority of SAH, and interval growth of an aneurysm >2 mm or change in aneurysm morphology (e.g., the development of a bleb or daughter sac) may suggest instability of the aneurysm and argue for intervention. The PHASES score is a scoring system including ethnic background, hypertension, age, aneurysm size, prior SAH, and site of the aneurysm. A 5-year cumulative rupture risk may be calculated from the total score.

Oral Boards Review—Diagnostic Pearls

1. A detailed history and careful review of angiographic anatomy are necessary in the evaluation of any intracranial aneurysm.
   a. The PHASES score offers an evidence-based estimate of 5-year cumulative rupture risk.
   b. Interval aneurysm growth >2 mm or development of daughter blebs suggests aneurysm instability and favors intervention.
2. The following aneurysm morphological parameters should be considered to facilitate treatment decisions:
   a. Neck width

b. Dome-to-neck ratio—the ratio between the maximum width of the dome divided by the width of the aneurysm neck

c. Aspect ratio—the ratio of the maximum height of the aneurysm divided by the width of the aneurysm neck

d. Other qualitative considerations—fusiform morphology, partial thrombosis, calcification of the aneurysm or parent vessels, and perforators or aberrant branches arising from the aneurysm dome

Questions

1. What factors are associated with increased risk of rupture for incidentally discovered aneurysms?

2. What attributes on surveillance imaging should prompt reconsideration of intervention?

Decision-Making

Once a decision is made to treat the aneurysm, careful consideration of both patient demographics and aneurysm morphology is needed to select the appropriate treatment modality. Several important studies, including ISUIA and the International Subarachnoid Aneurysm Trial, have demonstrated superior clinical outcomes with endovascular coiling compared to microsurgery in the treatment of intracranial aneurysms. For posterior circulation aneurysms, such as those arising from the basilar tip, the benefits of coiling may be even more apparent. For example, in the Barrow Ruptured Aneurysm Trial, patients with posterior circulation aneurysms, but not anterior circulation aneurysms, treated with endovascular coiling continued to have superior clinical outcomes at 6-year follow-up. As a result, many centers now favor endovascular treatment modalities over microsurgery, although with careful patient selection, endovascular and open microsurgical treatment may have equivalent outcomes.

The most common endovascular treatment option involves deployment of detachable coils to induce aneurysm thrombosis. In aneurysms with a wide neck (>4 mm or a dome-to-neck ratio of 1.5–2.0), balloon remodeling and placement of one or more stents often serve as important treatment adjuncts to prevent coil herniation into the parent artery and/or adjacent posterior cerebral arteries (PCAs). With ruptured aneurysms, balloon-assisted coiling is favored because stent placement requires dual antiplatelet therapy—most commonly aspirin and clopidogrel—to maintain stent patency. In patients with unruptured aneurysms and no contraindications to dual antiplatelet therapy, stent-assisted coiling with one or more stents is often preferred and is associated with lower rates of aneurysm recanalization and need for retreatment. Common stent configurations include a single stent spanning the upper basilar trunk into one of the proximal PCAs, a single horizontal stent that spans across the basilar apex from PCA to PCA (deployed via a posterior communicating artery [PCoA]), or two stents in Y-configuration in which each stent is deployed from the upper basilar trunk and into each proximal PCA. The optimal stent configuration must be determined on a case-by-case basis taking into account the relationship of the aneurysm neck with each PCA origin, the angle and caliber of each PCA with respect to its origin off of the basilar artery, perforator anatomy, and the presence and caliber of PCoAs joining the PCA P1–P2 segment. Even with complete aneurysm obliteration, endovascular coiling is still more likely to result in residual aneurysm or aneurysm recurrence requiring re-treatment, and aneurysms in the basilar tip are at higher risk for recanalization compared to other aneurysm locations. With long-term follow-up, large case series have shown that 26% of coiled basilar tip aneurysms require re-treatment. Rates of re-treatment are highest within the first year of treatment, but recanalization may occur in delayed fashion and annual rates of re-treatment are roughly 2.6%.

Despite the shift toward endovascular treatment of basilar artery aneurysms, microsurgical clipping remains a safe and durable treatment option for appropriately selected basilar tip aneurysms. Aneurysms with wide or complex neck configurations, smaller dome-to-neck ratios, and smaller aspect ratios (the ratio of the height of the aneurysm to the width of the neck) are less favorable for endovascular intervention and may favor clip ligation. Similarly, aneurysms that are large or giant, partially thrombosed, or with aberrant branches arising from the aneurysm dome may be better treated with open microsurgery. In addition to scrutiny of aneurysm morphology, the patient's medical comorbidities, age, and likelihood for re-treatment are important factors when considering treatment modalities. Although small, risks with endovascular intervention accumulate with each treatment and surveillance angiogram, and studies have consistently demonstrated greater durability with clip ligation.

Questions

1. What aneurysm morphologic parameters favor use of either balloon-assisted or stent-assisted coiling with endovascular treatment?
2. What patient or aneurysm characteristics favor microsurgical clipping?
3. What anatomic factors help guide approach selection when microsurgically treating aneurysms of the basilar apex?

Surgical Procedure

Open microsurgical clipping of basilar tip aneurysms is performed under general anesthesia with adequate intravenous access to facilitate rapid transfusion in the event of an intraoperative rupture. To ensure patient safety, the procedure should be performed with neuromonitoring, including both motor evoked potentials and somatosensory evoked potentials, and a coordinated effort between the neurophysiologist and the anesthesiologist is required to place the patient in burst suppression prior to aneurysm manipulation to minimize the deleterious consequences of any potential ischemic event.

Selection of the optimal surgical approach is determined by the position of the basilar tip aneurysm relative to the dorsum sellae, the direction of its projection, and the surgeon's experience. For the majority of basilar tip aneurysms, which are at or near the level of the dorsum sellae (such as in the current case), and for high-riding (above the dorsum sellae) aneurysms, an orbitozygomatic trans-sylvian approach is preferred (unless the aneurysm is completely in the third ventricle). For low-riding (below the dorsum sellae) aneurysms, the subtemporal approach is preferred.

The patient is positioned supine with a small bump under the ipsilateral shoulder, approached from the nondominant (usually right) side whenever possible. The head is affixed to a Mayfield head holder and then rotated 15–20 degrees toward the contralateral shoulder and extended roughly 20 degrees to make the malar eminence the highest point in the operative field. A curvilinear incision is made behind the hairline from the root of the zygoma to approximately the midline. The scalp is elevated using an interfascial technique to protect the frontalis branch of the fascial nerve, and both the scalp and the temporalis are reflected forward. Once exposed, a two-piece orbitozygomatic approach is used. First, a frontotemporal craniotomy is performed in standard fashion. Next, the orbitozygomatic unit is released as a second piece with a reciprocating saw. This is accomplished with a stereotypical series of cuts: (1) the zygomatic root, (2) the zygomatic body, (3) from the inferior orbital fissure to cut 2, (4) the medial orbital roof, (5) the posterior orbital roof, and (6) the lateral orbital wall. Once released, the lesser wing of the sphenoid is carefully shaved down to the superior orbital fissure, and the dura is opened.

The sylvian fissure is widely split, separating the frontal and temporal lobes. The temporal lobe is then further released through careful dissection and division of arachnoid adhesions and bridging veins along the middle fossa floor and the anterior temporal pole. Further dissection of the carotid and crural cisterns frees the temporal lobe and allows it to be retracted in a posterolateral dissection. Three operative corridors to the basilar apex are then identified: (1) the supracarotid triangle, (2) the optic–carotid triangle, and (3) the carotid–oculomotor triangle. The carotid–oculomotor triangle provides the widest corridor with medial displacement of the internal carotid artery (ICA) and is used most frequently. A series of anatomic steps are utilized to safely gain both proximal and distal control when accessing the basilar apex. First, the origin of the PCoA is identified and followed. The membrane of Liliequist is opened behind the posterior clinoid and medial to the oculomotor nerve, and the P1 segment of the PCA is identified. To further mobilize the ICA medially, the PCoA may be divided near its distal insertion at the P1–P2 junction of the PCA (Figure 12.2).

Once the basilar apex is visualized, access to the basilar trunk must be established for proximal vascular control. For a low-lying basilar apex, a posterior clinoidectomy or transcavernous exposure may be necessary. Adenosine cardiac arrest can also be used in conjunction with proximal control of the basilar trunk or as a standalone method for a short period of aneurysm deflation. After obtaining proximal and distal control, care and time must be spent to dissect free perforating arteries to prepare the neck of the aneurysm for clip application. Utilization of temporary clipping and/or intraoperative use of adenosine may soften the aneurysm dome to facilitate mobilization of the aneurysm and circumferential dissection of perforating arteries. Only after the perforators are identified and dissected free may the surgeon proceed with clip application (Figure 12.3A).

The optimal clip configuration depends on the aneurysm morphology, with emphasis on perforator and parent artery preservation, and it may require the use of fenestrated clips and/or multiple stacked clip configurations. Clip positioning should be immediately confirmed with intraoperative indocyanine green angiography. Alterations in neuromonitoring evoked potentials or absent or sluggish flow in perforators or parent PCAs warrant immediate clip repositioning. If doubts persist regarding aneurysm occlusion, an intraoperative angiogram may be warranted to confirm complete occlusion.

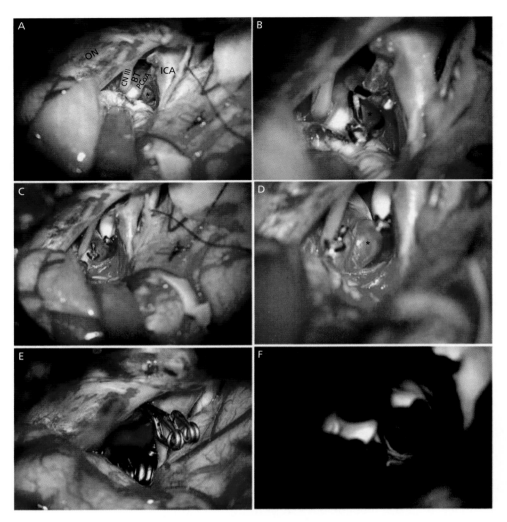

Figure 12.2 Intraoperative photographs showing the operative approach to surgical clipping of basilar tip aneurysms. (A) Following orbitozygomatic–pterional craniotomy and subarachnoid dissection, initial operative view through the optic–carotid triangle provides initial view of the basilar tip aneurysm (asterisk). BT, basilar trunk; CN III, third cranial nerve; ICA, internal carotid artery; ON, optic nerve; PCoA, posterior communicating artery. (B–D) To facilitate surgical access to the aneurysm, the PCoA is divided at the P1–P2 junction of the posterior cerebral artery (PCA). (B and C) Given the large size of the PCoA, arteriovenous malformation mini-clips were used to clip the PCoA proximally and distally. (D) The artery was subsequently divided to allow mobilization of the ICA. This provides better visualization of the aneurysm and facilitates circumferential dissection of thalamo-perforating arteries. (E) The complex aneurysm configuration was ultimately occluded with a "picket-fence" clipping strategy with multiple stacked straight aneurysm clips. (F) Complete occlusion of the aneurysm was confirmed with intraoperative indocyanine green angiography (ICG). Importantly, the ICG run confirmed patency of the posterior cerebral, superior cerebellar, and thalamo-perforating arteries. It is essential for complication avoidance that the surgeon immediately readjust clip position if perfusion of these arteries is sluggish or occluded on the ICG run.

Oral Boards Review—Management Pearls

1. Release of the temporal lobe and wide dissection of the arachnoid cisterns and sylvian fissure are necessary to allow surgical maneuverability when approaching aneurysms of the basilar apex.
2. Identification and dissection of thalamo-perforating arteries arising off of the proximal PCA are essential to avoid ischemic complications. Temporary clipping and/or intraoperative adenosine may soften the aneurysm dome to facilitate more complete visualization and dissection of arterial perforators to create a safe corridor for clip application.
3. Early proximal and distal control ensures safety and preparedness for unexpected intraoperative rupture. Adenosine should be readily available in case intraoperative rupture occurs without adequate control or if bleeding persists with temporary clipping.
4. Clip positioning should be immediately confirmed with indocyanine green angiography.

Pivot Points

1. If there are clinical concerns for subarachnoid or sentinel hemorrhage, such as worst headache of life, the patient should be emergently admitted to the hospital for prompt workup, blood pressure control, and intervention.
2. If there are clinical and radiographic signs of mass effect from the aneurysm dome, such as cranial neuropathy, or if the patient is aged 40 years or younger, microsurgical treatment may be considered.
3. If aneurysms of the basilar apex are located high above or below the dorsum sellae, alternative surgical approaches to the orbitozygomatic–pterional craniotomy should be considered.

Aftercare

Following completion of microsurgical clipping, patients should undergo close monitoring of their neurologic status for 1 or 2 days in the intensive care unit. Patients should be kept well hydrated with intravenous isotonic fluids to avoid hypotension. To help with retraction edema, patients are often treated with a short course of dexamethasone (<48 hours). In the absence of significant extra-axial or intraparenchymal blood products, routine prophylactic antiepileptic medications are not required. To minimize develop of deep venous thrombosis or pulmonary emboli, encourage early mobilization, sequential compression devices, and start chemical prophylaxis within 48 hours of the operation. Patients are treated with 24 hours of antibiotics to lessen the risk of surgical site infections.

A conventional angiogram or a CTA is obtained to confirm aneurysm occlusion and clip placement (Figure 12.3B). Surveillance digital subtraction angiography or CTA is performed 3–5 years following treatment to monitor growth of aneurysm

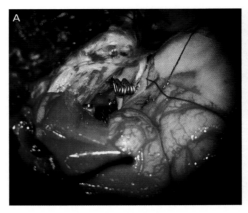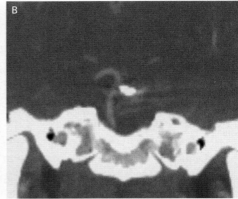

Figure 12.3 Intraoperative photograph and postoperative CTA confirming complete occlusion of the basilar tip aneurysm. (A) High-magnification view of the final clip confirmation to occlude the basilar tip aneurysm. (B) Postoperative CTA showing no residual filling in the basilar tip aneurysm but preservation of flow in bilateral posterior cerebral arteries. Improvements in clip technology have limited streak artifact, and a CTA may serve as an option for postoperative imaging in lieu of conventional catheter-based angiogram in appropriately selected patients.

residual and/or de novo aneurysm formation. Due to the greater recurrence rate with endovascular treatment, surveillance angiography or CTA is first performed 3–6 months post-treatment and then repeated 12–24 months and 3–5 years following treatment if no recurrence is detected. However, these are approximate guidelines, and surveillance imaging is often tailored to individual patients and treatment results.

Complications and Management

Microsurgical treatment of basilar tip aneurysms requires comfort working in narrow surgical corridors. Even with the most careful dissection, intraoperative rupture of the aneurysm may occur at any time. Early proximal and distal vascular control are tenets of cerebral aneurysm surgery and should be established prior to manipulation of the aneurysm. Should the aneurysm rupture, it is important for the surgeon to remain calm, in control, and effectively communicate with the anesthesiologist to ensure initiation of transfusion, if needed, and blood pressure control. Through a series of well-orchestrated steps, the surgeon should tamponade the site of hemorrhage, clear the operative field of blood with suctioning, apply temporary clips to slow bleeding, and permanently clip the aneurysm. If proximal or distal control has yet to be established or proves ineffective, intravenous administration of adenosine may provide temporary circulatory arrest and allow a narrow time period for the surgeon to visualize and clip the site of rupture. Clip positioning should be immediately confirmed and the clip repositioned as needed.

In addition to intraoperative rupture, complications from surgical treatment of basilar tip aneurysms include inadvertent occlusion of either the PCAs or the thalamoperforating arteries resulting in ischemic stroke, as well as oculomotor palsy from manipulation of the third nerve. Tremendous care should therefore be placed on the identification and dissection of thalamo-perforating arteries at the time of the operation (even at the expense of intraoperative rupture) to create a safe corridor for clip application. Patency should be confirmed with indocyanine green angiography to allow for immediate repositioning if perfusion is compromised. If clinical concerns for ischemia arise postoperatively, such as a new focal deficit and/or failure to rouse from anesthesia, patients should undergo immediate imaging to rule out an expanding mass lesion and evaluate for large vessel ischemia. If this is inconclusive, magnetic resonance imaging may demonstrate an isolated perforator artery infarct.

Oral Boards Review—Complications Pearls

1. Patients should be placed in burst suppression prior to proximal or distal temporary clip occlusion to minimize potential deleterious effects of any ischemia time.

2. Subarachnoid dissection should facilitate early proximal and distal control to help mitigate risks of intraoperative rupture. Temporary clips should be selected and loaded prior to manipulation of the aneurysm. Intraoperative adenosine may provide temporary circulatory arrest and allow a temporary period of visualization should bleeding continue with temporary clipping.

3. Infarction of thalamo-perforating arteries should be prevented with careful identification and dissection prior to clip placement, and preservation should be confirmed with intraoperative indocyanine angiography. Postoperatively, new focal deficits or depressed mental status should be evaluated with cranial imaging and permissive or induced hypertension.

Evidence and Outcomes

In experienced hands, microsurgical clipping of basilar tip aneurysms may offer a robust treatment option for aneurysms or patients less favorable for endovascular treatment. Contemporary data from several large centers have demonstrated that >75% of patients have good neurologic outcome as evidenced by modified or Glasgow outcome scales, with complete aneurysm occlusion in >95% of cases and a mortality rate <10%. Results improve with increasing experience, and in the era of dual-trained vascular neurosurgeons, open microsurgical treatment remains a viable option with appropriate patient selection.

Further Reading

Bender MT, Wendt H, Monarch T, et al. Small aneurysms account for the majority and increasing percentage of aneurysmal subarachnoid hemorrhage: A 25-year, single institution study. *Neurosurgery*. 2017;83(4):692–699.

Chalouhi N, Jabbour P, Gonzalez LF, et al. Safety and efficacy of endovascular treatment of basilar tip aneurysms by coiling with and without stent assistance: A review of 235 cases. *Neurosurgery*. 2012;71(4):785–794.

Greving JP, Wermer MJ, Brown RD Jr, et al. Development of the PHASES score for prediction of risk of rupture of intracranial aneurysms: A pooled analysis of six prospective cohort studies. *Lancet Neurol.* 2014;13(1):59–66.

Krisht AF, Krayenbuhl N, Sercl D, Bikmaz K, Kadri PA. Results of microsurgical clipping of 50 high complexity basilar apex aneurysms. *Neurosurgery.* 2007;60(2):242–250.

Sekhar LN, Tariq F, Morton RP, et al. Basilar tip aneurysms: A microsurgical and endovascular contemporary series of 100 patients. *Neurosurgery.* 2013;72(2):284–298.

Wide-Necked Large Ruptured Basilar Tip Aneurysm

Jacob F. Baranoski, Colin J. Przybylowski, Tyler S. Cole, Rami O. Almefty, Dale Ding, Felipe C. Albuquerque, and Andrew F. Ducruet

13

Case Presentation

A 57-year-old female with no significant past medical history is found unresponsive by her family soon after reporting a sudden-onset, severe headache. She is taken to a rural emergency room, where she is emergently intubated. After brain computed tomography (CT) shows significant intraventricular hemorrhage (IVH), with casting of the fourth ventricle and hydrocephalus (Figure 13.1), the patient is transferred to a tertiary center for further management. Upon arrival, she has a Glasgow Coma Scale of 4T, with equal and minimally reactive pupils. On exam, she exhibits extensor posturing to central stimuli, a gag reflex is present, and she is overbreathing the ventilator.

> ### Questions
>
> 1. What is the most likely diagnosis?
> 2. What is the most appropriate imaging modality?
> 3. What is the appropriate timing of the additional imaging workup? Should any interventions be performed prior to additional workup?

Assessment and Planning

The brain CT demonstrates a primary IVH, without significant intraparenchymal or subarachnoid hemorrhage (SAH). The differential diagnosis for a primary IVH includes (1) ruptured vascular lesions; (2) intraventricular tumors; and (3) spontaneous hemorrhage, which is more commonly seen in patients with uncontrolled hypertension and/or those on antiplatelet or anticoagulant medications.

The next step in the patient's workup is a CT angiogram (CTA) to look for an intracranial aneurysm or vascular malformation. The desire for definitive diagnosis must be balanced with initial stabilization of the patient, including treatment of acute hydrocephalus. In the current case, the patient already has radiographic and physiologic evidence of elevated intracranial pressure (ICP) and impending herniation. Therefore, prior to obtaining a CTA, a right frontal external ventricular drain (EVD) was placed, and

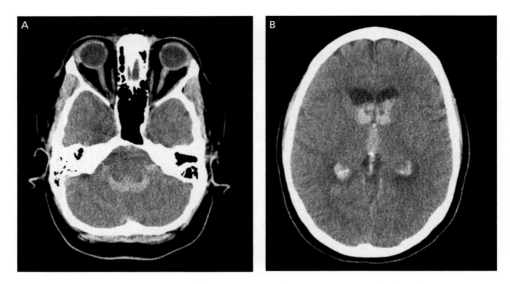

Figure 13.1 Noncontrast CT of the head demonstrates SAH in the basal cisterns (A) and lateral and third ventricles (B) with early hydrocephalus.

1 g/kg of mannitol was administered. The decision to place an EVD prior to obtaining vascular imaging should be made on a case-by-case basis. Early EVD placement can help treat ICPs; however, a CTA may help avoid an underlying vascular lesion (e.g., an arteriovenous malformation [AVM]) in the path of EVD placement.

In the current case, after EVD placement, the CTA demonstrated a wide-necked, giant basilar tip aneurysm and a small left middle cerebral artery (MCA) aneurysm (Figure 13.2).

Useful additional diagnostic studies and intervention at this point include laboratory studies if not already completed and blood pressure control to avoid hypertension. Antiepileptic medications may be administered for antiseizure prophylaxis.

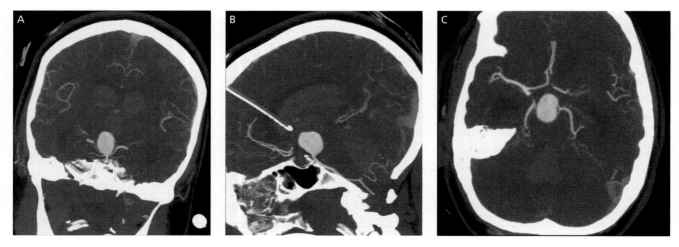

Figure 13.2 CTA of the head (coronal [A], sagittal [B], and axial [C] projections) demonstrates a wide-necked ruptured basilar tip aneurysm incorporating the origins of the bilateral posterior cerebral artery P1 segments.

Oral Boards Review—Diagnostic Pearls

1. Primary versus secondary IVH
   a. Primary: The blood products are almost exclusively confined to the ventricular system with little, if any, parenchymal or cisternal extension.
   b. Secondary: A large extraventricular component of blood is present (e.g., parenchymal or subarachnoid) with some subsequent extension of blood products into the ventricular system.
2. Causes of primary IVH
   a. Ruptured vascular malformations
      i. Aneurysms, especially those originating from the posterior inferior cerebellar artery or the basilar tip
      ii. Intraventricular or periventricular AVMs
      iii. Subependymal cavernous malformations
   b. Intraventricular tumors
      i. Ependymomas
      ii. Choroid plexus lesions
      iii. Intraventricular metastases
      iv. Adjacent parenchymal tumors
   c. Spontaneous hemorrhage
      i. Often associated with uncontrolled hypertension and/or antiplatelet or anticoagulant medication use
3. Acutely elevated ICP with concern for impending herniation should be suspected and addressed in patients with significant intraventricular blood due to obstructive hydrocephalus.
4. Multiple intracranial aneurysms are discovered in 15–35% of patients who present with aneurysmal rupture.
5. Giant aneurysms ($\geq$25 mm) represent only 3–5% of all intracranial aneurysms, with a female predominance (2:1). The most common presenting symptoms of these lesions are associated with the resultant mass effect (headaches and cranial neuropathies). Approximately 25% are diagnosed following intracranial hemorrhage, and up to 5% of patients may present with seizures.

Questions

1. How do these clinical and radiological findings influence treatment planning?
2. What is the most appropriate timing for intervention in this patient?
3. What options for treatment should be considered?

Decision-Making

Ruptured, giant basilar tip aneurysms represent a distinct and formidable subset of intracranial aneurysms. The natural history and outcomes following treatment for both unruptured and ruptured giant aneurysms are less favorable than those for smaller intracranial lesions. Accordingly, all viable microsurgical and endovascular treatment options should be considered, with evaluation of associated morbidities factored into the final treatment approach. We recommend that these cases be treated at centers with extensive experience in both endovascular and open microsurgical techniques, whenever possible.

Microsurgical options include clip reconstruction or distal basilar artery occlusion, with or without bypass (depending on the size of the posterior communicating arteries). Endovascular options include primary coiling with or without stent or balloon assistance, or the use of flow-diverting stents. Although the use of stents and flow diverters in the setting of aneurysm rupture has been described, the potential implications of dual antiplatelet therapy required after deployment of these devices still currently limit their widespread use in ruptured aneurysms.

In the current case, the CTA demonstrated both a wide-neck, giant basilar tip aneurysm and a small, left MCA aneurysm. Based on the location of the hemorrhage and the relative size and natural history of the two lesions in this case, it is more likely that the giant basilar tip aneurysm is the lesion that ruptured and, therefore, securing this lesion should be prioritized.

Careful study of the anatomical characteristics of the aneurysm and its relationship to the parent vessel is key. Certain characteristics (e.g., neck size, dome size, location, parent vessel angle, and rupture status) have been demonstrated to correlate with intraoperative complexity and rates of complications after endovascular intervention. For wide-necked aneurysms (i.e., dome-to-neck ratio <2:1 or neck width ≥4 mm), adjunctive techniques such as stent-assisted and balloon-assisted coiling have been demonstrated to be safe and effective techniques, resulting in improved obliteration and decreased recurrence.

The primary goal of the initial intervention in cases of ruptured, giant basilar tip aneurysms should be obliteration of the dome to decrease the risk of re-rupture, while preserving parent and branch vessel patency. The likely incidentally-discovered MCA aneurysm can be addressed in a delayed fashion after the patient is neurologically and clinically stabilized.

Questions

1. What endovascular devices/techniques should be prepared to be employed for coiling of this aneurysm?
2. Why is it important to assess the anterior cerebral circulation for this case?
3. What should be done if intraprocedural re-rupture of the aneurysm occurs?

Surgical Procedure

In general, endovascular therapy is the preferred modality for the vast majority of ruptured basilar tip aneurysms, and most centers adhere to this approach. The procedure is performed under general anesthesia with intraoperative neurophysiologic monitoring of somatosensory evoked potentials and brainstem auditory evoked potentials if available. Neurophysiologic monitoring can be helpful in these cases to alert the surgeon to changes in regional cerebral blood flow, particularly if balloon assistance is used.

In most cases, transfemoral access is achieved, and diagnostic angiography of the bilateral internal carotid arteries (ICAs) and dominant vertebral artery (VA) is performed to characterize the aneurysm and assess for collateral flow. Three-dimensional rotational cerebral angiography is performed through the appropriate VA to obtain the working projections that clearly elucidate the aneurysm neck, dome, and relationship to the parent vessel under high magnification (Figure 13.3). Identification of any perforating vessels, origins of the posterior cerebral and superior cerebellar arteries, relative caliber of the vertebral arteries, and the contribution of carotid blood flow to posterior cerebral circulation via the posterior communicating arteries are critical for this case. The size of the posterior communicating arteries is crucial if occlusion of the distal basilar artery is to be considered as a treatment option.

The patient is systemically anticoagulated with intravenous heparin at a loading dose of 70 U/kg (additional heparin is administered to achieve a goal activated clotting time of 200–250 seconds) immediately prior to intracranial catheterization, with protamine readily available for rapid reversal in case of intraoperative rupture. Some endovascular surgeons withhold systemic heparinization until the first coil (often called a framing coil) is deployed.

Once the working projections are obtained, the guide catheter is advanced into the dominant distal cervical VA. A coiling microcatheter is navigated over a micro guide wire to selectively catheterize the aneurysm dome. If balloon assistance is employed, it is usually navigated into place across the aneurysm neck prior to advancing the coiling microcatheter into the aneurysm dome. In general, the tip of the coiling microcatheter is advanced just past the midpoint of the aneurysm dome to avoid potential aneurysm perforation during catheterization.

The initial framing coil is then deployed to create a scaffold for the subsequent coils. The framing coil should outline the dome and neck of the aneurysm, and it represents a critical portion of the procedure because it can obviate the need

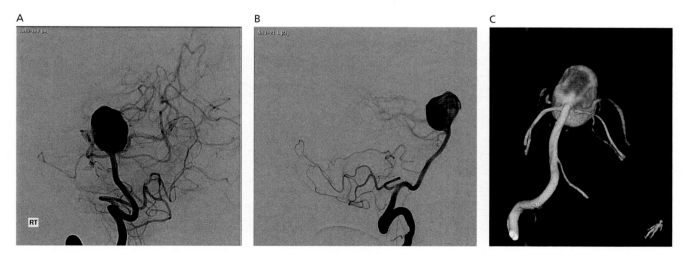

Figure 13.3 Diagnostic cerebral angiography of the right vertebral artery in the anterior–posterior (A) and lateral (B) projections and three-dimensional rotational angiography (C) demonstrate the anatomic detail of this wide-necked basilar tip aneurysm.

for balloon or stent assistance. Successive control angiograms are obtained while deploying additional filling coils to increase packing density and promote aneurysm thrombosis. In cases of coil prolapse or herniation, a balloon can be positioned across the aneurysm neck and inflated to remodel the neck and protect the normal vessels. The risk of balloon use, including vessel rupture and thromboembolic complications, must be considered. A stent could also be utilized to help keep the coil mass from protruding into the parent vessel, although this technique adds potential morbidity to ruptured aneurysm cases due to the need for dual antiplatelet therapy after the procedure.

After coiling, final angiograms should be performed to assess the degree of aneurysm embolization, parent vessel patency, and distal thrombosis (Figure 13.4).

Oral Boards Review—Management Pearls

1. Understanding the contribution of ICA supply to the posterior cerebral circulation via the posterior communicating arteries is critical for this case, especially if distal basilar artery occlusion is to be considered.

2. The microcatheter, microwire, and coils can all be sources of potential aneurysm wall perforation. Care should be taken to position the catheter in the optimal location for treatment but also to avoid microcatheter contact with the aneurysm wall.

3. For wide-necked aneurysms, the use of inflatable balloon- or stent-assisted coiling techniques can be helpful in achieving a good treatment result. In cases of ruptured aneurysms, stent-assisted coiling carries the risk of potential morbidity associated with dual antiplatelet therapy and ventriculostomy management.

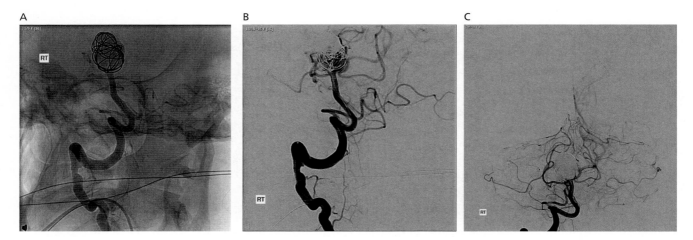

Figure 13.4 (A) An initial framing coil is placed into the aneurysm dome. (B) Control angiography is performed intermittently throughout coil embolization, and (C) final views are obtained to evaluate the remaining dome as well as the parent and daughter vessel patency.

> ## Pivot Points
>
> 1. Large, high-riding basilar tip aneurysms can cause obstructive hydrocephalus due to compression of the posterior third ventricle and cerebral aqueduct. These patients require cerebrospinal fluid diversion, the timing of which should be tailored to the rupture status of the aneurysm and the planned treatment strategy.
> 2. If the patient presents with an unruptured giant basilar tip aneurysm, additional treatment options can be considered, including stent-assisted coiling, use of flow diverting stents, and open surgical treatment with clip reconstruction or aneurysm trapping with high-flow bypass.

Aftercare

Following treatment, the patient should be transferred to the intensive care unit. The femoral puncture site and pedal pulses should be monitored for post-intervention hematoma and ischemia. Post-procedure hemoglobin levels should be monitored if there is concern for a potential retroperitoneal hemorrhage. Post-SAH symptomatic vasospasm, which develops in approximately 20–30% of patients, should be treated aggressively to reduce the risk of delayed cerebral ischemia. Follow-up angiography may be performed on post-bleed day 7 to assess for radiographic vasospasm and aneurysm occlusion status, although some centers rely on serial neurological examinations and transcranial Doppler ultrasonography. If concern for parent vessel stenosis or distal thromboses arose during the case, post-treatment magnetic resonance imaging can be useful to assess for evidence of infarction. Any sudden, unexpected change in neurologic exam or intracranial pressures should be assessed with an urgent brain CT and CTA (for hydrocephalus, aneurysm re-rupture, or vasospasm), although visualization of the vessels near the coiled aneurysm may be limited due to coil artifact.

Complications and Management

The most common and significant immediate complications of endovascular treatment for intracranial aneurysms are intraprocedural rupture and thromboembolism, which can be caused by coil migration or prolapse into the parent vessel. In addition to operative and angiographic findings, other ways to identify complications include examining hemodynamic and neurophysiological monitoring data. Obtaining these data requires good communication with the anesthesia team and close monitoring of vital signs, ICPs, EVD output, and neurophysiological monitoring (if employed).

Intraprocedural aneurysm rupture can occur during microcatheterization or coil placement, and it is recognized by observing active contrast extravasation or by a sudden and significant increase in ICP as well as Cushing response (hypertension and bradycardia). Timely recognition requires vigilant awareness of the location of the coils and conceptualization of the three-dimensional anatomy of the lesion, parent vessel, and coil mass.

When an intraprocedural rupture occurs, immediate recognition and action are required. Heparinization should be reversed using protamine. The ruptured aneurysm should be secured by quickly completing the coiling if possible. Temporary balloon inflation, if available, expeditiously achieves proximal control during aneurysm coiling. Rapid control of an intraprocedural rupture is a major advantage of coiling with balloon assistance, although overinflation of the balloon can rupture the parent or branch vessel. If a ruptured aneurysm cannot be adequately coiled, emergent surgical clipping or parent vessel sacrifice may be considered.

Thromboembolism is diagnosed by inspecting the distal vasculature on control and final angiograms and by being attentive to alterations in parent and branch vessel diameter. Small thromboembolisms may appear as lucencies within vessels, typically located at the coil–parent vessel interface or in the vessel territory distal to a balloon or microcatheter.

Thromboembolic complications are managed with intra-arterial or intraprocedural antithrombotic or antiplatelet medications such as additional heparin, abciximab, and eptifibatide; rarely, mechanical thrombectomy is necessary. The use of these medications is ideally reserved for after the aneurysm has been secured. Most minor cases of coil prolapse or herniation can be managed with postoperative aspirin. Rare instances of distal coil migration into a branch vessel necessitate coil retrieval, which can be performed with a snare or stent retriever.

Oral Boards Review—Complications Pearls

1. Aneurysm re-rupture, parent vessel stenosis/coil prolapse, and distal thrombus formation are all potentially devastating complications from endovascular intervention.
2. If intraprocedural re-rupture occurs, heparinization should be emergently reversed using protamine. If a balloon is present, it should be inflated to prevent further bleeding while the aneurysm is quickly coiled.
3. If coil prolapse is noted after the coil has already been detached, inflating a balloon and/or deploying a stent across the neck of the aneurysm may allow the coil to be pushed back into and secured within the aneurysm. These strategies may also permit the deployment of additional securing coils or stent placement to further ensure coils remain inside the aneurysm. Alternatively, coil removal can be attempted with a retrieval device if coil migration into the parent vessel is significant.

Evidence and Outcomes

Given the relative rarity of large and giant basilar tip aneurysms, high-quality long-term data for the treatment of these lesions are scarce. Left untreated, giant and wide-necked basilar tip aneurysms carry an overall poor prognosis due to both their high rupture risk and their mass effect upon critical adjacent neural structures such as the thalamus and brainstem. Open surgical intervention for these lesions carries a significantly increased risk of perioperative morbidity compared to that for aneurysms at other locations, which is attributable to their deep location and associated brainstem perforators. Conventional endovascular coil embolization of basilar tip aneurysm is associated with an increased risk of aneurysm recurrence, but overall, it has a more favorable safety profile than surgical treatment.

One study reported outcomes of endovascular coiling of 44 large and giant basilar tip aneurysms followed for a 12-year period. The study found a procedural and a permanent morbidity rate of 4.6% and 2.3%, respectively. In 31 patients with extended angiographic follow-up, 19 (61%) required re-treatment due to aneurysm recanalization.

Similarly, another study demonstrated that among basilar tip aneurysms treated with endovascular therapy, large aneurysm size (diameter >11 mm) was an independent risk factor for recanalization following treatment, and 8 of 9 aneurysms >14 mm in size had recanalization on angiographic follow-up.

The advent of flow diverters and aneurysm neck reconstruction devices may potentially improve obliteration rates for giant basilar tip aneurysms. A study of outcomes following a staged treatment strategy for ruptured giant aneurysms that included initial coiling followed by flow diversion in a delayed fashion demonstrated a complete occlusion rate of 58%, although basilar tip aneurysms represented only a portion of the studied cohort.

Further Reading

Brinjikji W, Piano M, Fang S, et al. Treatment of ruptured complex and large/giant ruptured cerebral aneurysms by acute coiling followed by staged flow diversion. *J Neurosurg.* 2016;125(1):120–127.

Ding D, Liu, KC. Management strategies for intraprocedural coil migration during endovascular treatment of intracranial aneurysms. *J Neurointerv Surg.* 2014;6(6):428–431.

Pierot L, Cognard C, Anxionnat R, Ricolfi F; CLARITY Investigators. Remodeling technique for endovascular treatment of ruptured intracranial aneurysms had a higher rate of adequate postoperative occlusion than did conventional coil embolization with comparable safety. *Radiology.* 2011;258(2):546–553.

Spiotta AM, Derdeyn CP, Tateshima S, et al. Results of the ANSWER trial using the PulseRider for the treatment of broad-necked, bifurcation aneurysms. *Neurosurgery.* 2017;81(1):56–65.

Tjahjadi M, Kim T, Ojar D, et al. Long-term review of selected basilar-tip aneurysm endovascular techniques in a single institution. *Interdisciplinary Neurosurg.* 2017;8:50–56.

Yang H, Sun Y, Jiang Y, et al. Comparison of stent-assisted coiling vs. coiling alone in 563 intracranial aneurysms: Safety and efficacy at a high-volume center. *Neurosurgery.* 2015;77(2):241–247.

Giant Cavernous-Segment Internal Carotid Artery Aneurysm Presenting with Cranial Neuropathy

Jacob F. Baranoski, Tyler S. Cole, Colin J. Przybylowski, Rami O. Almefty, Dale Ding, Andrew F. Ducruet, and Felipe C. Albuquerque

14

Case Presentation

A 79-year-old otherwise healthy female presented to her primary care physician with 1 month of headaches, dizziness, and diplopia. The patient has no personal or family history of intracranial pathology. On physical exam, the patient was noted to have a left abducens nerve palsy. Brain magnetic resonance imaging (MRI) with contrast showed a large, irregularly shaped, homogenously enhancing mass in the region of the left cavernous sinus extending laterally. The lesion did not have a dural tail or arise from a cranial nerve, nor extend into the sella or suprasellar space.

> ### Questions
>
> 1. What is the most likely diagnosis? What other etiologies should be considered in the differential diagnosis?
> 2. What is the next most appropriate imaging modality?
> 3. What is the appropriate timing of the additional imaging workup?

Assessment and Planning

The differential diagnosis includes a cavernous carotid aneurysm (CCA), cavernous sinus meningioma, or cranial nerve schwannoma. Brain computed tomography angiography (CTA) confirmed the diagnosis of a large left CCA. Intracranial aneurysms can present with cranial neuropathies as a result of cranial nerve compression from mass effect within the cavernous sinus or irritation by hemodynamic effects. CCAs represent approximately 2–9% of all intracranial aneurysms and are a unique class of aneurysms that, although intracranial, are predominantly extradural. CCA rupture is rare. When it occurs, it can cause carotid cavernous fistulas and potentially fatal epistaxis due to erosion through the sphenoid sinus. Uncommonly, CCAs can have an intradural component, and rupture can cause subarachnoid hemorrhage.

A diagnostic cerebral angiogram better characterizes this lesion to develop a treatment plan (Figure 14.1).

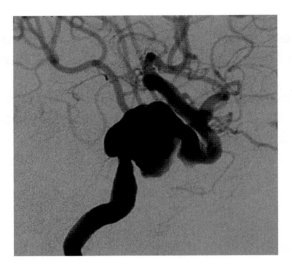

Figure 14.1 Cerebral angiography (lateral projection) demonstrates a giant, irregular CCA aneurysm.

Oral Boards Review—Diagnostic Pearls

1. CCAs can sometime be misdiagnosed as meningiomas or schwannomas. It is important to rule out the possibility of an aneurysm prior to planning surgery for resection of a presumed tumor.
2. Intracranial aneurysms, particularly CCAs, can present with cranial neuropathies due to either mass effect or hemodynamic effects.

Questions

1. How do these clinical and radiological findings influence the decision on whether or not to intervene?
2. What are the options for surgical intervention?
3. What are the options for endovascular intervention?

Decision-Making

Given their relatively benign natural history and low risk of intracranial hemorrhage, the decision to treat CCAs can pose a decision-making dilemma. In general, treatment is reserved for CCAs causing a cranial neuropathy or those that have ruptured. For asymptomatic CCAs, surgeons can attempt to extrapolate if the lesion has an intradural component based on anatomical and radiographic landmarks that may require intervention. Additional factors that warrant intervention for otherwise asymptomatic CCAs include sphenoid bone erosion and increase in aneurysm size over time.

For symptomatic aneurysms, as in the current case, intervention is warranted. Treatment options include surgery (primary clip reconstruction or internal carotid artery [ICA] occlusion with or without distal bypass) and endovascular options (parent vessel sacrifice, coil embolization, stent-assisted coiling, and flow diversion).

Surgical intervention carries a significant risk for procedural morbidity and mortality, which exceeds 30% in some series. Surgical treatment for large CCAs may require proximal ICA ligation with concomitant high-flow bypass. Due to the technical difficulty and operative risks of surgical treatment for CCAs as well as effective endovascular alternatives, this modality is rarely employed in the modern era.

For large or giant ICA aneurysms proximal to the posterior communicating artery, flow diversion has become the preferred treatment option at most cerebrovascular centers due to its favorable safety and efficacy data, particularly compared to surgical and conventional endovascular outcomes. Recent series have demonstrated high rates of improvement in cranial neuropathies following flow diversion, although they may persist despite adequate aneurysm occlusion.

Questions

1. What endovascular devices or techniques should be considered for treatment of this aneurysm?
2. If a flow-diverting stent is used, what medication should be prescribed prior to surgery?

Surgical Procedure

The patient was treated with flow diversion and adjunctive coiling. She was started on dual antiplatelet therapy (aspirin 325 mg and clopidogrel 75 mg daily) 1 or 2 weeks prior to flow diversion, and blood tests to verify antiplatelet response were performed before the procedure. In cases in which stent placement is unplanned and patients are not placed on preoperative dual antiplatelet therapy, an intraprocedural bolus of abciximab (0.125 mg/kg) is administered immediately following deployment of the stent, and the patient is subsequently loaded with aspirin (650 mg orally or 600 mg per rectum) and clopidogrel (300 mg orally) immediately after the procedure. All patients are maintained on dual antiplatelet therapy for at least 6 months after flow diversion. Depending on the results of the initial follow-up angiogram, which is typically performed 6 months after the procedure, most patients are continued on aspirin 81 or 325 mg daily indefinitely.

After transfemoral access, the guide catheter is positioned in the distal cervical ICA. Following arterial access, the patient is systemically heparinized with an intravenous loading dose of 70 U/kg, which is adjusted accordingly to a target activated clotting time of >250 seconds. Three-dimensional rotational angiography is performed to obtain the working projections under high magnification. In contrast to coil embolization cases, the aneurysm itself can be ignored in obtaining the working angles for flow diversion. Instead, the appropriately working angles should delineate the proximal and distal landing zones of the flow diverter. In general, the lateral projection is used to visualize the proximal landing zone, whereas the anteroposterior projection is used to visualize the distal landing zone. Appropriate sizing of the flow diverter is a crucial decision; a device that is too small will not properly appose the vessel wall, resulting in an endoleak, whereas a device that is too large will result in decreased flow diversion of the aneurysm due to widening of the stent interstices. The device length is chosen to allow for approximately 5 mm of stent on either side of the aneurysm neck. Longer devices are stiffer and therefore more difficult to advance through the microcatheter and to deploy. If there is a substantial mismatch between the diameter of the ICA at the proximal versus distal landing zones, one should consider deploying two devices. In these cases, the smaller distal device is deployed first, and then the larger proximal device is telescoped within the initial stent.

The microcatheter is navigated over a micro guide wire into the proximal middle cerebral artery M1 segment. When adjunctive coiling is being performed, a microcatheter is jailed in the aneurysm dome prior to deployment of the flow diverter because the tines of the stent cannot be crossed with a coiling microcatheter. The initial deployment of the flow diverter is an unsheathing maneuver to open the distal portion of the device. Once the device is unsheathed to the midpoint of the aneurysm neck, the operator begins to push the device out of the microcatheter, which closes the stent interstices across the neck to improve its flow-diverting properties. Finally, after the device is unsheathed proximal to the aneurysm neck, the remainder of the device is deployed. If adjunctive coiling is performed, the dome is loosely packed with large-diameter coils through the jailed coiling microcatheter (Figure 14.2). Following stent deployment, the microcatheter is then advanced along the delivery wire distal to the stent, which

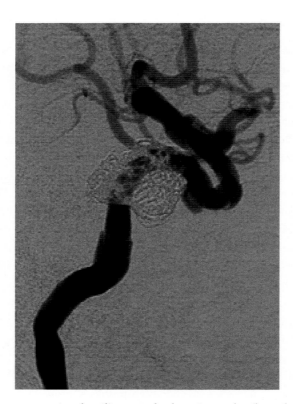

Figure 14.2 After stent-assisted coiling, cerebral angiography (lateral projection) demonstrates complete embolization of the aneurysm with preservation of the stented segment of the parent vessel.

facilitates subsequent angioplasty or deployment of a second stent, if necessary. Failure to recapture the delivery wire results in the operator having to navigate through the stent to obtain distal access, which carries the potential risk of stent displacement.

After stent deployment, final angiograms should be performed to assess for stent apposition, intra-aneurysmal contrast stasis, parent vessel patency, and distal thrombosis. Once satisfied with the final result, the catheter system is removed, and a closure device is deployed into the femoral arterial puncture site.

Oral Boards Review—Management Pearls

1. For large CCAs, the surgeon may consider coiling in addition to flow diversion.
2. During preoperative planning, patients who are scheduled to undergo flow diversion should be started on dual antiplatelet therapy and assessed for adequate antiplatelet response whenever possible.
3. Patients who are nonresponders to aspirin are switched to cilostazol 100 mg twice daily or dipyridamole 75 mg three times daily. Patients who are nonresponders to clopidogrel are switched to prasugrel 10 mg daily or ticagrelor 90 mg twice daily.

Pivot Points

1. If the patient presented with a large CCA that was asymptomatic, it would be reasonable to offer conservative management. Serial imaging could be obtained to assess for interval aneurysm growth.
2. If the ICA caliber appears markedly decreased after flow diversion or if there is evidence of an in-stent or distal thrombosis, immediate recognition is crucial. The neurointerventionalist must be prepared to perform salvage tactics including intra-arterial thrombolysis, mechanical thrombectomy, or angioplasty.
3. Adjunctive coiling during flow-diverting stent placement is considered to promote intra-aneurysmal thrombosis in aneurysms ≥10 mm in size.

Aftercare

Following treatment, the patient is monitored in the intensive care unit overnight, and with an uncomplicated postoperative course, the patient is discharged home the next day on a dual antiplatelet regimen. The femoral puncture site and pedal pulses should be monitored for post-intervention hematoma and ischemia. Post-procedural hemoglobin levels should be monitored, and an abdominal and pelvic CT should be obtained if there is concern for a retroperitoneal hematoma. We typically perform the first follow-up angiogram at 6 months. If the angiogram demonstrates progressive or complete aneurysm occlusion without significant in-stent stenosis, clopidogrel is discontinued, and the patient is maintained indefinitely on antiplatelet monotherapy with aspirin.

Complications and Management

The most frequent complication of flow diversion for CCAs is thromboembolic events, which can range in severity from small emboli in distal cortical arteries to ICA or branch vessel occlusion secondary to stent thrombosis. These events are diagnosed on control angiography by inspecting the distal vasculature, particularly in the branch vessel traversed by the delivery wire, being attentive to alterations in stent configuration and noting intraluminal thrombus or delayed flow through the parent vessel. Other ways to identify complications include examining clinical and neurophysiological monitoring data. Neurophysiological monitoring of changes in regional cerebral blood flow during endovascular treatment has also proved useful for early recognition of locoregional cerebral ischemia. In the event of nonocclusive thrombi or platelet aggregation, additional heparin and/or antiplatelet agents can be administered in order to stabilize the intraluminal thrombus. In rare instances of large vessel occlusion, mechanical thrombectomy may be necessary.

Device migration and prolapse into the aneurysm is a serious complication of flow diversion. It is best avoided by carefully sizing and accurately deploying the flow diverter. For large or giant aneurysms, multiple devices can be deployed in a telescoping fashion. In the event of device prolapse, if distal access can be attained across the stent, an additional device can be deployed to anchor the distal portion of the prolapsed stent to the distal landing zone. If this is not possible, parent vessel occlusion may be necessary, with or without surgical revascularization with a high-flow bypass, depending on the state of the collateral flow to the distal vasculature.

Infrequent, but potentially devastating, complications of flow diversion include delayed aneurysm rupture and ipsilateral intracranial hemorrhage. The underlying mechanisms for both these uncommon complications are incompletely understood. An analysis of the International Retrospective Study of Pipeline Embolization Device registry, which comprised 793 patients with 906 aneurysms, reported ipsilateral intracranial hemorrhage in 20 patients (2.5%) and delayed aneurysm rupture in 5 (0.6%).

A more common delayed complication is aneurysm recanalization. This is typically discovered on routine follow-up angiography, but the patient also may present with recurrent or new cranial neuropathies. Significant residual or recurrent aneurysms after flow diversion should be retreated with placement of additional flow diverter devices, usually if the aneurysm fails to obliterate in the first year after treatment. However, lesions that are completely obliterated by flow diversion have proven to be remarkably durable; few cases of aneurysm recurrence after complete occlusion by flow diversion have been reported.

Oral Boards Review—Complications Pearls

1. Aneurysm rupture, stent thrombosis, distal thromboemboli, and intraparenchymal hemorrhage are all potentially devastating complications from endovascular intervention for large or giant CCAs. Thromboembolic complications can be managed with intra-arterial thrombolysis with an antiplatelet agent (e.g., abciximab) or, less commonly, mechanical thrombectomy in cases of large vessel occlusions.

2. Delayed aneurysm rupture after flow diversion is uncommon, and adjunctive coiling may decrease its incidence by promoting intra-aneurysm thrombosis. Careful inspection of the flow diverter for its apposition to the parent vessel wall can detect an endoleak, which can result in persistent aneurysm filling and thromboembolic complications. Malapposition is treated with post-stenting balloon angioplasty.

3. For CCAs, delayed aneurysm recanalization is common. Recanalization can be detected on routine follow-up imaging or can result in new or recurrent neurological symptoms. Re-treatment should be considered, typically with deployment of an additional flow diverter, in CCAs that fail to obliterate at 1-year follow-up.

Evidence and Outcomes

The patient's abducens nerve palsy and diplopia completely resolved soon after treatment, and at 19-month follow-up, she remained neurologically intact. Follow-up angiography at 6 months demonstrated near-complete aneurysm occlusion.

Flow diversion has become the preferred treatment for symptomatic CCAs, with marked improvement of symptoms. A multicenter cohort study demonstrated that 72% of patients with oculomotor palsies improved following flow diversion of CCAs. These results are generally comparable to those following surgical or endovascular parent vessel occlusion, although some studies have suggested that proximal ICA occlusion may yield a higher rate of symptom improvement. However, deconstructive treatment with parent vessel occlusion carries a risk of ischemic stroke even if patients successfully pass balloon test occlusion.

Further Reading

Kim KS, Fraser JF, Grupke S, Cook AM. Management of antiplatelet therapy in patients undergoing neuroendovascular procedures. *J Neurosurg.* 2018;129(4):890–905.

Matouk CC, Kaderali Z, terBrugge KG, Willinsky RA. Long-term clinical and imaging follow-up of complex intracranial aneurysms treated by endovascular parent vessel occlusion. *AJNR Am J Neuroradiol.* 2012;33(10):1991–1997.

Moon K, Albuquerque FC, Ducruet AF, Crowley RW, McDougall CG. Resolution of cranial neuropathies following treatment of intracranial aneurysms with the Pipeline embolization device. *J Neurosurg.* 2014;121(5):1085–1092.

Park MS, Kilburg C, Taussky P, et al. Pipeline embolization device with or without adjunctive coil embolization: Analysis of complications from the IntrePED registry. *AJNR Am J Neuroradiol.* 2016;37(6):1127–1131.

Park MS, Nanaszko M, Sanborn MR, Moon K, Albuquerque FC, McDougall CG. Re-treatment rates after treatment with the Pipeline embolization device alone versus Pipeline and coil embolization of cerebral aneurysms: A single-center experience. *J Neurosurg.* 2016;125(1):137–144.

Szikora I, Marosfoi M, Salomvary B, Berentei Z, Gubucz I. Resolution of mass effect and compression symptoms following endoluminal flow diversion for the treatment of intracranial aneurysms. *AJNR Am J Neuroradiol.* 2013;34(5):935–939.

van Rooij WJ, Sluzewski M. Unruptured large and giant carotid artery aneurysms presenting with cranial nerve palsy: Comparison of clinical recovery after selective aneurysm coiling and therapeutic carotid artery occlusion. *AJNR Am J Neuroradiol.* 2008;29(5):997–1002.

Symptomatic Cervical Carotid Artery Stenosis

David Dornbos III, Brandon Burnsed, and Adam Arthur

15

Case Presentation

A 68-year-old African American male with a past medical history of hypertension presented with sudden onset of bilateral upper extremity shaking, followed by confusion, left facial droop, and left hemiparesis 2 hours prior to arrival in the emergency department. Neurological examination revealed orientation to person and place only, with significant dysarthria and confusion. Sensation was decreased on the left hemibody, with associated neglect of the left upper and lower extremities and a mild left hemiparesis. His National Institutes of Health Stroke Score was 6.

Questions

1. What is the likely diagnosis?
2. What are the most appropriate imaging modalities for further diagnostic workup?
3. What therapeutic measures are most appropriate in the immediate setting?

Assessment and Planning

Although the patient presented following a possible seizure, the persistent hemiparesis and confusion raises concern for possible transient ischemic attack (TIA), stroke, or a post-ictal (Todd's) paralysis. The most common stroke mimics include seizures, complicated migraines, neoplasms, metabolic derangements, sepsis, and syncope. Seizures, complicated migraines, and syncope can often be ruled out by the clinical history and physical examination. Patients suffering from complicated migraines will typically have a history of migraines, and the acute episode of hemiparesis will usually be accompanied by a severe headache, scintillating scotoma, and/or aura. Symptoms associated with a syncopal episode often overlap with those of a vertebrobasilar stroke, although typically without the cranial nerve findings expected with an ischemic insult to the brainstem. Neoplasms, sepsis, and metabolic derangements (e.g., hyper- or hypoglycemia, other electrolyte abnormalities, or hepatic encephalopathy) can be diagnosed with cranial imaging and blood tests.

The patient's initial presentation of possible seizure followed by sudden-onset hemiparesis, facial droop, and confusion was concerning for acute stroke. The persistent nature of the weakness led to the diagnosis of either stroke/TIA or a seizure with post-ictal paralysis. Cranial imaging (computed tomography [CT] head) ruled out the presence

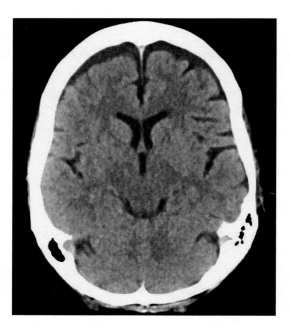

Figure 15.1 CT of the head, revealing no evidence of completed ischemic stroke or intracranial hemorrhage.

of a tumor, intracranial hemorrhage, or completed stroke, as shown in Figure 15.1. Treatment with intravenous tissue plasminogen activator (tPA) was initiated.

Although most studies have shown that treatment of stroke mimics (e.g., seizure) with intravenous tPA has minimal adverse sequelae, a small but significant risk of intracranial hemorrhage still exists. Given the urgency of treating acute ischemic stroke with tPA within 3–4½ hours of symptom onset, absolute confirmation of an ischemic etiology may not always be feasible, and aggressive early use of intravenous tPA is warranted in these cases.

CT angiography (CTA) of the head and neck was also performed to assess for a large vessel occlusion, intracranial atherosclerosis, and carotid disease. The patient was found to have 90% stenosis at the origin of the right internal carotid artery (ICA) without evidence of intracranial atherosclerotic disease or large vessel occlusion, as seen in Figure 15.2. Electroencephalogram (EEG) obtained soon thereafter identified moderate encephalopathy without evidence of seizures. The patient's confusion and hemiparesis completely resolved following administration of intravenous tPA, confirming the diagnosis of a treated ischemic stroke or TIA.

Oral Boards Review—Diagnostic Pearls

1. History and physical examination, in addition to cranial imaging, are often sufficient to distinguish between ischemic stroke and stroke-mimicking diagnoses.
   a. Ischemic stroke/transient ischemic attack: Patients may have a history of TIAs or prior stroke, and they often have associated comorbidities

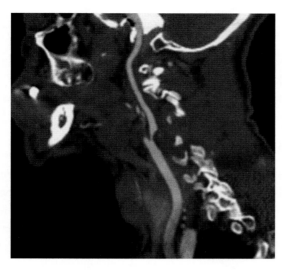

Figure 15.2 CTA of the neck, identifying 90% stenosis of the ICA at the carotid bifurcation.

(hypertension, hyperlipidemia, atrial fibrillation, and cardiac disease). Onset is typically sudden without preceding aura. Neurologic deficits depend on the affected vascular territory.

  b. Seizures: Although a post-ictal paresis or plegia is often seen following a seizure, the majority of patients will present with stereotypical motor movements or paresthesias. Unfortunately, the absence of such movements does not rule out a seizure, nor does their presence confirm diagnosis. Diagnosis is typically established with EEG. Nearly 10% of stroke patients may present with seizure.

  c. Complicated migraines: Migraines may be complicated with either hemiplegia or vertebrobasilar symptoms (ataxia, decreased consciousness, or vertigo). Patients will often have a personal or familial history of migraines, and these episodes are often accompanied by a headache and/or scintillating scotoma.

  d. Syncope: Symptoms of syncope may resemble vertebrobasilar ischemia, including loss of consciousness and vertigo. The lack of cranial nerve findings favors syncope over brainstem ischemia.

  e. Neoplasm: Intracranial neoplastic processes may present with stroke-like symptoms, such as in the case of seizure, intratumoral hemorrhage, or apoplexy, although presentation is often subacute or progressive. Cranial imaging establishes the diagnosis.

2. Initial diagnostic workup of a patient presenting with symptoms concerning for stroke/TIA or seizures should consist of cranial imaging (CT or magnetic resonance imaging), vascular imaging (CTA or magnetic resonance angiography of the head and neck), and potentially EEG.

Questions

1. How do these radiographic findings influence further surgical decision-making?
2. What is the most appropriate timing for intervention in this patient?

Decision-Making

The severe cervical carotid stenosis seen on vascular imaging was identified as the likely source of the patient's symptoms, given the lack of seizures and epileptogenic discharges on EEG. For this patient, the management of symptomatic carotid stenosis is relatively straightforward, although some debate exists regarding the timing and exact nature of treatment.

The indication for treatment of symptomatic carotid stenosis was established through the North American Carotid Endarterectomy Trial, in which patients suffering a TIA or nondisabling stroke and ipsilateral high-grade stenosis (>70%) received a significant benefit from carotid endarterectomy (CEA). CEA in this patient population reduced the absolute risk of subsequent stroke by 17% and death by 7% at 2 years compared to optimal medical management. This improvement in morbidity and mortality was substantially greater in patients with 90–99% stenosis.

Based on pooled data from several randomized trials evaluating outcomes following CEA for severe symptomatic carotid stenosis, patients treated within 14 days following a symptomatic event received greater benefit than those undergoing delayed treatment. As such, the American Heart Association official guidelines recommend that revascularization for symptomatic carotid artery stenosis should ideally occur within 14 days of an ischemic event.

Revascularization can be accomplished through either CEA or carotid artery stenting (CAS). Although several recent trials, including the Carotid Revascularization Endarterectomy versus Stenting Trial, have demonstrated no difference in composite outcomes when comparing CEA to CAS, current guidelines only recommend CAS for patients at high risk for CEA and with >70% stenosis. Patients may be classified as high risk for CEA based on numerous anatomic features and comorbidities. High-risk anatomic features include contralateral carotid occlusion or significant bilateral carotid stenosis, contralateral laryngeal nerve palsy, prior neck radiation therapy, surgically inaccessible carotid bifurcation, or restenosis following a prior CEA. Comorbidities that may preclude CEA include unstable angina, myocardial infarction within 6 weeks, congestive heart failure, left ventricular ejection fraction <30%, renal failure, and chronic obstructive pulmonary disease.

In this case, the patient had few comorbidities, no anatomic anomalies that would preclude CEA, and an echocardiogram demonstrating normal cardiac function with a left ventricular ejection fraction of 60%. A CEA was recommended.

Questions

1. What is the significance of the patient's lack of comorbidities and echocardiogram findings?
2. What adjunctive measures can be undertaken to detect potential ischemic complications during the procedure?

Surgical Procedure

Anesthesia may be general, regional, or local, and the incision may be transverse (typically oriented along a skin fold in the mid-neck starting 2 cm posterior to the mandibular angle, extending to 1 cm lateral to the midline) or longitudinal (along the anterior border of the sternocleidomastoid muscle).

Patients are typically started on 325 mg of daily aspirin prior to surgery, which is continued postoperatively, although some surgeons prefer additional perioperative clopidogrel. Intraoperative monitoring may include transcranial Doppler or EEG, depending on surgeon preference. Patients are typically placed under general anesthesia and positioned supine with the head rotated slightly away from the operative side. A shoulder roll may assist with a slight degree of extension to increase exposure.

A longitudinal incision is fashioned along the anterior border of the sternocleidomastoid muscle. This is carried down through the platysma, and a plane just medial to the anterior border of the sternocleidomastoid is identified and opened further through blunt dissection. A large transverse sensory nerve may be encountered and can be sacrificed to facilitate exposure, although the surgeon should be careful not to violate the parotid fascia. The neurovascular bundle involving the carotid artery can then be easily identified and palpated. Sharp dissection can be used to open the cervical fascia, and then blunt dissection can be performed. Exposure, as seen in Figure 15.3, should include the common carotid artery (CCA), carotid bifurcation, external carotid artery (ECA), and the ICA, whose distal exposure must extend well beyond the plaque, often to the level of the hypoglossal nerve. Often, the surgeon can feel and see normal artery distal to the plaque, the length of which must be able to comfortably accommodate the vessel loop and distal ICA clip.

Important structures encountered during this exposure include the common facial vein, omohyoid muscle, and hypoglossal nerve. The common facial vein, an anteriorly oriented branch of the internal jugular vein, often lies directly superficial to the carotid bifurcation and should be suture ligated and divided to facilitate exposure. The omohyoid muscle typically marks the inferior extent of the dissection and usually can be left intact. Running superficial to the ECA and ICA, the hypoglossal nerve must be identified and protected throughout the duration of the case to minimize risk of injury

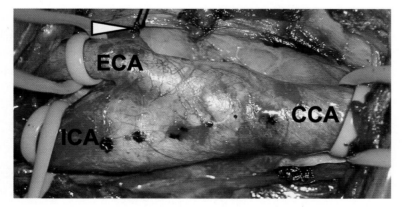

Figure 15.3 Pertinent vascular anatomy of the carotid bifurcation, including the common carotid artery (CCA), external carotid artery (ECA), internal carotid artery (ICA), and superior thyroid artery (arrowhead).

to this nerve. The vagus nerve and its superior laryngeal branch lie deep to the carotid and internal jugular vein, and care must be taken to avoid disruption of these structures when dissection below the carotid is needed. Damage to the superior laryngeal branch of the vagus nerve will result in significant postoperative dysphagia. Once an adequate distance along the CCA, ECA, and ICA is achieved, vessel loops can be placed around the ECA and ICA. The patient is then given 5000 IU of intravenous heparin, and attention can be turned to the arteriotomy.

A temporary aneurysm clip is often placed on the superior thyroid artery, which arises at the proximal ECA or distal CCA. Prior to further cross-clamping, mild hypertension (systolic blood pressure 160–180 mmHg) is induced by the anesthesiologist. Clamping of the carotid system then commences first with the ICA, followed by the CCA and then the ECA. Clamping in this order ensures that potential thromboembolic debris preferentially enters the ECA circulation. An arteriotomy is then performed with a No. 11 blade scalpel in the mid common carotid artery, which is extended into the ICA with Pott's scissors until normal intima is encountered. A shunt can be placed if clamping potentiates changes in intraoperative ischemic monitoring.

Circumferential dissection of the plaque is initiated proximally in the CCA. It is important to start the dissection below the bulk of the plaque and truncate the plaque sharply at the proximal extent of the arteriotomy. The plaque is then circumferentially dissected with a Penfield No. 4 up to the origin of the ECA and gently pulled out of the ECA with a hemostat. Finally, the dissection is carried distally into the ICA. Careful inspection of the intima is required to identify any residual debris or plaque material for removal. Particular attention must be paid to the distal end to ensure that no ledge or intimal flap is present because this significantly raises the risk of dissection. If the plaque does not come to a smooth end, it can be sharply cut and tacked down with sutures, although with adequate distal exposure this is rarely required. If tack-up sutures are needed, it is often prudent to employ a patch to obviate the possibility of residual stenosis at the distal end.

Primary arteriotomy closure is performed with 6–0 Prolene suture, starting at the distal ICA and run proximally until one-half or one-third of arteriotomy remains. A second suture is then started at the proximal CCA and run distally. Alternatively, a patch may be sewn into the arteriotomy site using an autologous saphenous vein or prosthetic material (e.g., Dacron). Sutures should be placed 1 mm apart and 1 mm deep to the arteriotomy edge. Prior to complete closure, the ICA clamp should be temporarily removed to allow backbleeding. The clamp is then replaced, and the CCA clamp is temporarily removed and then replaced. This maneuver facilitates removal of any air or surgical debris remaining within the lumen. The last few stitches are thrown, and the ECA and then CCA clamps are removed while the final knot is tied down. The ICA clamp is then removed.

Oral Boards Review—Management Pearls

1. Particular care must be paid to the distal site of the endarterectomy because a residual intimal flap or ledge can become an arterial dissection or the source of postoperative thromboembolism.
2. Transcranial Doppler, EEG, and other adjunctive measures may be used to monitor potential intraoperative ischemic complications.

Pivot Points

1. In patients presenting with symptomatic carotid stenosis of at least 70%, early surgical intervention within 14 days decreases the risk of recurrent ischemic events.

2. Development of significant changes in intraoperative monitoring concerning for cortical ischemia, if encountered soon after clamping, should prompt either aborting the procedure or placement of a carotid shunt to maintain perfusion during CEA.

Aftercare

Postoperative monitoring (including telemetry and blood pressure monitoring) should be performed in the intensive care unit. Strict blood pressure management, typically with a goal of approximately 20% reduction of the baseline blood pressure, is important to avoid cerebral hyperperfusion.

Postoperative antibiotics are only utilized for 24 hours. Early mobility and ambulation are encouraged the evening of surgery, and nearly all patients can be discharged on the first postoperative day.

Complications and Management

As mentioned previously, increased blood flow through the ICA may lead to cerebral hyperperfusion. Sustained elevations in blood pressure should be treated aggressively with intravenous β-blockers (labetalol) or vasodilators (hydralazine).

A postoperative decline in neurologic status raises concern for a thromboembolic event. An early postoperative deficit or decline in neurologic status demands an immediate response. Traditionally, such patients were returned to the operating room for immediate surgical exploration of the endarterectomy site. More recently, the preference has been to perform cerebral angiography instead, in case thrombectomy is required. A cone-beam CT of the brain can be obtained at the same time to assess for hemorrhage.

A neck hematoma is another significant, although rare, postoperative complication following CEA. This threat to the patient's airway constitutes a surgical and anesthetic emergency. When possible, immediate return to the operating room and awake fiberoptic intubation in a controlled setting are preferred. If imminent airway compromise and/or stridor are present, immediate opening of the wound may be necessary, even at the bedside. Once the airway has been secured, surgical exploration of the hematoma and arteriotomy can commence.

Oral Boards Review—Complications Pearls

1. Strict control of blood pressure in the postoperative setting can avoid cerebral hyperperfusion and potential secondary intracranial hemorrhage.

2. Early and significant postoperative neurologic decline should be addressed with immediate return to the operating room or neurointerventional suite.

> 3. Postoperative neck hematoma is a neurosurgical and anesthetic emergency, in which securing the airway is of utmost importance. Rarely, opening the wound at the bedside may be a necessary and life-saving maneuver.

Evidence and Outcomes

As previously discussed, numerous randomized controlled trials provide robust evidence in favor of CEA for symptomatic cervical carotid stenosis (>70%). Similar, but slightly worse, results can be seen in carotid stenting, which is why this is currently reserved for patients at high risk for CEA.

The risks associated with CEA are relatively low. Perioperative risk of stroke was 5.8–7.0% in several major trials, with perioperative mortality <1%. Cranial nerve deficits, most commonly transient vocal cord paralysis and/or dysphagia, can be seen in approximately 1% of patients, although these are rarely permanent. In summary, CEA provides a robust treatment for symptomatic severe carotid stenosis with relatively low morbidity and mortality and a substantial reduction in the risk of subsequent stroke or death.

Further Reading

Barnett HJ, Taylor DW, Eliaszie M, et al. Benefit of carotid endarterectomy in patients with symptomatic moderate or severe stenosis: North American Symptomatic Carotid Endarterectomy Trial Collaborators. *N Engl J Med.* 1998;339(20):1415–1425.

De Rango P, Brown MM, Chaturvedi S, et al. Summary of evidence on early carotid intervention for recently symptomatic stenosis based on meta-analysis of current risks. *Stroke.* 2015;46(12):3423–3436.

Ecker RD, Pichelmann MA, Meissner I, et al. Durability of carotid endarterectomy. *Stroke.* 2003;34:2941–2944.

Erdur H, Scheitz JF, Ebinger M, et al. In-hospital stroke recurrence and stroke after transient ischemic attack: Frequency and risk factors. *Stroke.* 2015;46(4):1031–1037.

Mantese VA, Timaran CH, Chiu D, et al. The Carotid Revascularization Endarterectomy versus Stenting Trial (CREST): Stenting versus carotid endarterectomy for carotid disease. *Stroke.* 2010;41(10 Suppl):S31–S34.

Randomised trial of endarterectomy for recently symptomatic carotid stenosis: Final results of the MRC European Carotid Surgery Trial (ECST). *Lancet.* 1998;351:1379–1387.

Reznik M, Kamel H, Gialdini G, et al. Timing of carotid revascularization procedures after ischemic stroke. *Stroke.* 2017;48(1):225–228.

Asymptomatic Cervical Carotid Stenosis

Kunal Vakharia, Sabareesh K. Natarajan, Hussain Shallwani, and Elad I. Levy

16

Case Presentation

A 77-year-old male with a medical history significant for hypertension, hyperlipidemia, and a coronary artery bypass graft was found to have a right-sided carotid bruit detected on auscultation during physical examination. His previous medical management consisted of lifestyle modifications, aspirin, and statin therapy. He had no referable symptoms, no history of ischemic or hemorrhagic stroke, and no signs of transient ischemic attack. Doppler ultrasound studies ordered by his primary care physician showed 70–99% stenosis of the right internal carotid artery (ICA). Subsequent magnetic resonance imaging and magnetic resonance angiography (MRA) of the carotid arteries showed 95–99% stenosis of the proximal right ICA. He was referred to us for further evaluation and management.

Questions

1. What are appropriate imaging modalities for the evaluation of asymptomatic carotid stenosis?
2. What is the best medical management and when is this appropriate?
3. When is surgical intervention warranted? What is the number needed to treat?

Assessment and Planning

Carotid stenosis is commonly found incidentally on physical examination during auscultation of the neck that reveals a carotid bruit or during evaluation for possible transient ischemic attacks. The typical modality used in a primary care setting is duplex carotid ultrasound imaging. The percentage of stenosis can be estimated from the ultrasound imaging based on the location in the common carotid artery (CCA) or ICA. The systolic and diastolic velocities measured with ultrasound imaging help clinicians judge the accuracy of the percentage. MRA and computed tomography angiography (CTA) are also useful studies to understand the plaque morphology as well as the location and extent of disease. Diagnostic cerebral digital subtraction angiography (DSA) is the "gold standard" for the evaluation of carotid disease and the true nature of a carotid plaque. Although CTA is nearly 90% as accurate and MRA is nearly 80% as accurate as DSA, diagnostic angiography allows for dynamic imaging and also for simultaneous comparison of the external carotid artery (ECA) and ICA circulations. The patient in this case had 90.7% stenosis on DSA (Figure 16.1). In cases in which it is difficult to determine the exact cause of stroke and potential for thromboemboli forming from a carotid plaque, MRA can help show the morphology of the plaque within the lumen of a vessel and show the irregularities of the plaque. Irregularities tend to indicate a higher risk of generating thromboemboli.

In addition to establishing the percentage of stenosis, clinically understanding the need to treat and the risks and benefits is critical when assessing and advising patients. The Asymptomatic Carotid Atherosclerosis Study (ACAS) and Asymptomatic Carotid Surgery Trial (ACST) found that patients with >60–70% stenosis had a 5-year stroke rate of 11–11.8% in the medical arm and 5.1–6.4% in the surgical arm (carotid endarterectomy [CEA]). Since the advent of these trials, medical management has significantly improved with the use of statin and antiplatelet therapies. There is no class I evidence estimating stroke rates associated with current best medical management. In addition to the literature surrounding CEA in asymptomatic carotid artery stenosis, there has been increasing literature and interest in carotid artery angioplasty and stenting (CAS), which is being evaluated in the four-armed parallel Carotid Revascularization and Medical Management for Asymptomatic Carotid Stenosis Trial (CREST-2). This study is a comparison of composite 30-day stroke and death outcomes between best medical therapy alone versus with CEA and best medical therapy alone versus with CAS. Understanding this risk profile will be important for future surgical planning and management for these patients. In addition, there is increasing interest and literature surrounding cognitive decline and its relation to asymptomatic carotid artery disease and whether surgical or endovascular revascularization can benefit cognitive decline.

For surgical planning, a detailed understanding of the arterial and venous anatomy and its association to bony landmarks is important. Understanding the location of the

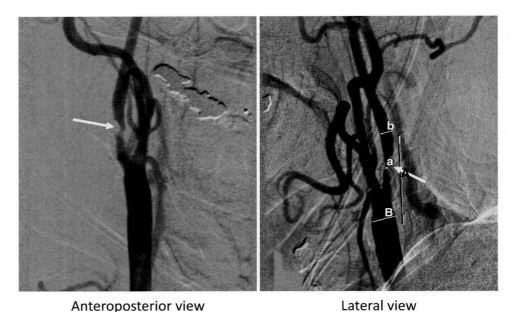

Anteroposterior view   Lateral view

Figure 16.1 DSA images (anteroposterior view and lateral view) confirming 90.7% stenosis of the proximal right internal carotid artery (arrows).

bifurcation of the common carotid artery and its relation to the angle of the mandible and also its bony landmarks in relation to the cervical spine allows for easier intraoperative exposure. In the current case, the lesion is at the level of the C4 vertebral body (Figure 16.2). In addition, cranial imaging is important in preoperative planning. Knowledge of the Circle of Willis helps one to distinguish sources of blood supply to the hemisphere ipsilateral to the stenosis. This allows a better understanding of potential collateral routes during clamp time while performing carotid endarterectomies. If there is an isolated middle cerebral artery supply from the ICA without adequate collaterals, there should be a higher suspicion and preparation for possible intraoperative shunting.

Oral Boards Review—Diagnostic Pearls

1. Physical examination and routine Doppler ultrasound studies are useful in screening for an underlying asymptomatic carotid stenosis.
2. MRA and CTA are good adjuncts to understand vascular anatomy and help in preoperative planning, but they are only 80% and 90% as accurate as cerebral angiography, respectively.
3. Cerebral angiography helps elucidate many different anatomical aspects of a carotid lesion, including the following:
   a. Bony landmarks and stenosis location
   b. Degree of stenosis and arterial flow limitation
   c. Tandem disease
   d. Cross-filling and patency of the circle of Willis
   e. Carotid kinking and tortuosity of the ICA in relation to the CCA

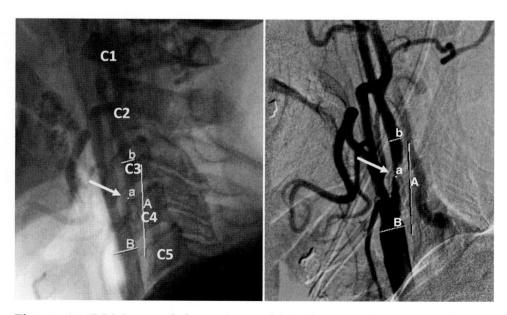

Figure 16.2 DSA images (left, unsubtracted lateral view; right, subtracted lateral view) of the cervical spine showing the lesion in the proximal internal carotid artery at the level of the C4 vertebral body (arrows).

Questions

1. Which other key radiographic features would increase the risk of periprocedural stroke?
2. Which studies can help differentiate plaque morphology and the likelihood that plaque is actively generating thromboemboli?
3. Which radiographic features can help determine the possible need for intraoperative shunting?

Decision-Making

After diagnosis, initiating the best medical therapy, including antiplatelet therapy, statin therapy, and lifestyle modifications, is warranted. Depending on the degree and location of the stenosis, CEA and CAS serve as complementary treatment modalities for revascularization. Currently in the United States, CEA has been the most studied modality and is the most widely accepted mode of treatment. Boxes 16.1 and 16.2 indicate high-risk features for CEA that may warrant CAS in place of microsurgical revascularization techniques.

The Carotid Revascularization Endarterectomy Versus Stenting Trial (CREST) was a randomized trial comparing the safety and efficacy of CAS versus CEA in patients with high-grade carotid stenosis. Asymptomatic patients were required to have >60% stenosis by angiography, >70% by ultrasound, or >80% by CTA or MRA if the stenosis on ultrasonography was 50–69%. Among 2,502 patients over a median follow-up period of 2½ years, there was no statistically significant difference in the estimated 4-year rates of the primary end point of stroke, myocardial infarction (MI), or death between the CAS group and the CEA group (7.2% and 6.8%, respectively; $p = 0.51$). The 4-year rate of stroke or death among asymptomatic patients between the stenting group and the endarterectomy group was 4.5% and 2.7%, respectively ($p = 0.07$). Periprocedural rates of individual components of the end points differed between the CAS group and the CEA group for death (0.7% vs. 0.3%, respectively; $p = 0.18$), stroke (4.1% vs. 2.3%, respectively; $p = 0.01$), and MI (1.1% vs. 2.3%, respectively; $p = 0.03$).

The patient in this case did not have high-risk features such as a lesion extending above C2, a neck with difficult access secondary to adipose tissue and other anatomical constraints, previous neck surgery (i.e., laryngectomy or tracheostomy) or radiation therapy, or other significant medical comorbidities. Given the low-lying bifurcation and thin and flexible neck, CEA was chosen for this patient.

Surgical Procedure

The current patient underwent routine preoperative evaluation and assessment, including medical clearance from his primary care physician. The patient was on 81 mg of aspirin daily, which was continued preoperatively. CEA is routinely performed under general anesthesia with endotracheal intubation. It is important to avoid overt hypotension during induction of the anesthesia to prevent hypoperfusion prior to surgery.

Box 16.1 US Food and Drug Administration Criteria for High-Risk Candidates for Carotid Endarterectomy

Significant Medical Comorbidities

- Class III or IV congestive heart failure
- Left ventricular ejection fraction <30%
- Recent myocardial infarction (>24 hours and <30 days)
- Unstable angina; Canadian Cardiovascular Society class III or IV
- Concurrent requirement for coronary revascularization
- Abnormal stress test
- Severe pulmonary disease
- Chronic oxygen therapy
- Resting minimum arterial O_2 partial pressure (PaO_2) <60 mmHg
- Baseline hematocrit >50% of normal

- Forced expiratory volume in 1 second or carbon monoxide lung diffusion capacity <500% of normal
- Age >80 years

Significant Anatomical Abnormalities

- Contralateral carotid artery occlusion
- Contralateral laryngeal palsy
- Previous radiation to head or neck
- Previous carotid endarterectomy with recurrent stenosis
- Surgically difficult to access high cervical lesions (high cervical lesions above the C2 vertebra or common carotid artery lesions below the clavicle)
- Severe tandem lesions
- Laryngectomy or tracheostomy
- Inability to extend head as a result of arthritis or other condition

Source: Adapted from the US Centers for Medicare and Medicaid Services (https://www.cms.gov/medicare-coverage-database/details/nca-decision-memo.aspx?NCAId=157&ver=29&NcaName=Carotid+Artery+Stenting+(1st+Recon)&bc=BEAAAAAAEAAA&&fromdb=true).

Neuromonitoring with somatosensory evoked potentials and continuous electroencephalography (EEG) is routinely performed. An arterial line is placed for strict blood pressure management.

The patient is positioned supine with the head slightly extended at the neck and chin and slightly rotated toward the opposite side of the lesion. A skin crease is used to plan a

---

Box 16.2 Centers for Medicare and Medicaid Services High-Risk Criteria for Carotid Endarterectomy

Significant Comorbid Conditions

- Class III or IV congestive heart failure
- Left ventricular ejection fraction <30%
- Unstable angina
- Contralateral carotid occlusion
- Recent myocardial infarction
- Previous carotid endarterectomy with recurrent stenosis
- Previous radiation treatment to the neck

Anatomical Risk Factors

- Recurrent stenosis and/or
- Previous radical neck dissection

Source: Adapted from the US Centers for Medicare and Medicaid Services (https://www.cms.gov/medicare-coverage-database/details/nca-decision-memo.aspx?NCAId=157&ver=29&NcaName=Carotid+Artery+Stenting+(1st+Recon)&bc=BEAAAAAAEAAA&&fromdb=true).

---

transverse incision to allow for appropriate cosmetic closure. The incision is marked from the midline crossing the sternocleidomastoid muscle (SCM) so that one-third of the incision is on the muscle and two-thirds of the incision lies medial. The skin is then prepared and draped in usual sterile fashion. Antibiotics are administered preoperatively. The skin incision is made over the medial border of the SCM while being mindful of the greater auricular nerve over the SCM because sectioning that nerve can lead to postoperative jaw and ear numbness. The platysma is split and undermined both above and below the incision to allow adequate exposure. The medial border of the SCM is identified, and the fascia medial to this is sharply dissected. The digastric muscle is exposed proximally; the omohyoid muscle is exposed distally. This leads to the carotid sheath. The common facial vein frequently crosses the middle of the surgical field and can be ligated and divided without concern. The ansa cervicalis runs superficial to the ICA and leads to the hypoglossal nerve, which is identified so for preservation during the operation. The superior thyroid artery, which is the first branch of the ECA, identifies the location of the ECA. The extent of ICA exposure beyond the plaque is determined by gentle palpation of the ICA.

At this point, the CCA, ECA, and ICA are exposed and carefully exposed. Heparin (5,000 units) is administered. Vascular loops are placed around each of the vessels. Burst suppression is induced, and the systolic blood pressure is elevated 20 mm above the patient's baseline. The order of clamp occlusion is ICA, CCA, and ECA. The arteriotomy is begun in the CCA with a No. 11 blade knife and extended into the ICA with a Potts scissors. A Penfield No. 4 is used to dissect the plaque from either side at the proximal end of the CCA, and the proximal end of the plaque is divided with the Potts scissors. The plaque is dissected toward the ECA orifice, and an eversion endarterectomy of the ECA orifice is done. Dissection is carried distally into the ICA, and the cranial end of the plaque is ideally removed *en bloc*. The inner lumen is flushed with heparinized saline, and any floating debris or intimal flaps are removed. Primary closure of the arteriotomy is done with running Prolene 6–0 suture. Before the arterial repair is completed, the ICA is backbled for approximately 10 seconds and the suture line is completed. The order of release of the clamps is ECA, CCA, and ICA. Doppler imaging is used to assess appropriate flow through the distal ICA and the repaired arteriotomy as well as the proximal and distal portion of the vessel to ensure no free flap is occlusive or limiting flow. The patient's blood pressure is lowered 20 mmHg below baseline after all clamps have been removed. Surgical is placed over the arteriotomy site, and meticulous hemostasis is achieved. The platysma is closed with 2–0 Vicryl. The skin is closed with subcuticular 4–0 Monocryl. Steri-Strips and a sterile dressing are applied.

Oral Boards Review—Management Pearls

1. Exposure to the angle of the mandible is important to confirm that clips are placed above the level of the plaque. This is also important for locating and preserving the hypoglossal nerve.
2. Division of the omohyoid muscle allows for adequate exposure in low bifurcation procedures.
3. Plaque removal ideally should begin at the lateral edge and be performed in a circumferential manner. A sharp dissection at the end of the plaque is useful to prevent plaque debris from remaining in the intimal layer.
4. Beginning the suture line with inside-out sutures allows for tacking of the plaque edge to the patent uninjured intimal layer to prevent flow stasis.
5. Placement of a shunt can sometimes be used in cases in which patients develop EEG changes early after clamping.
6. Be wary of atherosclerotic webs on the posterior margin of the vessel; these can create persistent stenosis after completion of the procedure. A single vertical stitch in the same fashion as a tacking suture can be used to hold and flatten the shelf of the web.

Pivot Points

1. Patients presenting with medical comorbidities requiring anticoagulation therapy need to be optimized preoperatively, and risk assessment needs to be done before stopping the therapy.
2. Intraoperatively, changes in continuous EEG warrant elevating blood pressure to help collateral supply, hastening plaque removal and vessel closure, and potentially using a shunt to temporarily restore blood flow.
3. If the patient has poor radiographic collaterals (e.g., lack of anterior and posterior communicating arteries), the surgeon should anticipate the need for shunting.

Aftercare

The patient is extubated and the systolic blood pressure is maintained 20 mmHg below his or her baseline for the next 24 hours. The patient is observed in the intensive care unit overnight and is maintained on 81 mg of aspirin on a daily basis.

Complications and Management

The current guidelines of the American Heart Association and the American Stroke Association have established a 3% upper limit perioperative risk for CEA in asymptomatic patients, assuming a life expectancy exceeding 5 years. Common complications associated with CEA include postoperative hematoma formation, ischemic complications, hemorrhagic complications, and cranial nerve injury.

Postoperative hematoma formation can occur secondary to a faulty suture line, with hematoma formation potentially occurring in a rapid fashion. An immediate return to the operating room and evacuation of the hematoma are critical to protecting the patient's airway. Venous bleeding can potentially cause significant postoperative hematomas and may warrant exploration if the hematoma is causing significant mass effect.

Ischemic complications after surgery tend to happen secondary to debris causing embolic strokes or carotid thrombus formation and carotid occlusion. Symptomatic carotid occlusion should prompt immediate return to the operating room for vessel exploration and possible thrombectomy and removal of the clot from the ICA. Direct suction aspiration in the vessel as well as the use of a Fogarty balloon to cross the thrombus with inflation of the balloon in the petrous or cavernous segment of the carotid artery with slow removal to the normal vessel can help in thrombus removal. Again, care should be taken because this maneuver can cause arterial dissections and predispose patients to the development of carotid cavernous fistulas.

Hemorrhagic complications tend to occur more frequently with severe stenotic lesions or pseudo-occlusions. Revascularization allows for return of blood flow into vasculature that has been in a low-flow state. Hyperperfusion syndrome is a recognized complication, and management with close neuromonitoring and blood pressure control is warranted in these patients. Slowly normalizing blood pressure over 24 hours postoperatively can avoid such complications.

Cranial nerve injuries can occur and are related to the dissection and exposure of the carotid artery. These injuries occur in 8–10% of cases, including injury to the ipsilateral hypoglossal nerve, which causes tongue deviation to the side of the injury; recurrent laryngeal nerve injury, which causes unilateral vocal cord paralysis; and marginal mandibular nerve injury, which causes loss of unilateral depressor motion of the lips.

Oral Boards Review—Complications Pearls

1. A postoperative, rapidly enlarging hematoma warrants opening the surgical site before intubating the patient. Tracheal deviation can cause difficulty with securing the airway; thus, decompression is the first step.
2. Direct suction aspiration and suction aspiration through shunt tubing can be used to recanalize a thrombotic occlusion of the carotid artery. The use of a Fogarty balloon to pass the thrombus and then slow removal of the balloon from the arteriotomy can be employed as a salvage maneuver.

Evidence and Outcomes

With the current understanding of the natural history of asymptomatic carotid stenosis, there is a risk of stratifying patients between medical and surgical management. Managing risks and working to medically optimize patients and revascularize those who have significant stenosis can significantly reduce the risk of stroke, as seen in ACAS and ACST. With the increasing popularity and ease of CAS, CREST has shown that CAS and CEA are nearly equivocal therapies for treating carotid artery disease. Surgical management along with best medical therapy requires an understanding of anatomical nuances and preparation for all possible eventualities. In addition, current studies such as CREST-2 will shed light on the results of long-term follow-up for CAS versus CEA in asymptomatic disease. The patient discussed in this chapter did well and was discharged on postoperative day 1. He has since had 2 years of follow-up with carotid Doppler studies and continues to do well. Ongoing studies are examining the association between carotid revascularization for asymptomatic carotid disease and the prevention of cognitive decline. Further studies are needed to understand the influence of revascularization on cognition.

Acknowledgments

We thank Paul H. Dressel for preparation of the figures and W. Fawn Dorr and Debra J. Zimmer for editorial assistance.

Further Reading

Antonopoulos CN, Kakisis JD, Sfyroeras GS, et al. The impact of carotid artery stenting on cognitive function in patients with extracranial carotid artery stenosis. *Ann Vasc Surg.* 2015;29:457–469.

Brott TG, Hobson RW 2nd, Howard G, et al. Stenting versus endarterectomy for treatment of carotid-artery stenosis. *N Engl J Med.* 2010;363:11–23.

Executive Committee for the Asymptomatic Carotid Atherosclerosis Study. Endarterectomy for asymptomatic carotid artery stenosis. *JAMA.* 1995;273:1421–1428.

Halliday A, Mansfield A, Marro J, et al. Prevention of disabling and fatal strokes by successful carotid endarterectomy in patients without recent neurological symptoms: Randomised controlled trial. *Lancet.* 2004;363:1491–1502.

Mantese VA, Timaran CH, Chiu D, et al. The Carotid Revascularization Endarterectomy Versus Stenting Trial (CREST): Stenting versus carotid endarterectomy for carotid disease. *Stroke.* 2010;41:S31–S34.

Sacco RL, Adams R, Albers G, et al. Guidelines for prevention of stroke in patients with ischemic stroke or transient ischemic attack: A statement for healthcare professionals from the American Heart Association/American Stroke Association Council on Stroke: Co-sponsored by the Council on Cardiovascular Radiology and Intervention: The American Academy of Neurology affirms the value of this guideline. *Circulation.* 2006;113:e409–e449.

Acute Middle Cerebral Artery Occlusion

Phillip A. Bonney, Parampreet Singh, Benjamin Yim, and William J. Mack

17

Case Presentation

A right-handed female in her 80s with atrial fibrillation presented with wake-up symptoms of left arm and face weakness. Neurological exam demonstrated a left lower facial droop, left arm pronator drift, and weakness (National Institutes of Health Stroke Scale of 9). She was last seen normal the previous night, 9 hours prior to presentation. A computed tomography (CT) scan was obtained 5 hours after waking up (Figure 17.1).

> ### Questions
>
> 1. What is the likely diagnosis?
> 2. What additional imaging studies are warranted?

Assessment and Planning

The clinical presentation is typical of an acute ischemic stroke, likely due to large vessel occlusion. The symptoms are sudden in onset in a patient with multiple stroke risk factors. In particular, the findings are concerning for a right middle cerebral artery (MCA) territory stroke. CT scan excludes intracerebral hemorrhage and most other mass lesions and makes the diagnosis of ischemic stroke more likely. Subtle cortical ischemic changes are also present, increasing suspicion of a large vessel occlusion.

Acute ischemic stroke is common in elderly patients, particularly those with cardiac risk factors or atherosclerotic disease. It is a leading cause of morbidity and mortality in older patients in developed countries. Increasing attention is being paid to early triage of patients with large vessel occlusions because many of these patients benefit from reperfusion via both intravenous thrombolytics and mechanical thrombectomy.

Additional vascular imaging, such as CT angiography (CTA) and magnetic resonance angiography, is urgently indicated to assess for an occlusion amenable to thrombectomy. CT perfusion imaging is also valuable in identifying patients who will benefit from thrombectomy, especially in patients presenting more than 6 hours after symptom onset. CTA is shown in Figure 17.2, and CT perfusion imaging is shown in Figure 17.3.

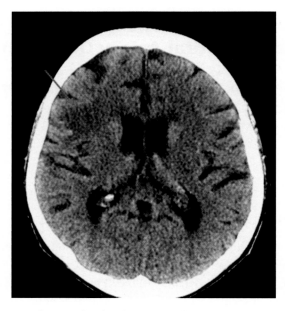

Figure 17.1 CT scan 9 hours after last known well time and 5 hours after wake-up time demonstrates hypodensity in the right posterior frontal lobe (arrow) for an ASPECTS of 9.

Oral Boards Review—Diagnostic Pearls

1. Noncontrast CT scan is important not only for excluding hemorrhage but also for establishing the extent of early ischemic change. The Alberta Stroke Program Early CT Score (ASPECTS) is a commonly used tool to evaluate the degree of ischemic changes on initial CT. ASPECTS divides the MCA territory into 10 regions, and 1 point is subtracted for each region with hypodensity. Patients with extensive early infarction (ASPECTS ≤5) are less likely to improve significantly after thrombectomy and may have a higher rate of reperfusion hemorrhage.

2. The optimal lesion for thrombectomy is a distal internal carotid artery (ICA) or M1 segment occlusion, although more distal MCA occlusions and posterior circulation occlusions can often be treated as well.

3. Perfusion imaging is an important adjunct to guide decision-making. This modality is used to evaluate for both the ischemic core and the hypoperfused region ("penumbra"), which is at risk for future infarction. Perfusion imaging is based on the rate at which contrast enters and leaves the vasculature. Automated software algorithms are used to determine volumes of ischemic core and hypoperfused regions. The difference in these volumes (the "mismatch") is a surrogate for ischemic penumbra. Patients with significant mismatch are most likely to benefit from thrombectomy procedures, especially when presenting between 6 and 24 hours after symptom onset.

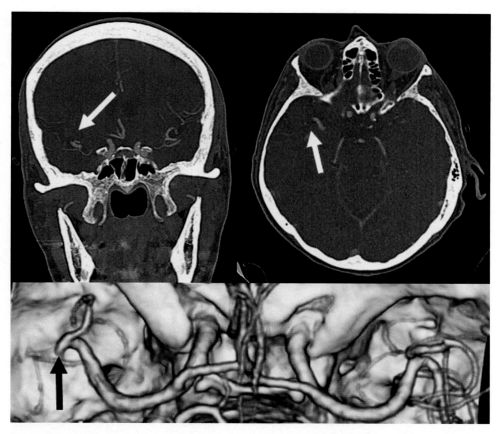

Figure 17.2 CTA demonstrates a right M1 occlusion distal to the anterior temporal artery (arrows). (Top) Coronal (left) and axial (right) reconstructions. (Bottom) Three-dimensional reconstruction.

Questions

1. What lesion is evident on CTA?
2. What information is added by the CT perfusion study?

Decision-Making

The constellation of clinical and imaging findings must be assessed to formulate an individualized treatment plan. In general, patients with an occlusive thrombus of the M1 segment will benefit from thrombectomy if there is salvageable brain tissue. In patients with large ischemic cores, demonstrated by ASPECTS on initial CT scan or by perfusion imaging, the benefit may be less. If there is no mismatch and hence no penumbra, the stroke is effectively completed, and thrombectomy is unlikely to be beneficial.

The patients most likely to benefit from thrombectomy have a large at-risk territory with little or no ischemic core. As the core volume increases, the chance of achieving functional independence decreases with or without endovascular treatment, but patients receiving thrombectomy are still more likely to have a good clinical outcome. Similarly,

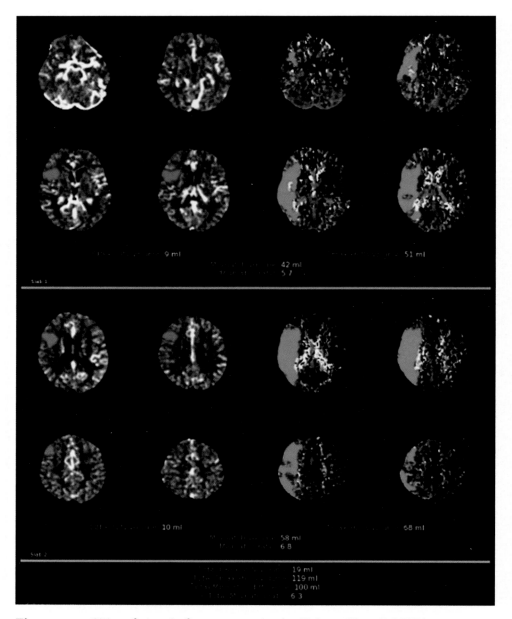

Figure 17.3 CT perfusion (software processing by iSchemaView RAPID) demonstrates a large mismatch between the ischemic core (purple) and the area of hypoperfusion (green), resulting in a large penumbra.

older patients, especially those older than age 80 years, have lower rates of good outcome after large vessel stroke, although thrombectomy has still been shown to be beneficial in this age group.

During assessment, the CTA should first be evaluated for large vessel occlusive thrombus. Figure 17.2 shows a right M1 segment occlusion. It is beneficial to evaluate the cervical carotid artery for significant stenosis as well. Although this does not preclude thrombectomy, it may require angioplasty with or without stenting to advance working catheters through a significant stenosis. Additional information that can be gleaned from the CTA includes the presence or absence of anterior communicating and posterior communicating arteries, vessel tortuosity, and intracranial stenosis.

CT perfusion can be used to assess for mismatch between completed infarction and at-risk penumbra. In this case, there is a fairly small ischemic core in the right inferior frontal lobe. At-risk territory encompasses the majority of the right MCA territory. The difference in these volumes is significant, leaving a large volume that may be potentially salvaged. Treatment may be offered on the basis of these findings in patients presenting 6–24 hours after presentation.

Questions

1. What are contraindications to thrombectomy?
2. What methods may be used to achieve thrombectomy?

Surgical Procedure

There are no absolute contraindications to mechanical thrombectomy. Importantly, alteplase and other coagulopathies do not preclude intervention. Although impaired renal function should be taken into account, the benefit of thrombectomy is so significant that intervention should proceed even in patients with poor kidney function.

There are many ways to approach mechanical thrombectomy; these are classified under the main categories of clot retrieval devices, aspiration systems, combination retrieval–aspiration systems, and balloon-assisted systems. Most operators perform the procedure through the femoral artery, with the patient under conscious sedation. A diagnostic angiogram is performed initially to confirm the lesion or to establish the presence of a lesion if none is evident with noninvasive angiography. The initial diagnostic angiogram can also be useful in better identifying arch anatomy to aid in selection of intermediate catheters. Intravenous heparinization is considered in patients who have not received preoperative intravenous alteplase.

The stent retriever technique was used in the initial pivotal trials demonstrating the efficacy of thrombectomy within 6–8 hours of symptom onset. The setup for use of stent retrievers often involves a triaxial catheter system. A long sheath or balloon guide catheter (typically 8 Fr) is first advanced into the common carotid artery or ICA of interest. Next, many operators advance an intermediate catheter into the ICA via the long sheath over a microcatheter and microwire. The intermediate catheter is advanced as far distally as possible (usually to the ICA terminus or proximal M1) for maximal support to the microcatheter system, which is then advanced over the microwire through and distal to the site of occlusion. The microwire is removed, and an angiogram may be performed via the microcatheter to confirm correction positioning distal to the thrombus. A stent retriever is placed through the microcatheter and deployed to span both the distal and proximal ends of the occlusive thrombus. The device is left to engage with the thrombus for approximately 5 minutes and then removed. During removal, aspiration through the intermediate catheter or guide catheter (with or without proximal guide catheter balloon occlusion) may be used to prevent distal embolization. If the occlusion is persistent, the process is repeated.

The grading system for evaluating success of thrombectomy, Thrombolysis in Cerebral Infarction (TICI), is based on the percentage of restored distal angiographic territory. TICI 2B or TICI 3 recanalization is considered adequate, meaning that >50% (TICI 2B) or all (TICI 3) of the distal territory is opened. In this case, a stent retriever was used to achieve TICI 3 recanalization (Figure 17.4).

Oral Boards Review—Management Pearls

1. Time is critically important in stroke management, and systems of care quality measures are aimed at minimizing time to intervention. However, many patients with delayed presentation will still benefit from thrombectomy. Although the cutoff time was previously 6–8 hours after last known well, this

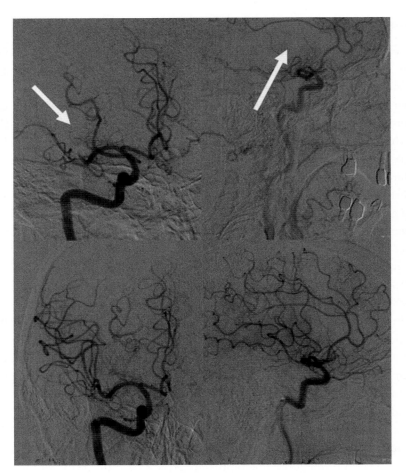

Figure 17.4 (Top) Pre-thrombectomy catheter angiography demonstrates right MCA cutoff distal to the anterior temporal artery (left, anterior–posterior [AP] view; right, lateral view). Arrows show the region of absent MCA branches. (Bottom) After stent retriever thrombectomy, TICI 3 recanalization was achieved with a stent retriever (left, AP view; right, lateral view). The patient was discharged back to her assisted living center with slight weakness of left face and arm (modified Rankin Score of 2).

has been extended to 16–24 hours based on data from recent randomized trials.

2. Thrombectomy can be performed using several methods, most commonly with a stent retriever device or direct aspiration. Challenging cases may require multiple techniques to achieve thrombectomy.

3. There is considerable debate regarding whether patients undergoing thrombectomy should receive conscious sedation or general anesthesia. Early publications suggested conscious sedation improved outcome, presumably due to shorter reperfusion times and avoidance of hypotension, but recent trials have suggested no difference between the two approaches or even a potential benefit to general anesthesia.

Pivot Points

1. Rarely, significant vascular disease in the femoral artery or descending aorta will preclude access from the groin. With tortuous arch anatomy, the common carotid artery may be inaccessible even with shaped intermediate catheters. In these cases, radial, brachial, or direct carotid access may be necessary.

2. Significant cervical carotid stenosis may require angioplasty with or without stenting prior to attaining access of the ipsilateral intracranial carotid. In some cases, access across the circle of Willis (e.g., through the anterior or posterior communicating artery) is necessary.

3. If initial thrombectomy attempts fail, it may be reasonable to attempt other techniques other methods. For example, if a stent retriever has been unsuccessful in three attempts, direct aspiration, a different stent retriever, or a combination technique could be tried. The risk of complication increases with increasing thrombectomy attempts. In cases of refractory occlusion, there may be diminishing returns in which the risks of continued intervention outweigh the benefits.

Aftercare

A CT scan may be obtained after thrombectomy to assess for hemorrhagic conversion, progression of ischemic infarct, or other changes. This may be used to serve as a baseline for subsequent studies. Importantly, standard CT may not distinguish between intracranial hemorrhage and parenchymal or subarachnoid contrast as a result of the thrombectomy procedure; in such cases, dual-energy CT scanners can eliminate contrast staining to better detect actual hemorrhage, or follow-up CT scans can be obtained.

Two important considerations after thrombectomy relate to antiplatelets/anticoagulation and blood pressure goals. The timing of starting antiplatelet therapy and/or therapeutic anticoagulation depends in part on the extent of post-procedure infarct and the presence of hemorrhagic conversion. It is not uncommon to wait up to 7 days to start therapeutic anticoagulation if there is evidence of hemorrhage or if the infarct size is large. Many providers are comfortable starting aspirin and deep vein thrombosis chemoprophylaxis immediately after the procedure if the post-procedure scan is stable. Antiplatelet agents should be avoided within 24 hours if the patient received intravenous alteplase.

The primary consideration of systolic blood pressure is to prevent hypotension and promote cerebral perfusion while avoiding significant hypertension, which may be a risk factor for hemorrhage in acute infarction. A common systolic blood pressure goal is 140–220 mmHg, or 140–180 mmHg if the patient received alteplase, although this may vary considerably depending on the patient's baseline blood pressure, the post-procedure CT findings, and provider preference.

Complications and Management

The most feared procedure-related complication is intracranial arterial perforation, which may occur during navigation of the microwire beyond an occlusive lesion or upon deployment of the stent retriever. Arterial perforation is associated with significant morbidity, particularly in patients who received alteplase and/or heparin. Management strategies include inflating a balloon catheter proximal to the perforation and waiting several minutes with the hope that clotting will take place. Vessel sacrifice may be necessary in uncontrollable cases.

A more common complication is thromboembolic events, which may occur from arterial dissection or clot fragmentation and distal embolization. To reduce the likelihood of this complication, the stent retriever is typically withdrawn while manual or pump aspiration is applied to either the intermediate or the guide catheter.

Additional complications include access site complications, such as femoral pseudoaneurysm, retroperitoneal hematoma, or distal ischemia, which in severe cases may be limb threatening. In such cases, consultation with vascular surgery may be needed.

Oral Boards Review—Complications Pearls

1. The most important complications for thrombectomy procedures include arterial injury (perforation and dissection) and thromboembolic events. The greater the number of thrombectomy passes, the greater the risk of intracerebral complication. Use of aspiration and/or balloon catheters may decrease the risk of distal thromboembolic events.
2. Postoperative imaging is important to assess for hemorrhagic conversion. Management of blood pressure and antiplatelets/anticoagulation should be guided by extent of infarction and the presence of intracranial hemorrhage.
3. Significant hypotension after the thrombectomy procedure should prompt evaluation for retroperitoneal hematoma, including CT of the abdomen and pelvis, with vascular surgery consultation if necessary.

Evidence and Outcomes

The evidence for the benefit of thrombectomy in large vessel occlusions is resounding, with seven well-conducted, randomized controlled trials since 2015. The effect of the treatment is significant, and the number needed to treat to achieve functional independence is fewer than three patients, based on the selection paradigms used in these studies. These trials establish a clear functional benefit within 6 hours of symptom onset and up to 24 hours if mismatch is present on CT perfusion imaging. Further work is needed to investigate the benefit of additional indications, including strokes with large ischemic cores, more distal MCA occlusions, and lower clinical stroke severity. However, given the safety of the procedure and the effectiveness of thrombectomy in carefully selected patients, most providers do not withhold treatment to patients judged to potentially benefit.

Further Reading

Albers GW, Marks MP, Kemp S, et al. Thrombectomy for stroke at 6 to 16 hours with selection by perfusion imaging. *N Engl J Med*. 2018;378(8):708–718. doi:10.1056/NEJMoa1713973

Campbell BCV, Mitchell PJ, Kleinig TJ, et al. Endovascular therapy for ischemic stroke with perfusion-imaging selection. *N Engl J Med*. 2015;372(11):1009–1018. doi:10.1056/NEJMoa1414792

Jovin TG, Chamorro A, Cobo E, et al. Thrombectomy within 8 hours after symptom onset in ischemic stroke. *N Engl J Med*. 2015;372(24):2296–2306. doi:10.1056/NEJMoa1503780

McTaggart RA, Ansari SA, Goyal M, et al. Initial hospital management of patients with emergent large vessel occlusion (ELVO): Report of the Standards and Guidelines Committee of the Society of NeuroInterventional Surgery. *J Neurointerv Surg*. 2017;9(3):316–323. doi:10.1136/neurintsurg-2015-011984

Nogueira RG, Jadhav AP, Haussen DC, et al. Thrombectomy 6 to 24 hours after stroke with a mismatch between deficit and infarct. *N Engl J Med*. 2018;378(1):11–21. doi:10.1056/NEJMoa1706442

Symptomatic Intracranial Arterial Stenosis

*Rajeev D. Sen, Basavaraj Ghodke, Michael R. Levitt,
and Laligam N. Sekhar*

18

Case Presentation

A 55-year-old right-handed male presents with transient episodes of left-sided weakness during the past 6 months. The episodes involve weakness in the left upper and lower extremity and sustain for 30 seconds before self-resolving. He tends to have a cluster of episodes within a period of days followed by episode-free periods. More recently, he describes instances of left leg spasm and confusion and altered mental status that last several seconds. He denies vision changes, speech or balance disturbance, dizziness, or headaches. He has a history of medically controlled type 2 diabetes, hyperlipidemia, and hypertension. He has never smoked and occasionally drinks alcohol. He has no family history of stroke. Detailed neurological examination is unremarkable with intact cranial nerves; normal funduscopic exam; full strength in all extremities; and a normal, steady gait.

Questions

1. What is the differential diagnosis?
2. What is the most appropriate imaging modality?
3. What is the appropriate timing of imaging workup?

Assessment and Planning

The neurosurgeon suspects that the patient has been having transient ischemic attacks (TIAs). The differential diagnosis for a patient presenting with abrupt-onset, episodic, focal neurologic deficits includes seizure; tumor; psychogenic behavior; and stroke including ischemic, hemorrhagic, or venous infarcts. Stroke is by far the most common, accounting for approximately 95% of such presentations. Of these cases, approximately 85% are due to ischemic infarction.

When there is concern for TIAs, further workup is urgently indicated. This is because 10–15% of patients with TIA have a completed stroke within 3 months of the event, which can result in permanent neurologic deficit such as hemiparesis or aphasia. Evaluation for stroke involves a combination of clinical information as well as radiographic studies. Key components to the clinical assessment are identifying the time of the patient's last known normal neurological exam, the duration of symptoms, and an accurate neurological exam. Upon presentation with stroke symptoms, a noncontrast

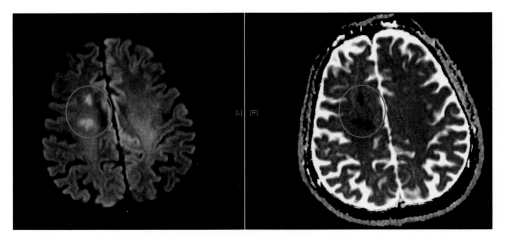

Figure 18.1 Brain MRI showing diffusion restriction (left) correlating with diminished signal on apparent diffusion coefficient (right) consistent with ischemic infarct.

head computed tomography (CT) scan should be done immediately to rule out hemorrhage or other mass lesions that may be causing the symptoms. Conventional magnetic resonance imaging (MRI) can also be used to diagnose areas of diffusion restriction, indicative of infarction, even if symptoms resolve spontaneously (Figure 18.1). Vascular imaging including either CT angiography (CTA) or MR angiography (MRA) of the head and neck vessels should be performed to evaluate for extracranial or intracranial vascular compromise.

In cases of intracranial arterial stenosis (IAS), such as this case, the main radiological finding on CTA or MRA is substantial narrowing or a focal gap of signal intensity loss along an arterial segment (Figure 18.2). Cerebral angiography may be performed to confirm the diagnosis. Angiography provides the high-resolution images of intracranial vessels and, therefore, has the highest sensitivity and specificity for stenosis. Angiography can also diagnose specific types of IAS, such as those associated with moyamoya vasculopathy, for which treatment differs from atherosclerotic IAS. Although

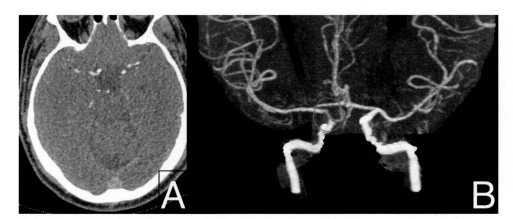

Figure 18.2 CTA demonstrates severe stenosis of the supraclinoid right internal carotid artery in the axial plane (A) and on three-dimensional reconstructions (B).

angiography is considered an invasive test, in experienced hands, the risk of stroke-related complications is <1%. Another major advantage of angiography is that it affords the opportunity to perform endovascular intervention when indicated.

Questions

1. How do these clinical and radiographic findings influence management?
2. What is the most appropriate timing for intervention in this patient?

Oral Boards Review—Diagnostic Pearls

1. Transient neurologic deficit can have a variety of etiologies.
   a. TIA: Abrupt onset, temporary, focal neurologic deficit caused by ischemia. The deficit tends to be at its peak at the time of onset. Symptoms may take up to 60 minutes to resolve.
   b. Hemiplegic migraine: Unlike TIA, hemiplegic migraine tends to be progressive over a period of minutes to hours. It is commonly accompanied by headaches and associated with nonfocal, sometimes vague auras.
   c. Seizure: Similar onset and focal nature of TIAs but commonly associated with a prodrome and latency in recovery such as Todd's paralysis.
2. Transcranial Doppler ultrasonography can be used to evaluate for intracranial thromboembolic events. Although its efficacy is largely operator dependent, it can be a rapid, noninvasive test for both intracranial arterial velocity and microemboli that may portend repeated events.

Decision-Making

Primary treatment of symptomatic IAS begins with aggressive medical management, including antiplatelet medications, and the mitigation of vascular risk factors, including hypertension, hyperlipidemia, diabetes mellitus, and smoking cessation. Upon his initial presentation, the current patient was started on dual antiplatelet therapy with aspirin and clopidogrel, a statin to manage his hyperlipidemia, and metformin for his diabetes. However, after more than 6 months of medical management, including optimization of blood pressure, hemoglobin A1C, and cholesterol, the patient continued to be symptomatic and was referred for surgical management.

The Stenting Versus Aggressive Medical Management for Preventing Recurrent Stroke in Intracranial Stenosis (SAMMPRIS) trial compared endovascular stenting with aggressive medical management of risk factors with antiplatelet therapy and found that there was a significantly lower rate of stroke and death in the medical arm for patients with a high degree of IAS (>70%). This remained true for both short- and long-term follow-up and was due to the unexpectedly high complication rates associated with stenting.

However, there remains a role for endovascular management in cases of recurrent ischemia due to hemodynamic impairment that does not respond to medical management because the collateral blood supply is insufficient. Stenting also plays a role in cases of recurrent thromboembolic events due to unstable plaque that has failed medical management, as in the current patient.

This discussion would be incomplete without addressing the role of extracranial–intracranial (EC–IC) artery bypass surgery for IAS. Popularized by Yasargil in 1967, the EC–IC bypass functions to augment intracranial blood flow. In 1985, a large, randomized study involving 1,377 patients with symptomatic ICA or MCA stenosis compared EC–IC bypass surgery with medical therapy and found that despite 96% bypass graft patency, the surgical group experienced earlier and more frequent strokes. There have been several criticisms of this study, the most important of which is that the study failed to distinguish between thromboembolic strokes and hemodynamic strokes. A study in 2011 randomized patients with symptomatic atherosclerotic internal carotid artery occlusive disease to EC–IC bypass surgery with medical therapy compared to medical therapy alone. This trial was terminated early due to futility because the 2-year stroke rate was equal but the 30-day stroke rate was significantly higher in the surgical group (14.4% vs. 2%, respectively). Other than patients with moyamoya vasculopathy, EC–IC bypass surgery is reserved for rare IAS patients with poor hemodynamic reserve who cannot tolerate endovascular treatment, and it should not be offered as a primary treatment for IAS.

Questions

1. What are the components of "best medical management" of symptomatic IAS?
2. In which cases of IAS is endovascular stenting indicated?

Surgical Procedure

Intracranial angioplasty and stenting are performed under general anesthesia or conscious sedation with access through the common femoral artery. Patients are often already taking dual antiplatelet agents as part of medical management, but in rare cases of emergency stenting, patients are loaded with aspirin and clopidogrel. Heparinization is used to achieve a target activated coagulation time of 250–350 seconds. A guide catheter is navigated into the parent vessel, and diagnostic angiography is performed usually including three-dimensional angiography spins with reconstructions to generate working-angle views (Figure 18.3A). An exchange-length microwire is then navigated across the site of stenosis. To initially dilate the region of stenosis, a noncompliant angioplasty balloon is introduced and is inflated to 80–90% of the normal parent artery diameter. The length of the balloon should match the length of the stenosis. In the current case, a 2 × 9-mm Gateway balloon was inflated up to 8 atm for 1 minute and 30 seconds across the stenosis within the right supraclinoid internal carotid artery (Figure 18.3B). Then, a Wingspan stent is advanced over the exchange wire to the region of stenosis, and the stent is deployed (Figure 18.3C). Post-stent deployment runs are used to rule out contrast extravasation, new vessel wall abnormalities such as aneurysms or dissections, or acute stent thrombosis.

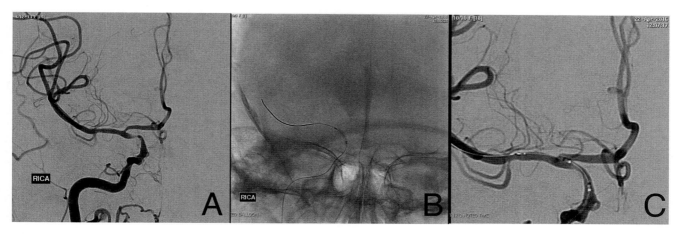

Figure 18.3 (A) Cerebral angiography of the right internal carotid artery shows supraclinoid stenosis. (B) Balloon angioplasty is performed. (C) Stenosis is alleviated after placement.

Oral Boards Review—Management Pearls

1. Medical management includes treatment of modifiable risk factors.
   a. Hypertension: The most powerful and treatable risk factor. Both systolic and diastolic blood pressures are independently associated with risk of stroke.
   b. Tobacco smoking cessation.
   c. Hyperlipidemia: Statins are used to reach a goal low-density lipoprotein level of <70 mg/dL.
   d. Alcohol: Heavy consumption is associated with increased risk of stroke. However, moderate use may be protective against stroke.
2. Generally, a stent does not apply enough radial force to expand an atherosclerotic intracranial vessel on its own. Therefore, prior to stenting, balloon angioplasty is performed using an undersized balloon at low inflation pressures.
3. It is important to maintain exchange-length microwire access beyond the stenotic lesion even after the stent is deployed. In case of a dissection or thrombosis complication, this is often the only way to permit microcatheter or balloon access distal to the lesion for complication management.

Pivot Points

1. In patients who exhibit hemodynamic impairment and inadequate collateral circulation, more timely intervention is indicated. These patients may not have enough time for medical management to take effect.
2. In cases of non-atherosclerotic intracranial stenosis such as in moyamoya vasculopathy, EC–IC bypass surgery may be indicated.

Aftercare

After completion of the procedure and withdrawal of catheters, hemostasis is achieved using a sealing device for the access site in the femoral artery. A noncontrast head CT is obtained to rule out any hemorrhage. The patient is observed overnight in the intensive care unit with frequent neurological examinations. Assuming no complications, the patient is discharged the next day. Postoperative antiplatelet regimens vary, but typically patients are instructed to continue dual antiplatelet therapy for 6 months and then aspirin 325 mg daily indefinitely.

Complications and Management

Perioperative complication rates for intracranial artery stenting range from 5% to 10%. Stent-related complications can be categorized as ischemic and hemorrhagic. The former is due to in-stent restenosis (ISR), perforating vessel occlusion, or thromboembolism; the latter is due to guide wire perforation or reperfusion injury.

Ischemic complications are most commonly due to perforating vessel occlusion, either from arterial dissection or from atherosclerotic plaque migration. Clinical implications can range from asymptomatic to permanent neurologic deficit depending on the territory of the occluded vessel. This complication can be minimized by submaximal (rather than maximal) angioplasty and by selecting the shortest possible stent length to address the stenotic segment. Management varies, but it often involves systemic anticoagulation with heparin in the acute postoperative period. Risk factors for ischemic events are nonsmokers, prior non-perforator strokes, and old infarcts on baseline imaging.

Rates of long-term ISR range from 7.5% to 29.7%, and patients with ISR are largely asymptomatic. When symptomatic, they generally present with recurrent TIAs or stroke and require re-treatment. Re-treatment is not always straightforward due to the open-cell design of the stent and its relatively low metal surface area coverage, which allows for inadvertent passage of the microwire between the stent and the vessel wall. There are no clear guidelines for the management of asymptomatic ISR and no data supporting additional or more frequent imaging outside of standard follow-up.

Post-procedure hemorrhage can be potentially devastating due to the dual antiplatelet therapy, which likely exacerbates the hemorrhage. However, dual antiplatelet therapy is necessary to maintain patency of the stent and avoid stent thrombosis. Hemorrhage can be caused by guide wire perforation or reperfusion injury. Whereas some cases of hemorrhage can be managed expectantly with blood pressure control, some are severe and may require surgical decompression. Risk factors for post-procedure hemorrhage are higher grade stenosis, rapid clopidogrel loading, and intraprocedural activated clotting time >300 seconds.

Given the relatively high rate of complications, stenting for intracranial artery stenosis should be restricted to medically refractory, high-grade lesions with a high risk of recurrent stroke and should be performed by experienced operators.

Oral Boards Review—Complications Pearls

1. Angioplasty should be carefully tailored to the diameter of the target vessel, and slightly submaximal balloon inflation is recommended to reduce the incidence of perforator occlusion and dissection.
2. Maintenance of a distal wire beyond the stenosis over which the balloon or stent can be navigated ensures that if angioplasty-related occlusion occurs, distal wire access (and thus subsequent rescue stenting) can be performed.

Questions

1. What is the most common cause of ischemic strokes after intracranial stenting?
2. How can occlusion of perforating vessels be avoided?
3. What are the two main mechanisms of postoperative hemorrhage?

Evidence and Outcomes

The SAMMPRIS trial demonstrated that aggressive medical management including antiplatelet medication and risk factor modification was superior to stenting with regard to the primary outcomes of stroke and death. This seminal study highlighted the importance of medical management in intracranial artery stenosis. More recently, the Vitesse Intracranial Stent Study for Ischemic Stroke Therapy trial confirmed the superiority of medical management over stenting by finding that 36% of the stented patients reached the primary outcome of stroke or death within the first year compared to only 15.1% of the medically managed patients.

Despite these results, there remains a role for endovascular intervention. Such intervention should be considered on a case-by-case basis, and patient selection as well as operator experience are essential for good outcomes. Stenting should be considered only in patients for whom medical management has failed and symptoms continue or in rare cases in which rapidly progressive symptoms occur due to an unstable atherosclerotic plaque.

Further Reading

Chimowitz MI, Lynn MJ, Derdeyn CP, et al.; SAMMPRIS Trial Investigators. Stenting versus aggressive medical therapy for intracranial arterial stenosis. *N Engl J Med.* 2011;365(11):993–1003.

Derdeyn CP, Chimowitz MI, Lynn MJ, et al.; SAMMPRIS Trial Investigators. Aggressive medical treatment with or without stenting in high-risk patients with intracranial artery stenosis (SAMMPRIS): The final results of a randomised trial. *Lancet.* 2014;383(9914):333–341.

EC/IC Bypass Study Group. Failure of extracranial–intracranial arterial bypass to reduce the risk of ischemic stroke: Results of an international randomized trial. *N Engl J Med.* 1985;313(19):1191–1200.

Fiorella D, Derdeyn CP, Lynn MJ, et al.; SAMMPRIS Trial Investigators. Detailed analysis of periprocedural strokes in patients undergoing intracranial stenting in Stenting and Aggressive Medical Management for Preventing Recurrent Stroke in Intracranial Stenosis (SAMMPRIS). *Stroke*. 2012;43(10):2682–2688.

Powers WJ, Clarke WR, Grubb RL Jr, et al.; COSS Investigators. Extracranial–intracranial bypass surgery for stroke prevention in hemodynamic cerebral ischemia: The Carotid Occlusion Surgery Study randomized trial. *JAMA*. 2011;306(18):1983–1992.

Wong KS, Chen C, Fu J, et al.; CLAIR Study Investigators. Clopidogrel plus aspirin versus aspirin alone for reducing embolisation in patients with acute symptomatic cerebral or carotid artery stenosis (CLAIR study): A randomised, open-label, blinded-endpoint trial. *Lancet Neurol*. 2010;9(5):489–497.

Zaidat OO, Fitzsimmons BF, Woodward BK, et al.; VISSIT Trial Investigators. Effect of a balloon-expandable intracranial stent vs medical therapy on risk of stroke in patients with symptomatic intracranial stenosis: The VISSIT randomized clinical trial. *JAMA*. 2015;313(12):1240–1248.

Moyamoya Vasculopathy Presenting with Transient Neurological Deficit

Denise Brunozzi, Sepideh Amin-Hanjani, and Fady T. Charbel

19

Case Presentation

A 23-year-old female presented to the emergency department with intermittent recurrent episodes of right arm numbness lasting a few minutes, occurring up to three times per day during the past month. She denies any other neurological symptoms, headache, or seizure activity, and she reports no current symptoms at the time of evaluation. The patient has a past medical history of surgical repair for ventricular septal defect in infancy. There is a family history of fatal stroke in her maternal grandfather. The patient denies any history of tobacco, alcohol, or illicit drug abuse. Detailed neurological examination is unremarkable.

Questions

1. What is the likely diagnosis?
2. What is the most appropriate imaging modality?
3. What are the most appropriate anatomical areas to image and why?
4. What is the appropriate timing of the diagnostic workup?

Assessment and Planning

Transient repetitive symptoms raise concern for transient ischemic attacks (TIAs) or focal seizures. Any new focal neurological deficit warrants computed tomography (CT) or magnetic resonance imaging (MRI) of the brain to rule out major differential diagnostic considerations, such as brain tumor, infection, or hemorrhage, and should be performed as an urgent assessment. For evaluation of suspected TIA, MRI is more sensitive than CT to evaluate for evidence of acute stroke on diffusion-weighted sequences. In addition, symptoms consistent with TIA warrant cerebrovascular imaging; MRI combined with head and neck MR angiography (MRA) are appropriate as a workup for suspected ischemic symptoms. A pattern of acute/subacute or chronic infarcts, especially in watershed areas, points toward a hemodynamic mechanism of stroke from stenosis or occlusion of a major intracranial vessel of the anterior circulation.

In pediatric patients, moyamoya vasculopathy or moyamoya disease (MMD) is a cause of cerebrovascular stenosis involving the anterior circulation vessels, particularly the distal internal carotid artery (ICA) and its main branches. The differential diagnosis also includes vasculitis, carotid dissection, reversible cerebral vasoconstriction syndrome, or vessel occlusions caused by cardiogenic emboli. Although MMD is a relatively rare disease, more frequently occurring in Asian countries, ischemic symptoms in young adults should prompt its consideration.

Although MRA can show characteristic findings of vessel stenosis, and MRI may demonstrate collateral vessels as multiple small flow voids in deep and basal ganglia structures, digital subtraction angiography (DSA) is the gold standard for MMD diagnosis and characterization. The characteristic angiographic pattern shows stenosis or occlusion in bilateral ICAs or their main branches associated with enlarged perforators distributed to the white deep matter of the basal brain in a classically hazy angiographic appearance. The DSA appearance of the affected vessels, graded according to the Suzuki grading system, does not always correlate with the clinical severity and the evolution of the disease. Although MMD is classically a bilateral disease, patients can also present with unilateral findings.

Oral Boards Review—Diagnostic Pearls

1. Differential diagnosis for subacute–chronic unilateral facial, arm, and leg numbness includes a wide spectrum of disease associated with different underlying etiologies:
   a. Vascular: cardiogenic emboli, carotid dissection, moyamoya
   b. Mass effect: extra-axial or intra-axial tumors
   c. Epileptogenic: seizure
   d. Infectious: bacterial or viral encephalitis, cerebral abscess
   e. Autoimmune: cerebral vasculitis, neurosarcoidosis, multiple sclerosis
2. Presentation of MMD disease is mainly ischemic in children, related to ICA steno-occlusion, and additionally hemorrhagic in adults, related to collateral vessel fragility and rupture. Headache, seizure, cognitive impairment, and involuntary movements are other possible clinical manifestations.
3. Characteristic DSA features are steno-occlusion of distal ICAs or their proximal branches, associated with fine perforator collateral networks organized in a hazy pattern, and relative sparing of the posterior circulation. MMD diagnosis requires findings of bilateral cerebrovascular involvement on MRI or MRA or findings of unilateral involvement associated with the typical collateral network on DSA (previously known as "possible moyamoya").
4. Moyamoya syndrome is a typical moyamoya pattern secondary to a non-idiopathic condition such as intracranial atherosclerosis; radiotherapy; autoimmune disorders; immunosuppressive therapy; infectious disease; and genetic disorders including sickle cell disease, protein C and S deficiency, Downs syndrome, and neurofibromatosis type I.
5. Functional MRI (fMRI) and quantitative MRA (QMRA), or other perfusion imaging, under basal conditions and with provocative testing assesses cerebrovascular reserve and helps guide the decision-making process about treatment.

Although standard MRI helps localize and date hemorrhagic and ischemic lesions in the brain parenchyma and MRA is used as an alternative noninvasive method to screen

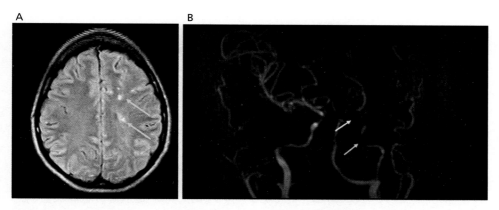

Figure 19.1 (A) Axial projections of T$_2$-weighted fluid attenuated inversion recovery sequences of MRI demonstrating frontoparietal subacute infarction (yellow arrows). (B) MRA reconstruction showing left petrous ICA stenosis (yellow arrow) and supraclinoid ICA likely occlusion (white arrow).

for cerebrovascular angiopathy, additional imaging for the assessment of hemodynamic reserve is also important. Such assessment can be performed with a variety of imaging modalities, including single-photon emission tomography, CT perfusion or MR perfusion with Diamox challenge to assess cerebrovascular reserve. This evaluation can also be done with fMRI to evaluate global and regional cerebrovascular reserve, in addition to phase-contrast QMRA to directly measure intracranial vessel blood flow at baseline and under physiologic challenges. A lack of hemodynamic reserve suggests a higher risk of ischemic events and may prompt preventative treatment.

In the current case, MRI/MRA demonstrated distal left ICA stenosis, left leptomeningeal collaterals, and subacute watershed infarcts in the left frontoparietal periventricular white matter (Figure 19.1). These findings prompted further evaluation with DSA (Figure 19.2).

Questions

1. How do these clinical and radiological findings influence surgical planning?
2. What is the most appropriate timing for intervention in this patient?
3. How should surgery be approached?

Decision-Making

Conservative management of MMD with antiplatelet medication, especially in symptomatic patients, is not generally effective in preventing recurrent cerebral infarction. The treatment of choice is surgical revascularization, aimed at improving cerebral blood flow and vascular reserve, performed either through direct or indirect cerebrovascular bypass. Treatment is typically offered to patients with clinical or radiologic evidence of TIAs or ischemic stroke, and it can be considered in asymptomatic patients with evidence of impaired hemodynamics. MMD may also present with hemorrhage, related to the friable moyamoya collaterals. Hemorrhagic MMD has been shown to benefit from revascularization with

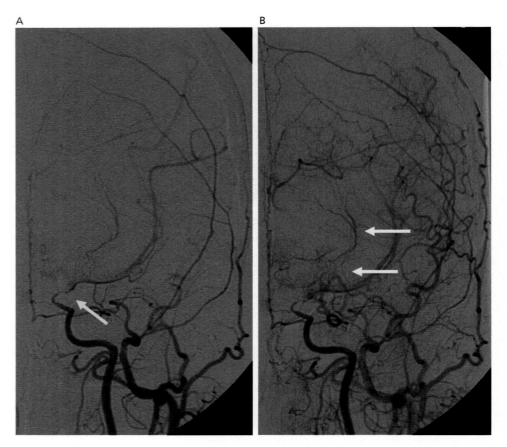

Figure 19.2 Anterior–posterior DSA projections of left ICA showing supraclinoid ICA and M1 severe stenosis (A, yellow arrow) and moyamoya enlarged and hazy collaterals (B, white arrows).

direct bypass aimed at providing an alternate route for blood flow and reducing the hemodynamic stress on the intrinsic collaterals, which are prone to hemorrhage.

Direct superficial temporal artery–middle cerebral artery (STA–MCA) bypass and indirect bypass such as encephaloduroarteriosynangiosis are often used in adults as a combined revascularization strategy to gain the advantages of immediate postoperative flow augmentation carried by the direct bypass with the long-term development of collaterals generated by the indirect bypass. Surgery is performed in an expeditious manner following presentation, but in the setting of recent infarct, revascularization is typically delayed 2–6 weeks or more to reduce the risk of post-bypass hyperperfusion hemorrhage.

The current patient presented with recurrent TIAs associated with radiologic signs of cerebral infarction (Figure 19.1). The cerebrovascular reserve assessment with fMRI (Figure 19.3) showed reduced reserve in the left ICA territory after hypercapnic challenge and absent activation of the left motor and somatosensory areas during standard task performance, indicating reduced regional reserve in anterior cerebral artery and MCA territories.

QMRA (Figure 19.4) at baseline showed diffuse diminutive anterior circulation flow on the left side, associated with reduced cerebrovascular reserve after the vasodilatory challenge with Diamox. The patient was referred for STA–MCA bypass.

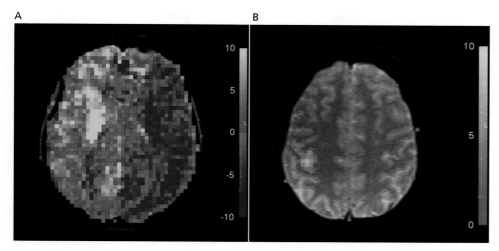

Figure 19.3 (A) fMRI global blood oxygenation level-dependent activation after hypercapnic challenge showing reduced left hemisphere reserve (blue) compared to contralateral normal reserve (red). (B) Compromised regional reserve in somatosensory and motor areas on the left side, indicating decreased anterior circulation reserve.

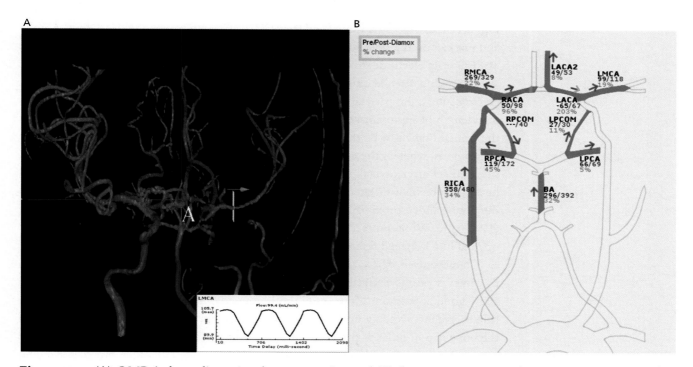

Figure 19.4 (A) QMRA three-dimensional reconstruction and (B) flow measurements prior to surgery. Intracranial arterial blood flow map at baseline (numbers in black) and after Diamox challenge (numbers in blue) and respective percentage increase/decrease (numbers in orange) are shown. Green arrows indicate the direction of flow. Left ICA flow is under QMRA detection threshold. After vasodilatation challenge, anterior and posterior circulation, already compromised at baseline, showed only mild flow increase.

> **Questions**
>
> 1. What factors influence performing a direct versus indirect revascularization surgery?
> 2. How is perioperative risk of stroke or hemorrhage reduced?

Surgical Procedure

The revascularization surgery is performed under general anesthesia. In order to reduce the risk of perioperative ischemia during anesthesia induction, systemic blood pressure should be kept at or above the patient's baseline values, and it is advisable to admit the patient the night prior to surgery to ensure intravenous hydration. Full-dose aspirin should be started preoperatively and continued after the procedure to improve graft patency, and aspirin sensitivity can be verified by platelet function assays.

During the procedure, constant monitoring of invasive blood pressure and normocapnia helps maintain normal brain perfusion. Intraoperative neuromonitoring with electroencephalography (EEG) is helpful to alert for signs of cerebral ischemia; both hemispheres should be monitored. EEG also verifies the achievement of burst suppression during the temporary vessel occlusion required for direct STA–MCA bypass.

Following induction of anesthesia, the patient is placed supine, with head turned in the lateral position to expose the affected side. In preparation for a combined direct and indirect bypass, the STA frontal and parietal branches are mapped with a Doppler probe and marked on the skin from the root of the zygoma to the vertex prior to placement of EEG scalp electrodes to avoid accidental injury.

Through a straight skin incision made with either a scalpel or needle tip bovie electrocautery, the parietal branch of the STA is exposed using blunt dissection for a total length of approximately 8–10 cm. The incision may be curved anteriorly, allowing the frontal branch to be dissected. The frontal branch is usually utilized for the direct anastomosis, whereas the continuity of the parietal branch is typically preserved for in situ indirect arteriosynangiosis and helps reduce the risk of scalp necrosis and wound healing problems associated with dual STA branch harvesting. The frontal branch is cut distally, occluded proximally with a temporary clip, and flushed with heparin solution (10 U/mL). While protecting the STA branches, the temporalis muscle and fascia are opened in a T-shaped fashion below the parietal branch in order to access the cranium.

Craniotomy is performed in standard fashion with a power drill, paying attention to center it on the parietal branch (usually approximately 6 cm above the zygoma) to allow good apposition of the vessel on the underlying brain for indirect bypass; attention is given to avoiding injury to the middle meningeal artery (MMA) while elevating the bone flap in order to preserve dural vasculature, which serves as a source of indirect bypass. Similarly, the dura opening, performed in cruciate fashion, is aimed at avoiding MMA and major dural branches.

An arachnoid knife is used under the microscope to dissect the chosen recipient M4 MCA vessel, ideally central in the surgical field and matching the size of the STA donor (Figure 19.5A). If the cortical vessels are found to be of very small caliber (<1 mm), as often encountered in infant or pediatric patients, direct bypass is less feasible and indirect bypass alone is performed. Otherwise, the distal portion of the frontal branch is then

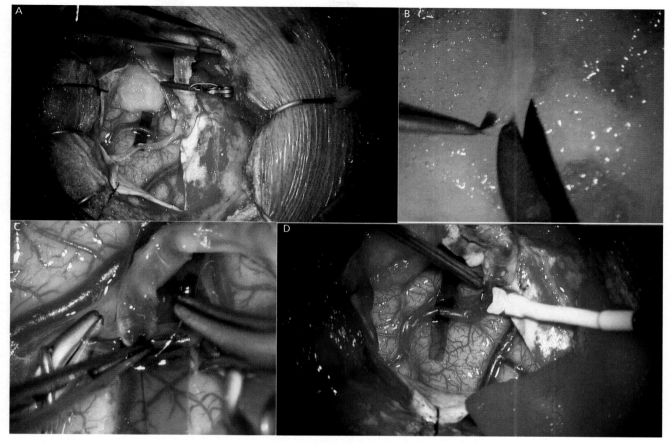

Figure 19.5 Intraoperative images of the procedure. (A) The cruciate dural opening; the microsurgical clip is positioned at the proximal segment of the harvested left STA that has already been dissected and freed from cuff tissue at its distal portion. The green rubber dam helps isolation of the recipient vessel from the underlying brain and surrounding arachnoid to facilitate the anastomosis step. (B) Fish-mouthing of the STA distal edge with microscissors. (C) Suturing of the end-to-side STA–MCA anastomosis with 10–0 nylon. Vessel edges are marked to help visualization. (D) The final result of the direct bypass and intraoperative ultrasonic bypass flow measurement with Transonic Charbel Micro-Flowprobe.

freed from its surrounding cuff of tissue using microscissors, and it is opened in a fish-mouth shape (Figure 19.5B). The recipient vessel is prepared by exposing at least 1 cm of length, cauterizing any small perforators along its length, and applying proximal and distal temporary clips. Arteriotomy on the recipient vessel, performed with combination of a fine microblade and microscissor, is customized to the size of the distal aspect of the donor vessel. The anastomosis is performed with a 10–0 nylon suture in a running or interrupted fashion, according to the surgeon's preference (Figure 19.5C). Intraoperative measurements of bypass flow are obtained with the ultrasonic transit-time flow probe (Transonic Charbel Micro-Flowprobe; Figure 19.5D), and the ratio to the cut flow (flow measurement of the free flow from the cut end of the harvested donor prior to anastomosis) serves as a useful predictor of bypass outcome.

The indirect bypass is performed by suturing the cuff of the parietal STA branch to the arachnoid of the brain surface (encephaloarteriosynangiosis). In addition, inverting the cut dural leaflets onto the brain surface under the craniotomy creates the substrate for encephalodurosynangiosis.

The use of the temporalis muscle as an indirect source of collaterals (encephalomyosynangiosis), although feasible, requires larger craniotomy and involves higher risk of postoperative hematoma and cosmetic issues.

Oral Boards Review—Management Pearls

1. It is important to avoid hypotension, hypovolemia, and hypocapnea during anesthesia induction and during the procedure; invasive blood pressure, carbon dioxide end-tidal, and EEG monitoring helps detect cerebral hypoperfusion.
2. Careful attention should be paid to preserve the integrity of STA and MMA branches during the opening of the procedure.
3. Papaverine-soaked cottonoids can be applied temporarily to relieve possible vessel vasospasm caused by dissection and manipulation.
4. Donor-to-recipient anastomosis is the most critical part of the surgical procedure. It is performed under burst suppression, verified on EEG, in order to decrease brain oxygen demand and consequent risk of infarction.
5. During the anastomosis, check for possible back wall catching. After the anastomosis, check carefully for any leakage, which might require gentle pressure or additional stitches, or for any thrombus formation, which might be managed with gentle massage to help dislodgment.
6. Avoid STA strangulation during final bone flap replacement or accidental suture catching during skin closure.

Pivot Points

1. Young patients with symptoms of TIAs or stroke should undergo immediate workup for possible cerebral vascular stenosis or occlusion.
2. Although MRI and MRA are useful noninvasive tools for screening, DSA is the gold standard for cerebral vessel status assessment and preoperative planning.
3. Symptomatic MMD patients, and potentially asymptomatic MMD patients with reduced cerebrovascular reserve, are managed with surgical revascularization, performing direct and indirect bypass to combine the advantages of both techniques.

Aftercare

Postoperative observation in the intensive care unit for the first 24–48 hours is recommended, and tight control on systemic blood pressure targeted to the patient's baseline range is important. Full-dose aspirin should be continued. Postoperative imaging includes head CT to rule out hemorrhagic complications, QMRA to assess bypass patency and flow (Figure 19.6), and CTA or DSA as a baseline reference (Figure 19.7).

Reassessment of hemodynamics with imaging and neuropsychological testing is recommended at 6 weeks, 6 and 12 months, and annually thereafter. Ongoing monitoring

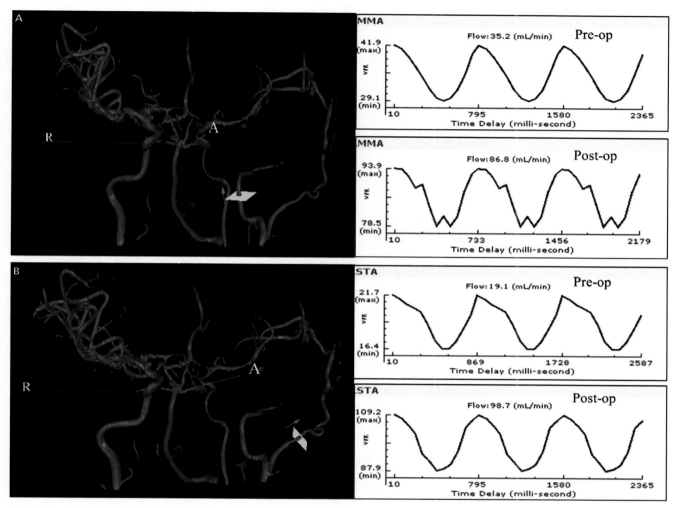

Figure 19.6 (A) Left MMA and (B) left STA QMRA three-dimensional reconstruction and blood flow comparison before and after revascularization surgery. Increase of flow in the left MMA and the left STA after surgery is evident.

for contralateral side MMD development should be performed in case of unilateral disease. Contralateral surgery, if needed, often requires at least 4–6 weeks' delay.

The current patient's procedure was uneventful, and she was discharged home after 24 hours. At 2 weeks' clinical follow-up, the patient was asymptomatic and was cleared to return to work. At 6 months' follow-up, the patient was asymptomatic and fMRI showed improved activation in left primary motor, somatosensory, and supplemental motor areas.

Complications and Management

In addition to the risk for perioperative ischemic stroke, direct bypass surgery might increase the risk of postoperative hyperperfusion or reperfusion hemorrhage. As mentioned previously, perioperative systemic blood pressure control within a tight range based on the patient's baseline values is crucial to avoid excess in either direction.

Dual harvest of both STA branches required for combined direct–indirect bypass technique entails an increased risk of wound dehiscence or infection due to greater

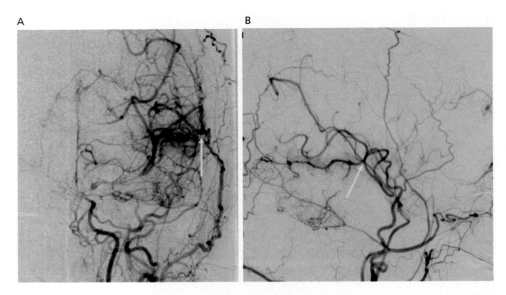

Figure 19.7 Postoperative DSA, left CCA injection: (A) anterior–posterior projection and (B) lateral projection. Yellow arrows indicate the anastomotic point between STA and MCA.

devascularization of the scalp tissue compared to single branch direct or indirect technique. Preserving the continuity of the posterior branch of the STA is usually sufficient to avoid scalp necrosis.

Oral Boards Review—Complications Pearls

1. Careful perioperative management of systemic blood pressure is important to reduce risk of hyperperfusion.
2. A close clinic follow-up visit after hospital discharge is warranted to verify incision healing, particularly after harvest of both STA branches.
3. Regular follow-up hemodynamic imaging and neurocognitive reassessment should be performed to evaluate long-term outcome and possible contralateral MMD development in patients presenting with unilateral disease.

Evidence and Outcome

Although surgical revascularization has demonstrated better long-term outcome compared to conservative therapy for symptomatic patients, the ideal surgical technique is still controversial. Indirect revascularization alone seems to be more effective in the pediatric population than in adult patients; direct or combined bypass surgery has proven to be an effective treatment to prevent stroke recurrence in the adult population with MMD. However, class I evidence for the comparative efficacy of the combined technique compared to indirect or direct procedures alone is still lacking.

Further Reading

Amin-Hanjani S, Du X, Mlinarevich N, Meglio G, Zhao M, Charbel FT. The cut flow index: An intraoperative predictor of the success of extracranial–intracranial bypass for occlusive cerebrovascular disease. *Neurosurgery*. 2005;56(1 Suppl):75–85.

Amin-Hanjani S, Singh A, Rifai H, et al. Combined direct and indirect bypass for moyamoya: Quantitative assessment of direct bypass flow over time. *Neurosurgery*. 2013;73(6):962–968.

Charbel FT, Meglio G, Amin-Hanjani S. Superficial temporal artery-to-middle cerebral artery bypass. *Neurosurgery*. 2005;56(1 Suppl):186–190.

Houkin K, Yoshimoto T, Kuroda S, Ishikawa T, Takahashi A, Abe H. Angiographic analysis of moyamoya disease—How does moyamoya disease progress? *Neurol Med Chir (Tokyo)*. 1996;36:783–788.

Jeon JP, Kim JE, Cho WS, Bang JS, Son YJ, Oh CW. Meta-analysis of the surgical outcomes of symptomatic moyamoya disease in adults. *J Neurosurg*. 2018;128(3):793–799.

Kim JS. Moyamoya disease: Epidemiology, clinical features, and diagnosis. *J Stroke*. 2016:18(1):2–11.

Miyamoto S, Yoshimoto T, Hashimoto N, et al. Effects of extracranial–intracranial bypass for patients with hemorrhagic moyamoya disease: Results of the Japan Adult Moyamoya Trial. *Stroke*. 2014;45(5):1415–1421.

Cerebral Venous Sinus Thrombosis Presenting with Altered Mental Status

Arvin R. Wali, Vincent Cheung, David R. Santiago-Dieppa, J. Scott Pannell, and Alexander A. Khalessi

20

Case Presentation

A 28-year-old female presents to a local emergency room with altered mental status and decreased responsiveness. Earlier that day, the patient developed slurred speech and confusion when talking on the phone with her family. She additionally had complained of headaches and nausea, which began several days prior. Due to her nausea, the patient had decreased intake of food and water. The patient has no notable past medical history. The patient occasionally drinks and smokes and has been taking an oral contraceptive agent for 6 months. The patient has no known family history of neurological disorders. The patient is afebrile and hemodynamically stable. On initial examination, the patient's eyes are closed and she is moaning. Her pupils are equal in size and briskly reactive to light, but ophthalmoscopic examination demonstrates mild papilledema. The patient is unable to answer questions and does not follow commands, but she withdraws symmetrically in all extremities to pain.

Questions

1. What is the differential diagnosis?
2. What are the most appropriate diagnostic steps to take next?

Assessment and Planning

An emergent medical workup is initiated. The differential diagnosis for progressively worsening altered mental status in an otherwise healthy young woman is broad and can include stroke/cerebrovascular accident, vasculitis, subarachnoid hemorrhage, brain trauma, cerebral sinus thrombosis, delirium, seizure, cardiopulmonary disorders, psychiatric disturbance, metabolic disturbance (e.g., electrolyte abnormality, hypoglycemia, toxin ingestion, illicit drug use, and alcohol withdrawal), endocrine disturbance (e.g., thyroid disorder and pituitary apoplexy), meningitis, brain abscess, systemic infections, and brain tumor. However, in the context of the patient's female gender, oral contraceptive usage, current smoking, and recent poor oral intake, cerebral venous sinus thrombosis (CVST) must be suspected.

Initial diagnostic workup for altered mental status must be sufficiently broad to evaluate for conditions requiring emergent intervention and should include computed tomography (CT) of the head, chest X-ray, electrocardiogram, cardiac enzymes, serum electrolyte panel, liver function panel, blood glucose, complete blood count, prothrombin time/international normalized ratio, partial thromboplastin time (PTT), blood cultures, urinalysis/urine culture, urine toxicology screen, and arterial blood gas. If there is a high clinical suspicion for ischemic stroke due to large vessel occlusion, then CT angiography can rapidly evaluate such a lesion. If there is a high clinical suspicion for meningitis, then a lumbar puncture can be performed and broad-spectrum intravenous (IV) antibiotics empirically administered. For patients suspected of having CVST, an elevated D-dimer yields a positive predictive value of 99.6% and a negative predictive value of 55.7% to help confirm diagnosis. However, D-dimer elevation is a nonspecific finding and therefore not a definitive test for CVST.

Oral Boards Review—Diagnostic Pearls

1. Red flags in the patient's history and physical exam should build the clinical suspicion for cerebral venous thrombosis. Since the introduction of oral contraceptives, women have come to comprise 70–80% of new cases of CVST. Smoking, dehydration, and a family history of thrombophilia are all associated with an increased risk of CVST.

2. CT of the head with or without contrast can rapidly differentiate among competing etiologies, such as ischemic or hemorrhagic stroke, subarachnoid hemorrhage, traumatic intracranial hemorrhage, hydrocephalus, or a mass lesion.

3. Characteristic signs of CVST that may be present on a CT scan include the following:
   a. Cord sign (noncontrast CT): Hyperdense thrombus within an occluded vein.
   b. Empty delta sign (contrast CT): Lack of contrast filling within an occluded cerebral vein. Although this is regarded as a "classic" sign of CVST, it is present in only 20–30% of cases of CVST.
   c. Augmented venous drainage through collateral pathways may result in contrast enhancement of the tentorium or transcortical medullary veins.
   d. Cerebral edema and loss of gray–white differentiation within brain parenchyma may develop due to venous infarction. Thrombus within the cerebral sinuses may lead to inadequate venous drainage resulting in increased intracranial pressure and the development of cytotoxic or vasogenic edema. Hemorrhagic conversion of infarcted brain parenchyma can occur.

4. Catheter-based cerebral angiography is the gold standard diagnostic study for the evaluation of CVST. If noninvasive vascular imaging, such as magnetic resonance venography or CT venography, is equivocal, then a diagnostic cerebral angiogram may be indicated to confirm the diagnosis and determine the location and extent of the thrombus.

The patient undergoes standard evaluation and workup in the emergency department as described previously. A noncontrast CT scan demonstrates a hyperdense cord sign

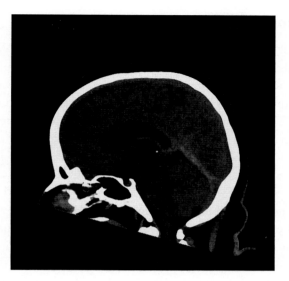

Figure 20.1 Noncontrast sagittal CT scan demonstrating a hyperdense cord sign indicative of a thrombosed straight sinus.

indicative of a thrombosed straight sinus (Figure 20.1). Bilateral thalamic hypodensity indicates infarction due to compromise of the deep venous drainage system (Figure 20.2).

Questions

1. What treatment options are available for the patient?
2. What is the appropriate timing for intervention?
3. How would the presence of intracerebral hemorrhage affect the role of systemic anticoagulation in the treatment of this patient?

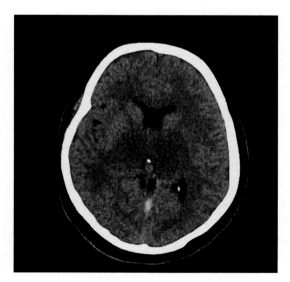

Figure 20.2 Noncontrast axial CT scan demonstrating bilateral thalamic hypodensity indicating infarction due to compromise of the deep venous drainage system.

Decision-Making

CVST in clinically stable patients can often be managed medically with generous IV hydration and implementation of systemic anticoagulation. Options for systemic anticoagulation include IV unfractionated heparin or low-molecular-weight heparin. If using IV unfractionated heparin, some authors recommend targeting a therapeutic PTT that is double the pretreatment PTT, thereby preventing expansion of the thrombus and promoting recanalization of the occluded sinus. However, specific laboratory value goals may vary depending on institution. Treatment should be initiated urgently to prevent subsequent neurologic worsening associated with expansion of the thrombus.

Patients who present with an intracerebral hemorrhage secondary to CVST have increased mortality overall. However, the presence of intracerebral hemorrhage should not be regarded as an absolute contraindication to therapeutic anticoagulation. Further clinical discretion weighing the risks and benefits of anticoagulation may be necessary if the patient has a recent history of major hemorrhage or other risk factors.

Endovascular treatment of CVST with mechanical thrombectomy and/or targeted fibrinolytic administration is typically reserved for patients who present in extremis or decompensate despite medical therapy. Endovascular options for the treatment of CVST include balloon-assisted thrombectomy, aspiration catheter thrombectomy, and targeted administration of fibrinolytic agents. In some cases, mechanical thrombectomy with aspiration or balloon assistance may be used to initially reduce clot burden, thereby decreasing the degree of systemic anticoagulation required to treat the thrombus. In general, endovascular techniques are able to remove thrombus from dural venous sinuses but not cortical veins. Therefore, even after endovascular treatment, continued systemic anticoagulation is necessary as a synergistic strategy to restore and preserve flow through cortical veins. If drainage from cortical veins into dural venous sinuses is not restored, the dural venous sinuses may not remain patent after mechanical thrombectomy.

In severe cases, patients who have intractable intracranial hypertension due to cerebral edema or a large intracerebral hematoma may require decompressive craniectomy for definitive management of intracranial pressure. Surgical evacuation of a large intracerebral hematoma may be required for patient stabilization prior to initiation of therapeutic anticoagulation.

Surgical Procedure

The patient was brought to the neurointerventional surgery suite and positioned supine on the procedure table. The procedure was performed under monitored anesthesia care without endotracheal intubation. Treatment with IV heparin was initiated prior to the start of the procedure. The patient was prepped and draped for femoral access. Percutaneous access to the right femoral artery was obtained, and then a 5 Fr femoral sheath was introduced into the femoral artery using the modified Seldinger technique. A 4 Fr diagnostic catheter and 0.35-inch glide wire were introduced into the femoral sheath and used to catheterize the internal carotid arteries and vertebral arteries selectively. Baseline angiographic images were obtained, which demonstrated non-opacification of the straight sinus and right transverse sinus, indicative of occlusive

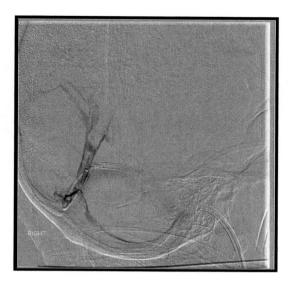

Figure 20.3 Diagnostic angiogram (lateral view), with the aspiration catheter positioned in the straight sinus. Contrast filling defect demonstrates thrombus burden within the vessel.

thrombus at those locations. Next, percutaneous access to the right common femoral vein was obtained under ultrasound guidance, and using the modified Seldinger technique, a 6 Fr guide catheter (Neuron Max 088) was advanced over an LT guide wire into the right internal jugular vein under fluoroscopic guidance. We then introduced a triaxial system consisting of an ACE60 reperfusion catheter, 3MAX reperfusion catheter, and Fathom microwire. Further diagnostic angiograms were obtained by contrast injection of the right internal carotid artery, and venous phase images were used as overlay guidance for navigation of the triaxial system into the right transverse sinus and then into the straight sinus thrombus. The 3MAX catheter and Fathom wire were removed from the ACE60, and then the ACE60 was slowly withdrawn through the straight sinus and right transverse sinus while mechanical aspiration was performed (Figure 20.3). Follow-up angiography demonstrated reduced clot burden within the straight sinus and right transverse sinus. This process was repeated until consistent flow through these vessels was restored. After successful treatment of the sinus thrombosis, the catheters were removed and the vascular access sites were closed and dressed in a sterile manner. The patient was subsequently transported to the neurological intensive care unit for further care. The patient remained on an IV heparin drip.

Oral Boards Review—Management Pearls

1. Medical management with IV fluids and anticoagulation is the mainstay of CVST treatment.
2. Endovascular techniques include mechanical thrombectomy and local administration of fibrinolytics, but they are typically reserved for patients who are refractory to medical therapy.

Pivot Points

1. Therapeutic anticoagulation remains the mainstay of treatment for CVST even if there is hemorrhagic conversion of a venous infarct.
2. Intracranial hypertension due to cerebral edema or intracranial hemorrhage may necessitate craniotomy for hematoma evacuation or decompression. In this case, maintenance of anticoagulation is recommended despite surgery to maximize the chances of sinus patency.

Aftercare

Current guidelines for the management of long-term anticoagulation in patients with CVST are extrapolated from observational studies. No randomized clinical trials are available to guide management. Commonly used agents for long-term anticoagulation include warfarin and other vitamin K pathway antagonists.

Patients can be classified into three categories based on their risk for recurrent CVST. Patients who develop CVST in the context of a modifiable risk factor such as smoking or oral contraceptive use may undergo anticoagulation for a 3- to 6-month course. Patients who have idiopathic CVST may undergo anticoagulation for a 6- to 12-month course. Patients with congenital thrombophilia or recurrent CVST may undergo life-long anticoagulation.

Comprehensive evaluation is important to identify an underlying hypercoagulable state. Acquired hypercoagulable states include malignancy, surgery, trauma, pregnancy, immobilization, dehydration, and oral contraceptive usage. Congenital hypercoagulable states include protein C or S deficiency, factor V Leiden thrombophilia, antithrombin III deficiency, prothrombin G20210A mutation, and hyperhomocysteinemia.

Complications and Management

Patients with CVST may have secondary neurologic symptoms related to focal edema or intracerebral hemorrhage that require additional treatment. A portion of patients may develop seizures that require the ongoing use of antiepileptic agents.

Acetazolamide administration may be beneficial in CVST patients with symptomatic intracranial hypertension. Hydrocephalus may develop from intracranial hemorrhage or reduced cerebrospinal fluid (CSF) absorption due to compromised venous drainage. CSF removal with serial lumbar punctures, lumbar drain placement, or ventricular drain placement may also be helpful in the management of intracranial hypertension, but these interventions carry elevated risk in anticoagulated patients.

After the acute phase, patients who develop worsening headache, nausea, visual disturbance, focal neurologic deficits, or mental status changes should be promptly evaluated to rule out the expansion or recurrence of CVST.

Oral Boards Review—Complications Pearls

1. CVST may lead to secondary neurologic symptoms, such as seizure or hydrocephalus, that require additional treatment.
2. Seizures may be caused by cerebral edema or hemorrhage.
3. Hydrocephalus may be caused by compromised venous drainage or by intracranial hemorrhage.
4. Hydrocephalus may be managed medically with acetazolamide or with CSF drainage.
5. It is important to remain vigilant for potential recurrence or expansion of CVST.

Evidence and Outcomes

Existing clinical evidence supports the use of systemic anticoagulation for the acute management of CVST as a first-line treatment in the neurologically stable patient. In cases with a coexisting asymptomatic intracerebral hemorrhage, systemic anticoagulation is still associated with improved outcomes. There is no definitive evidence that demonstrates the relative superiority of either low-molecular-weight heparin or unfractionated heparin. There is no definitive evidence to delineate the role of antiplatelet agents or novel anticoagulants in the treatment of CVST. No randomized controlled trials exist regarding long-term anticoagulant management in CVST.

There are no randomized controlled trials examining the use of endovascular techniques in the treatment of CVST. Existing practice patterns have developed around large, single-center case series. Nonetheless, a meta-analysis of 185 patients concluded that mechanical thrombectomy may be safe and clinically appropriate in patients who have medically refractory CVST. Given the rapid advancement of endovascular technology, future device development may increase the role of endovascular techniques in the treatment of CVST.

Further Reading

Chiewvit P, Piyapittayanan S, Poungvarin N. Cerebral venous thrombosis: Diagnosis dilemma. *Neurol Int.* 2011;3(3):13.

Ferro JM, Canhão P, Stam J, Bousser M-G, Barinagarrementeria F. Prognosis of cerebral vein and dural sinus thrombosis. *Stroke.* 2004;35(3):664–670.

Gosk-Bierska I, Wysokinski W, Brown R, et al. Cerebral venous sinus thrombosis: Incidence of venous thrombosis recurrence and survival. *Neurology.* 2006;67(5):814–819.

Rao K, Knipp HC, Wagner EJ. Computed tomographic findings in cerebral sinus and venous thrombosis. *Radiology.* 1981;140(2):391–398.

Saposnik G, Barinagarrementeria F, Brown RD, et al. Diagnosis and management of cerebral venous thrombosis. *Stroke.* 2011;42:1158–1192.

Siddiqui FM, Dandapat S, Banerjee C, et al. Mechanical thrombectomy in cerebral venous thrombosis. *Stroke.* 2015;46(5):1263–1268.

Incidental Unruptured Arteriovenous Malformation

Nicholas C. Bambakidis and Jeffrey T. Nelson

21

Case Presentation

A left-handed 42-year-old female with newly diagnosed right-sided Bell's palsy undergoes magnetic resonance imaging (MRI) of the brain without contrast in workup of the disease. The study is remarkable only for a small subcortical white matter hyperintensity (WMH) in the left frontal lobe. An MRI brain scan with and without contrast is ordered to rule out a neoplasm. The left frontal WMH does not enhance; however, a 1-cm contrast-enhancing lesion is noted in the cingulate sulcus along the medial right frontal lobe concerning for a vascular lesion (Figure 21.1). Referral is made to a neurosurgeon. The patient has a history of hypertension, hypothyroidism, migraines, depression, and attention-deficit/hyperactivity disorder; there is no history of seizures. Detailed neurological examination reveals only mild residual right lower motor neuron facial droop.

Questions

1. What is the differential diagnosis?
2. Is further diagnostic workup required for this patient?
3. What other studies may help establish a diagnosis?
4. What is the appropriate timing of the diagnostic workup?

Assessment and Planning

An enhancing lesion on an MRI brain scan with the appearance of a tangle of blood vessels without an associated solid or cystic mass is likely a cerebral arteriovenous malformation (AVM). The differential diagnosis includes other vascular lesions, such as developmental venous anomaly, and hypervascular tumors, such as hemangioblastoma and metastasis of renal cell carcinoma, papillary thyroid carcinoma, melanoma, or cholangiocarcinoma. An AVM is a tangle of abnormal blood vessels connecting the arterial and venous vasculature without intervening capillaries. Cerebral AVMs are rare, affecting <0.1% of the population, but they often present with rupture, sometimes with devastating effects.

Further diagnostic workup is needed for accurate diagnosis. Because the MRI suggests the presence of hypervascularity, approaching this lesion unprepared, by either stereotactic biopsy or open resection, can lead to catastrophic hemorrhage. Cerebral digital subtraction angiography (DSA) is the gold standard for imaging AVMs of the

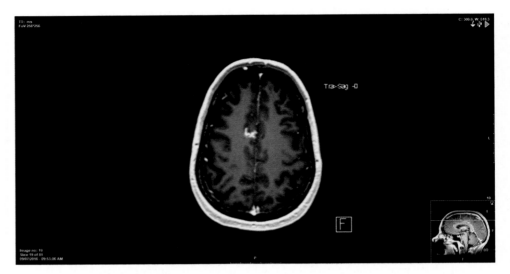

Figure 21.1 T_1-weighted MRI of the brain with contrast demonstrates a serpiginous enhancing lesion in the right medial frontal lobe, extending to the midline.

brain and is the most appropriate next step in the diagnostic workup of this patient. CT or MR angiography do not provide the dynamic visualization of blood flow or spatial resolution required for accurate diagnosis and planning of further treatment.

Oral Boards Review—Diagnostic Pearls

1. Unruptured cerebral AVMs can be symptomatic and cause seizures or focal neurological deficit, but unruptured low-grade AVMs are most commonly found incidentally when neuroimaging is obtained for another reason, such as headache or trauma.
   a. On a noncontrast CT scan of the head, an AVM is generally isodense to slightly hyperintense to the surrounding brain parenchyma.
   b. On an unenhanced MRI scan of the head, AVMs are most easily spotted by flow voids on T_2-weighted imaging.
2. Cerebral AVMs are most often discussed in reference to their Spetzler–Martin grade, which classifies AVMs by their surgical morbidity based on the following three factors:
   a. Size of the nidus: 1 point for <3 cm in diameter, 2 points for 3–6 cm in diameter, and 3 points for >6 cm in diameter
   b. Pattern of drainage: 0 points for exclusive superficial drainage and 1 point for any component of deep drainage
   c. Location: 0 points if the nidus is in a noneloquent brain region and 1 point if it is in an area of eloquence (primary motor, somatosensory, and primary visual cortex; language centers; hypothalamus; thalamus; internal capsule; brainstem; cerebellar peduncles; and deep cerebellar nuclei)
3. Low-grade cerebral AVMs are Spetzler–Martin grade 1 and 2.

The key diagnostic features of an AVM on cerebral angiography are the presence of a nidus of abnormal vessels and the presence of an early draining vein—that is, contrast opacifying a vein prior to the venous phase of the study. The nidus of an AVM may be either compact, also known as glomerular, or diffuse, also called proliferative, and it may have both compact and diffuse components. An early draining vein emanating from the cortex without a nidus is indicative of a pial arteriovenous fistula. A diffuse nidus without the presence of an early draining vein is seen in cerebral proliferative angiopathy. An abnormal venous structure that fills during the normal venous phase is consistent with a developmental venous anomaly.

In addition to establishing the diagnosis of cerebral AVM, DSA shows many attributes of an AVM necessary to make further management decisions. The size of the nidus is measured, the pattern of venous drainage is noted, and the arterial feeding vessels are characterized. The presence of aneurysms of feeding vessels or within the nidus is determined. For large AVMs with high-volume arteriovenous shunts, the blood supply to the normal brain is often disrupted; angiography also shows how the normal brain parenchyma is supplied. The precise location of an AVM is also important in management decisions; a thin-slice gadolinium-enhanced MRI of the brain, with functional MRI imaging and/or diffusion tensor imaging tractography where indicated, is the most accurate study for determining location.

In the current patient, a cerebral angiogram is ordered. She is found to have a 1-cm tangle of blood vessels supplied by branches of the right anterior cerebral artery draining via a single dilated vessel superiorly to the superior sagittal sinus. This is a Spetzler–Martin grade 1 lesion (Figure 21.2).

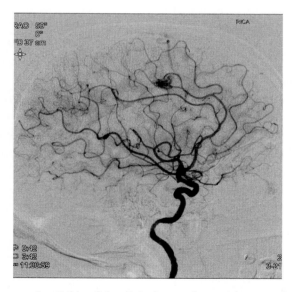

Figure 21.2 Preoperative DSA of the right internal carotid artery (lateral projection) demonstrates an AVM with supply primarily from the right anterior cerebral artery and also superficial venous drainage into the superior sagittal sinus.

Questions

1. Does this patient require treatment, or would observation be appropriate?
2. What are the treatment options for the patient's lesion?
3. How likely is treatment of the lesion to prevent future hemorrhage?

Decision-Making

Because of the relatively low incidence of cerebral AVMs along with a significant heterogeneity between lesions, the natural history and risk of rupture are not definitively established. The best estimate of overall rupture rate is approximately 3% or 4% per year. Unruptured AVMs have a slightly lower yearly risk of rupture at 2% or 3%, whereas previously ruptured AVMs have a 4% or 5% yearly risk of rupture, at least initially. Certain factors have been shown to increase the risk of rupture, including exclusively deep venous drainage, deep nidus location, and associated aneurysms. Other factors increase the complication risk with treatment: deep venous drainage, size of the nidus, and location of the nidus in an area of eloquence in the brain (e.g., motor cortex or language areas). Patient symptoms are also taken into consideration, particularly in the case of intractable seizures or focal deficit from oligemia secondary to "steal" phenomenon of the AVM. The decision to observe or treat must be made individually, taking into account the lifetime risk of the lesion, the risk of treatment, and the patient's symptoms.

Microsurgical resection and radiosurgery are the main treatment options. Endovascular embolization is used as an adjunct to these procedures, except in rare cases such as a small, deep lesion with a single feeding artery adjacent to critical structures. Partial embolization has been shown to increase rupture risk, likely secondary to change in blood flow dynamics.

Microsurgical resection is the definitive treatment of cerebral AVMs, with a >95% rate of obliteration. Radiosurgery is less invasive; however, it often takes three or more years for the lesions to become obliterated. Until total obliteration, the rupture risk is similar to that of untreated lesions. Obliteration rate after radiosurgery is dependent on the AVM size; lesions <3 mm have obliteration rates of 75–80%, whereas larger lesions have obliteration rates of 30–70%. Overall, complication rates of both microsurgical resection and radiosurgery are 5–7%; surgical complication rates for resection of low-grade AVMs are lower at 2% to 3%.

The current patient has a 40+-year life expectancy, so despite the fact that she is currently asymptomatic, the risk of rupture over her lifetime is high. Treatment is recommended.

Questions

1. When should preoperative embolization be considered?
2. During surgery, when should the draining vein(s) be coagulated or clipped?

Surgical Procedure

Microsurgical resection of cerebral AVMs is one of the most challenging procedures encountered in neurosurgical practice. Preoperative familiarization with the individual patient's AVM and normal anatomy is imperative to plan the appropriate resection strategy and prevent complications.

After induction of general anesthesia, the patient's head is fixed in a Mayfield head holder (radiolucent if intraoperative angiography is planned) and positioned for the appropriate craniotomy. AVMs can occur anywhere in the brain, and choosing the approach depends on the size, location, and drainage of the AVM. Head positioning also takes into account the effect of gravity on the adjacent tissues; gravity can assist or impede retraction during surgery.

A wide craniotomy is made to expose the AVM and surrounding brain tissue so as to provide complete visualization of the AVM throughout the surgery with an unencumbered working corridor. Meticulous subarachnoid dissection is employed to localize the draining vein and feeding arteries. In a superficial, low-grade AVM, the primary draining vein will be directed superficially, and as in all AVM surgeries, it must be preserved until the end of the resection. Feeding arteries are coagulated and divided at the border of the AVM; "en passage" arteries, which contribute small feeders but also supply normal brain tissue, are skeletonized, and patency of the main trunk is preserved to prevent infarction. As more feeding arteries are coagulated, the draining vein slackens and eventually darkens in color (Figure 21.3). After the AVM has been divided from the surrounding tissue, the nidus resembles a pedicle on a stalk created by the draining vein. Finally, the draining vein is clipped and divided, hemostasis is achieved in the resection bed with careful inspection for residual nidus, and the resection is complete.

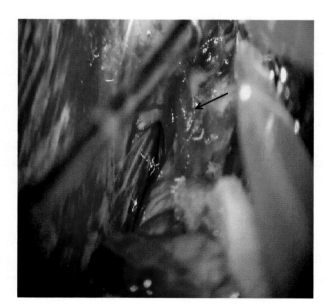

Figure 21.3 Surgical view of the medial surface of the right hemisphere (via interhemispheric exposure) demonstrates the AVM's single draining vein prior to resection (arrow).

Oral Boards Review—Management Pearls

1. A wide craniotomy is necessary to ensure adequate visualization and provide unencumbered access to the AVM even in the face of brain swelling or relaxation.
2. Keeping a bloodless working field is paramount; all bleeding should be controlled before advancing further with the resection.
3. The main draining vein must be identified and preserved until the end of the resection. It will be similar in color to the feeding arteries due to shunting of arterial blood, but it will be identifiable by its larger diameter and lack of muscular tunica media layer.
4. AVM rupture during resection of low-grade AVMs is rare with meticulous dissection and preservation of the main draining vein. If it does occur, the resection must progress rapidly; a bleeding AVM cannot be packed or tamponaded.
5. Anesthesia should be instructed to maintain systolic blood pressure strictly below 140 mmHg throughout the case and, importantly, during extubation. A gentle extubation must occur without allowing the patient to cough uncontrollably.

Pivot Points

1. If the low-grade AVM is located in eloquent tissue (i.e., an AVM <3 cm with a superficial draining vein that is present in an eloquent region), the patient must be counseled that temporary or even permanent disability is a risk of surgery, however small. Radiosurgery may be considered, although deficits can occur after radiosurgery due to gliosis or radiation necrosis.
2. The vast majority of cerebral AVMs are solitary and not inherited in a genetic pattern. If multiple AVMs are discovered, syndromic association with hereditary hemorrhagic telangiectasia (Osler–Weber–Rendu syndrome) or Wyburn–Mason syndrome should be considered.
3. Preoperative embolization may be considered if feeding arteries to the deep surface of the AVM are present and accessible with a microcatheter.

Aftercare

An initial postoperative CT scan of the head without contrast is obtained to rule out hemorrhage and act as a baseline in the event of postoperative neurologic decline. The patient is monitored in an intensive care unit with nursing staff trained to recognize changes in the neurological exam. Nursing staff is instructed to notify the physician at the first sign of a neurological exam change. Close monitoring of blood pressure is maintained; hypertension is avoided to prevent hemorrhage in the AVM nidus resection bed.

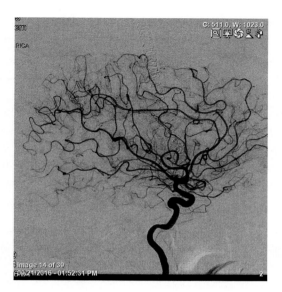

Figure 21.4 Preoperative DSA of the right internal carotid artery (lateral projection) demonstrates no residual AVM or early draining vein.

A postoperative cerebral angiogram is obtained to confirm complete resection of the AVM (Figure 21.4). Residual nidus or persistent early draining is rare, but if encountered, it should be treated during the hospitalization. In such a case, the patient is taken back to the operating room for re-exploration and total obliteration. Delaying repeat surgery can allow time for scar tissue formation, and opting for radiosurgery puts the AVM at risk of rupture for another several years.

A totally obliterated AVM will not recur in adult patients after microsurgical resection. After a routine postoperative visit, patients may be seen on an as-needed basis. In the pediatric population, recurrence does occur even with radiographically confirmed obliteration, so routine follow-up imaging is recommended until adulthood.

Complications and Management

Major complications after resection of unruptured low-grade cerebral AVMs are rare; >95% of patients have a good long-term outcome after surgery.

Preoperative seizures can occur in up to one-third of patients with cerebral AVMs. After resection, 75% of those patients will no longer have seizures. New seizures after microsurgical AVM resection occur in approximately 3% of patients. If a patient had seizures preoperatively, antiepileptic drugs (AEDs) are continued throughout the perioperative period. In general, AEDs are not started prophylactically.

In the event of postoperative neurological deterioration, an emergent noncontrast CT head scan is obtained to rule out intracranial hemorrhage, hydrocephalus, or subacute infarct. Positive findings are dealt with in the appropriate manner (e.g., intracranial hemorrhage evacuation, craniectomy, and ventriculostomy). Postoperative seizure should be suspected with a negative scan. If the neurological change was transient and has resolved, AEDs should be held while prolonged electroencephalography (EEG) is in place; an appropriate AED is started if subsequent seizure activity is seen on the EEG.

If the patient continues to have neurological deficit with a negative CT head scan, the patient should be loaded on an appropriate AED immediately without waiting for the EEG leads to be placed. Other systemic causes of neurological deterioration, such as hypercarbia, narcotic overdose, and infection, should be investigated concurrently if suspected.

Perioperative ischemic stroke is rare, but it should be kept on the differential when investigating causes for an acute neurological decline, particularly for patients with atrial fibrillation in whom anticoagulation was held for surgery. Symptoms consistent with large vessel occlusion may warrant a CT angiogram of the head and subsequent mechanical thrombectomy if appropriate. Intravenous recombinant tissue plasminogen activator is contraindicated in patients with recent intracranial surgery.

Oral Boards Review—Complications Pearls

1. Monitoring of patients in a specialized neurosurgical intensive care unit, or at least with specialized nursing care trained to recognize neurological deficits, will allow for more immediate recognition of postoperative complications.
2. Continuous monitoring of arterial blood pressure with strict protocols to keep systolic blood pressure below 140 mmHg should be maintained until postoperative day 1 to prevent fragile arteries in the resection bed from bleeding after surgery. Normal perfusion pressure breakthrough, although rare, can cause postoperative hemorrhage even without blood pressure spikes.

Evidence and Outcomes

Due to the relative rarity of cerebral AVMs and heterogeneity of the lesions, high-quality data in the management and outcomes of patients with AVMs are lacking. Most of our knowledge of the disease derives from large, retrospective case series and, more recently, prospectively maintained registries.

Data from randomized controlled trials are preferred, but the disease process does not lend itself to such trials. The dangers of a poorly designed randomized trial have been observed. The Randomized Trial of Unruptured Brain AVMs was an effort to determine if unruptured AVMs should be observed or treated. After 223 patients had been enrolled, the trial was halted early due to higher rates of stroke and death in the treatment arm versus the medical arm. Criticisms of the trial include significant selection bias because fewer than one-third of patients screened were enrolled, higher than expected complication rates, a large percentage of patients treated with embolization alone, and lack of long-term follow-up to account for the lifetime of expected risks in the conservative arm. Only 17 patients were treated with microsurgery, with or without embolization.

Particularly in the case of unruptured low-grade AVMs, few physicians would elect to enroll patients in a clinical trial with an observational arm. Microsurgical resection of these lesions has an obliteration rate that approaches 100% and a 2% or 3% incidence of complications, whereas the neurological effects can be potentially devastating from a rupture if the AVM is left untreated.

Further Reading

Bambakidis NC, Cockroft KM, Hirsch JA, et al. The case against a randomized trial of unruptured brain arteriovenous malformations: Misinterpretation of a flawed study. *Stroke.* 2014;45(9):2808–2810.

Gross BA, Du R. Natural history of cerebral arteriovenous malformations: A meta-analysis. *J Neurosurg.* 2013;118(2):437–443.

Potts MB, Lau D, Abla AA, Kim H, Young WL, Lawton MT. Current surgical results with low-grade brain arteriovenous malformations. *J Neurosurg.* 2015;122(4):912–920.

Spetzler RF, Martin NA. A proposed grading system for arteriovenous malformations. *J Neurosurg.* 1986;65(4):476–483.

van Beijnum J, van der Worp HB, Buis DR, et al. Treatment of brain arteriovenous malformations: A systematic review and meta-analysis. *JAMA.* 2011;306(18):2011–2019.

Unruptured Eloquent Arteriovenous Malformation Presenting with Seizure

Philip G. R. Schmalz, Raghav Gupta, and Christopher S. Ogilvy

22

Case Presentation

A 36-year-old male presented after a motor vehicle collision in which he was the driver and sole occupant of the vehicle. He lost consciousness due to a suspected seizure while driving, suffering a mild traumatic brain injury. A thorough trauma evaluation revealed no other injuries. Initial neurological examination revealed a well-developed young man with mild confusion and right upper extremity weakness. No other neurological abnormalities were apparent. A noncontrast computed tomography (CT) scan of the head was obtained, which demonstrated faint cortical subarachnoid hemorrhage in a non-aneurysmal pattern as well as a left hemispheric, perirolandic, hypoattenuating structure. Neurosurgical consultation was requested, and the patient was admitted to the hospital and placed in a monitored bed. During the next several hours, the patient's mentation and right upper extremity weakness improved; however, the weakness did not completely resolve, suggesting an initial Todd's paralysis with underlying structural lesion. As the patient's examination improved, a more detailed history revealed a history of rare generalized seizures for the past year that had not been evaluated with imaging or by consultation with a neurological specialist. There was no prior history of seizures in childhood or as a young adult. There was no history of antiepileptic medication use, and the patient was started on oral anticonvulsants. A magnetic resonance imaging (MRI) study of the brain was obtained, which demonstrated a T_2 hyperintense region in the left parietal lobe extending deep toward the lateral ventricle with associated hypervascularity and an enlarged superficial draining vein (Figure 22.1).

Questions

1. What is the most likely diagnosis? What other entities should be considered?
2. What imaging modalities are available, and what is the most appropriate imaging evaluation?
3. Given the presence of subarachnoid hemorrhage, even with the history of recent trauma, what important anatomical features of the primary lesion must be evaluated?
4. What is the appropriate timing of the imaging evaluation? Is there urgency to evaluating this lesion?

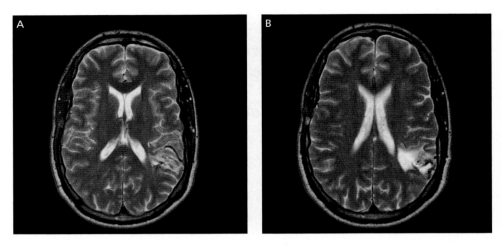

Figure 22.1 Axial T$_2$-weighted MRI demonstrates flow voids in the left parietal lobe (A) as well as a region of periventricular encephalomalacia and cortical vessels (B).

Assessment and Planning

The cerebrovascular neurosurgical consultant suspects an arteriovenous malformation (AVM). Other diagnostic considerations include a large developmental venous anomaly with or without an associated cavernous malformation, dural arteriovenous fistula, or pial arteriovenous fistula (AVF). The T$_2$ hyperintensity in this case is atypical of developmental venous anomalies, which are generally thought to be benign lesions. In addition, no imaging features suggest a cavernous malformation. Although dural and pial AVFs can cause enlargement of cortical veins, they generally do not cause parenchymal change that extends toward the ventricular system as in this case. Cerebral proliferative angiopathy can mimic AVMs; however, this disease state is notable for a large, diffuse nidus that can involve an entire hemisphere.

An understanding of the exact etiology of AVMs remains incomplete. They are assumed to occur in fetal life or early growth and development while continuing to enlarge after birth, although AVMs are rarely detected in utero or in infancy. They are rare lesions, with estimates of their prevalence in the general population ranging from 0.005% to 0.6%. The development of AVMs is associated with several hereditary conditions, including familial AVM syndromes, hereditary hemorrhagic telangiectasia (Rendu–Osler–Weber syndrome), Wyburn–Mason syndrome, and Sturge–Weber syndrome. Hemorrhage remains the most common clinical presentation, and seizures are the next most frequent, occurring in 20–25% of cases. As seen in this case, a temporal or parietal lobe location is more likely to result in seizures than AVMs in other locations, and these seizures are more likely to have a focal semiology as opposed to frontal AVMs. Natural history estimates for hemorrhage range from less than 2% to 17.8% risk of rupture per year. Most studies of patients without prior hemorrhage suggest an annual hemorrhage risk of 2–4% per year.

Computed tomography is the most sensitive imaging technique to detect hemorrhage from an AVM; however, noncontrast CT can be negative in unruptured lesions. The sensitivity of CT scanning is improved with CT angiography or contrasted CT, which demonstrates hypervascularity and enlarged venous varices. MRI remains the most sensitive noninvasive imaging modality and is often useful for detecting subtle lesions. In addition, MRI often shows perilesional atrophy and provides precise anatomical localization. Noninvasive imaging has a limited ability to detect associated feeding vessel or intranidal aneurysms, particularly when aneurysm diameter is less than 5 mm. In addition, noninvasive imaging provides a static image and little information about the detailed angioarchitecture and lesion hemodynamics, which is best evaluated with catheter angiography. Catheter angiography provides extremely sensitive and complementary information to noninvasive imaging and remains the gold standard for AVM evaluation. Many authors recommend catheter angiography for all patients presenting with AVMs and especially those presenting with associated hemorrhage, which may obscure subtle findings on noninvasive studies.

Oral Boards Review—Diagnostic Pearls

1. Differential diagnosis of AVM includes developmental venous anomaly with or without associated cavernous malformation, pial AVF, and dural AVF.
2. Noninvasive imaging modalities, including CT/CT angiography and MRI, are valuable for the initial assessment and are complementary to catheter angiography in the evaluation of patients with AVMs. Catheter angiography is recommended for most patients with AVMs, especially in the setting of hemorrhage, to better elucidate the angioarchitecture and to diagnose feeding vessel or intranidal aneurysms.
3. Hemorrhage is the most common presentation in patients with AVMs. The risk of hemorrhage is approximately 2–4% per year. Patients with a recent AVM hemorrhage are at an increased risk of rebleeding of approximately 7% in the first year after hemorrhage. The risk decreases to the baseline rate after 3–5 years.
4. Certain anatomic features have been associated with a higher risk of hemorrhage, including deep or impaired venous drainage or outflow restriction, the presence of associated aneurysms, and infratentorial location.

This patient underwent CT angiography as well as catheter angiography at the time of initial hospitalization. Despite the patient's history of recent trauma from a motor vehicle accident, the cortical location of both the suspected AVM and the subarachnoid hemorrhage raised suspicion for feeding vessel aneurysm. For this reason, a digital subtraction angiogram was completed, which confirmed a left parietal AVM measuring 3 cm with principal arterial supply from the superior division of the left middle cerebral artery (MCA). No intranidal or feeding vessel aneurysm was found. Venous drainage was through the superficial venous system predominantly to the vein of Trolard, with additional drainage through the vein of Labbé (Figure 22.2).

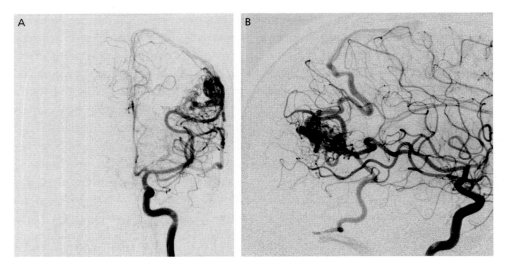

Figure 22.2 Preoperative digital subtraction angiography of the left internal carotid artery in the anterior–posterior (A) and lateral (B) projections demonstrates an AVM supplied by branches of the MCA, with superficial venous drainage superiorly (through the superior anastomotic vein of Trolard, onward to the superior sagittal sinus) and inferiorly (through the inferior anastomotic vein of Labbé, onward to the transverse–sigmoid sinus junction).

Questions

1. What are the medical, neuro-interventional, surgical, and radiosurgical options for this patient?
2. How do the anatomic and angiographic findings in the imaging studies influence management in this case?
3. What are the risks and benefits of treatment in this patient and how will treatment alter the natural history of the disease (positively or negatively)? What tools are available for surgical risk stratification?

Decision-Making

Multiple treatment options exist for patients with AVMs, including observation, surgical resection or radiosurgery with or without pretreatment embolization, and embolization alone. Treatment of unruptured AVMs remains one of the most controversial and debated topics in the neurosurgical and neurological literature.

With regard to successful obliteration of the lesion, surgical resection remains the most efficacious treatment modality. Surgery has the advantage of immediate lesion obliteration without a latency period during which the patient is exposed to rupture risk. However, patients treated surgically have taken their risk "up front" as opposed to a lower risk profile spread out over their remaining life span. Obliteration rates for Spetzler–Martin grade I–III AVMs range from 94% to 100%. Surgical obliteration rates for larger AVMs are more difficult to define because many of these lesions, if treated, are often addressed using multimodality treatment of embolization and surgical resection or radiosurgery. The overall morbidity of surgical resection is related to AVM grade (using the Spetzler–Martin or newer grading systems). Overall postoperative mortality for surgical treatment is approximately 3–5%, and morbidity is 8–38%. For patients with grade I–III lesions, permanent morbidity is approximately 5%. In patients with grade IV and V lesions, rates of morbidity and mortality are substantially higher. For patients presenting with seizures, surgical treatment has been shown to reduce or eliminate seizures in approximately 50–80%.

Radiosurgery with or without pretreatment embolization is an effective treatment strategy for certain AVMs. The major advantages of radiosurgical treatment are that it is noninvasive; relatively low-risk, especially for larger lesions; and useful for AVMs in eloquent cortex or in areas that are technically challenging to access surgically. The major disadvantages of radiosurgery are reduced chance of complete obliteration and effect latency up to 3 years. Larger lesions are also difficult to treat without off-target dosing to normal brain parenchyma. Radiosurgical techniques include gamma knife, linear accelerator systems, and proton beam accelerator systems. The end result of radiation, regardless of delivery system, is endothelial damage to AVM vessels with resultant proliferation of myofibroblasts and collagen deposition. This causes progressive stenosis and eventual involution of the feeding vessels and nidus. Outcomes with radiosurgery are generally favorable, with angiographic cure rates of 75–95% for lesions 3 cm or smaller. Efficacy decreases for larger lesions to approximately 70% for those greater than 3 cm, although staged or multimodality procedures may increase this rate. Radiosurgery has also been shown to decrease seizure frequency in patients with pretreatment epilepsy at rates comparable to surgery. The overall permanent complication rate for radiosurgery is approximately 5%, generally related to edema and radionecrosis of brain parenchyma.

In the United States, embolization of AVMs remains largely an adjunctive treatment to surgical resection or radiosurgical treatment. Complete AVM obliteration with embolization alone occurs in approximately 10–20% of cases and is likely appropriate only for AVMs with a single pedicle and relatively small nidus. Despite this limitation as monotherapy, embolization is a valuable adjunct to surgical treatment, particularly in cases with deep arterial feeders that will be inaccessible until late in the operation. In these cases, presurgical embolization can reduce blood loss, improve visualization and thereby lower overall surgical risk, and may make a surgically high-risk AVM much more amenable to safe resection. Embolization prior to radiosurgery, as in presurgical embolization, can reduce the volume of the nidus and facilitate radiosurgical targeting. In addition, embolization can be used to eliminate high-risk AVM features, such as feeding vessel aneurysms, to reduce the risk of rupture during the latency period. However, pre-radiosurgical embolization may reduce the overall AVM obliteration rate, possibly due to radiation scatter from radio-opaque embolic material or hypoxia-induced local angiogenic activity. Like many topics surrounding this disease, the effect of embolization on radiosurgical efficacy remains controversial, and practice varies widely from center to center. Despite this risk, certain AVMs, particularly larger AVMs with significant intervening normal brain parenchyma or those with high-risk angiographic features, are likely to benefit from preoperative embolization.

Neurosurgeons and their patients with unruptured AVMs are faced with a challenging and controversial situation without clear guidance from high-quality prospective clinical trials. A careful and frank discussion between patient and surgeon is critical to assess patient values and risk preferences (up-front risk with surgery vs. prolonged, cumulative risk with observation or delayed or incomplete obliteration with radiosurgery) and to arrive at a treatment strategy that is most congruent with both the best available data and patient preferences. In this case, the patient was young and otherwise healthy, and she was suffering from generalized seizures. The tissue surrounding the lesion was abnormal, suggesting there was a reasonable margin of nonfunctional neural tissue around the nidus. A deep MCA feeding vessel arising from the posterior ramus of the sylvian fissure was noted, which, although accessible, would require dissection of the posterior aspect of the fissure on the left side. In light of the patient's desires, surgical accessibility of the AVM, and deep arterial supply in close proximity to eloquent cortex, a strategy of presurgical embolization of the major MCA feeding vessel followed by surgical resection was developed.

Questions

1. How can the risks of embolization be mitigated?
2. What are the key aspects of patient positioning and cortical exposure when planning a craniotomy for an AVM?
3. How should draining veins be managed during the initial dissection?
4. How can early entry of the nidus be managed?
5. What techniques are available for managing deep bleeding or small arteriolar hemorrhage at the base of the resection?

Surgical Procedure

Surgical resection of an AVM with presurgical embolization is a complex and relatively high-risk undertaking, particularly when the AVM is associated with eloquent brain regions. AVM surgery has been compared to a military battle with the corollary mapping, battle plan, execution of the plan, and escape strategy. In this case, we planned for preoperative embolization of the MCA feeding artery prior to definitive treatment. Presurgical embolization is usually performed under general anesthesia within a short window prior to operation because there is some concern that embolization can "destabilize" the AVM. Although most neurointerventionalists perform embolization under anesthesia, in select patients with at-risk en passage vessels, selective provocative testing using sodium amytal or methohexital can be useful, particularly for lesions near the spinal cord or brainstem. Liquid embolic agents such as n-BCA (Trufill) or ethylene vinyl alcohol copolymer in dimethyl sulfoxide solution (Onyx) are used to occlude deep pedicles and can often penetrate the nidus.

Patients are positioned on the angiographic table, and general anesthesia is induced. Particular attention should be paid to hemodynamic stability throughout the procedure, and arterial line placement should be considered. After baseline angiographic runs are completed, a guide catheter is positioned along with an intermediate catheter (if required), and road map working views are obtained. Access to the pedicle of interest is established with an embolic-compatible microcatheter, and embolization is completed under continuous fluoroscopic guidance. Distal pedicles can be accessed using 0.010-inch wires and extra-long microcatheters or flow-directed microcatheters. Particular care should be exercised when reflux is noted along the microcatheter to avoid the complication of a retained microcatheter. The risk of a retained microcatheter can be mitigated with care to reduce reflux and the use of detachable-tip embolization catheters, which may be later removed during surgery in the event of tip detachment. After embolization is complete, the microcatheter is withdrawn, and follow-up low-magnification runs are completed. The patient is awoken with particular care to avoid hemodynamic changes and examined for neurologic deficit.

In this patient's case, a single MCA feeding vessel was embolized using Onyx liquid embolic. To allow time for recovery from his closed head injury, the procedure was performed 3 months after initial diagnosis. Pre-embolization angiography indicated that this feeding vessel terminated in the AVM nidus and was a safe target for embolization. Low-magnification anterior–posterior and lateral angiographic views after embolization demonstrate abrupt termination of the feeding vessel within the sylvian fissure and reduction in venous outflow through the superior anastomotic vein (Figure 22.3).

The goal of surgical resection of an AVM is complete excision of the nidus and elimination of arteriovenous shunting. Surgery is carried out under general anesthesia with continuous hemodynamic monitoring using an arterial catheter to monitor blood pressure and robust venous access with two large-bore peripheral IVs or a combination of peripheral and central venous access. Given the potential for significant blood loss, matched blood products should be available during the procedure. The patient is positioned such that the AVM and the overlying craniotomy flap are at the highest point of the skull to facilitate circumferential dissection. The use of a neuronavigation console with MRI and merged CT angiography can be extremely helpful when planning the craniotomy. For lesions in language areas or other eloquent cortex, preoperative

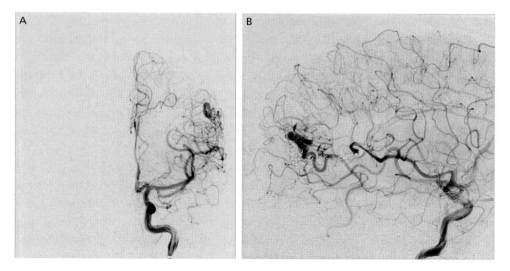

Figure 22.3 Post-embolization digital subtraction angiography of the left internal carotid artery in the anterior–posterior (A) and lateral (B) projections demonstrates reduction in arterial filling of the AVM nidus and slowed venous drainage in the early arterial phase. Embolization material is seen in a major branch of the MCA supplying the AVM.

functional MRI and tractography studies can be merged with navigational scans to improve situational awareness and avoid injury. In contrast to the smaller exposures that have become common in aneurysm surgery, resection of an AVM is safest with wider exposure. The craniotomy should expose the entire nidus with a wide margin, as well as all feeding vessels and draining veins so that they can be identified early in the dissection and preserved.

After the bone flap is removed, the dura should be opened with particular care taken to avoid damage to enlarged cortical venous varices. These vessels should be dissected free with utmost care and preserved until the nidus is devascularized. Damage to these vessels before feeding vessels are disconnected will result in engorgement of the nidus from outflow restriction, making safe dissection difficult, and it can even result in rupture of the nidus. After the dura is opened, the arachnoid planes surrounding the AVM, associated sulci, and all feeding arteries and draining veins should be identified and dissected free. Once these components are identified, dissection of the AVM can begin in a circumferential, spiral-type pattern progressing from the cortical surface toward the deep apex of the lesion. Frequently, a gliotic tissue plane surrounds the lesion, facilitating dissection. Early entry of the nidus should be avoided. If the nidus is entered prematurely, the surgeon should resume dissection superficially and re-establish a dissection plane outside of the nidus in the gliotic plane or surrounding parenchyma. Early coagulation of the nidus after early entry is ineffective.

Particular care should be exercised at the deep apex of the lesion near the ventricular surface. The deep arterial supply is often composed of multiple small arteriolar vessels with high flow. Their high flow resists coagulation, and they often retract into deep parenchyma, making their control difficult with bipolar cautery. Packing these regions with cottonoids is not advised because this can direct hemorrhage into deep parenchyma or the ventricular system with disastrous results. If feasible and safe, preoperative embolization can reduce their number, and small AVM clips can be used to arrest flow and facilitate effective electrocauterization of these arterioles.

After the apex of the lesion is devascularized and freed, the venous drainage can be coagulated and divided. Often, the color of venous outflow can give a visual aid to gauge the amount of remaining arteriovenous shunting. After the nidus is removed, the resection bed should be carefully examined for residual AVM nidus, and meticulous hemostasis should be attained with cautery and topical hemostatic agents. Continuous or difficult-to-control bleeding often indicates residual nidus and should be carefully inspected and addressed.

After hemostasis is achieved, the dura and bone flap are closed in the standard fashion. Particular care should be exercised during the procedure and particularly during awakening and extubation to prevent hemodynamic changes that can predispose to hemorrhage within the cavity. Postoperative angiography, completed either immediately postoperatively or soon thereafter, is required to ensure complete obliteration of the AVM. Immediate postoperative or intraoperative angiography is ideal because residual AVM can be immediately addressed.

In this case, the patient underwent presurgical embolization 3 months after his initial closed head injury to allow for recovery. Surgical resection was completed on the following day. The patient was positioned supine with a large shoulder roll and the head rotated over the right shoulder. Three-point head fixation was attached, and

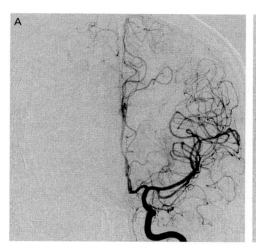 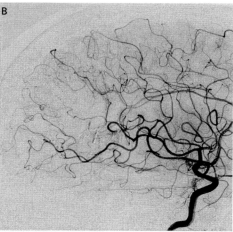

Figure 22.4 Postoperative digital subtraction angiography of the left internal carotid artery in the anterior–posterior (A) and lateral (B) projections demonstrates complete resection of the AVM, with no residual nidus or early draining vein.

neuronavigation was used to plan the craniotomy. A wide frontoparietal craniotomy was turned, and the dura opened in a cruciate fashion. The cortical venous drainage was easily identified because it was superficial, and resection was completed without issue. A wide gliotic plane was present around the AVM nidus, as suggested by the patient's preoperative MRI studies, facilitating dissection. After wound closure, the patient was maintained under general anesthesia and transported directly to the angiography suite, where a catheter angiogram demonstrated complete lesion resection without residual AVM (Figure 22.4). After angiography, the patient was awakened, extubated in the angiography suite, and thereafter transported to a neurosciences intensive care unit.

Oral Boards Review—Management Pearls

1. The goal of AVM surgery is complete excision of all AVM nidus and elimination of arteriovenous shunting.
2. Embolization prior to surgery can aid in control of deep arterial feeders and reduce blood loss and overall risk.
3. Venous drainage should be preserved until sufficient control and reduction in arterial supply have been achieved. Compromised venous outflow can make dissection difficult and can result in AVM rupture.
4. Meticulous hemostasis and careful hemodynamic management during surgery and extubation are critical to prevent postoperative bleeding.

Pivot Points

1. Patients presenting with aneurysmal rupture from a feeding vessel aneurysm associated with an AVM require urgent treatment to prevent aneurysmal re-rupture, just as do patients presenting with conventional aneurysmal

> subarachnoid hemorrhage. Securing the aneurysm can be performed concurrently with AVM surgery, as a separate surgical procedure prior to AVM management, or endovascularly with coil embolization or feeding vessel sacrifice.
> 2. Patients presenting with AVM hemorrhage, unlike those with aneurysmal bleeding, may be safely treated in a delayed fashion to allow recovery of the patient and liquefaction of dense fresh clot. Unlike with aneurysm rupture, the annual rate of AVM rebleeding is sufficiently low (6% in the first 6 months and then 2.4–4% thereafter) to permit delayed surgery or even radiosurgical management.

Aftercare

After AVM resection, patients should be monitored closely in an intensive care setting, ideally a neurosciences intensive care unit, with continuous arterial line monitoring and robust venous access. Careful management of blood pressure should continue for 24–48 hours after the procedure, depending on the size and complexity of the AVM. In certain patients, normotension or slight hypotension may be desirable to reduce the risk of postoperative bleeding. A noncontrast CT scan obtained the morning after operation can be helpful in the early identification of worrisome complications such as hematoma formation or cerebral edema. After 24–48 hours, the Foley catheter and arterial lines may be removed, and the patient may be transferred to an acute care unit and begin to ambulate. In the absence of significant neurologic deficit or other complications, many patients may be discharged 5–7 days after the operation.

Complications and Management

The most feared early postoperative complication of AVM surgery is hemorrhage, either from residual AVM or from the resection bed. The overall incidence of re-hemorrhage within the first week of operation is approximately 2%. Risk factors for re-hemorrhage include higher grade AVM, residual AVM, and the presence of lenticulostriate feeding vessels. In severe cases with neurological decline from hematoma and mass effect, reoperation is required to evacuate the hematoma and control bleeding. Early detection by frequent neurological monitoring in an intensive care unit setting is recommended. The risk of early hemorrhage can be mitigated by early postoperative angiography to ensure lesion obliteration and strict blood pressure control both during surgery and in the early postoperative period. Surgeons tackling higher grade AVMs should be particularly vigilant about this complication.

New-onset seizures occur in 5–20% of patients after AVM surgery and are more likely in patients who presented with seizures. Even in patients without a history of epilepsy, we recommend the routine prophylactic administration of anticonvulsants during the perioperative period, particularly for large lesions given the hemodynamic changes that can accompany convulsions.

Cerebral edema due to altered hemodynamics occurs in 3–5% of patients after AVM treatment and can occur after either resection or embolization. The condition may first present in the operating room and up to 7–10 days after intervention. Two theories exist as to its cause: normal perfusion pressure breakthrough and occlusive hyperemia. The brain parenchyma around AVMs can be subject to chronic ischemia due to steal phenomenon, and thus the vasculature is dilated to the maximum amount by disordered autoregulatory mechanisms. Removal of the shunt thus exposes this tissue to normal perfusion pressures that "break through" the disordered autoregulatory system, causing hyperperfusion and edema. Occlusive hyperemia can result from obstruction of venous outflow by resection of venous varices draining the AVM, resulting in venous hypertension and edema. Avoidance of cerebral edema is accomplished by careful blood pressure control and preservation of venous structures not associated with the AVM nidus. In addition, standard measures to control symptomatic edema should be implemented, including elevation and neutral positioning of the head; mannitol and hypertonic saline administration; ventriculostomy; and, rarely, intubation and mechanical ventilation with decompressive craniectomy in severe cases.

Less frequent complications include retrograde arterial thrombosis and vasospasm, which can be mitigated by minimizing arterial dissection when not needed for vascular control and elimination of subarachnoid blood by saline lavage.

Oral Boards Review—Complications Pearls

1. Early re-hemorrhage is the most severe complication after a successful operation and can be minimized by complete lesion obliteration confirmed by angiography, meticulous hemostasis of the resection cavity, and careful hemodynamic control in the perioperative period. Large hematomas require emergent exploration for clot evacuation and control of bleeding.
2. Prophylactic anticonvulsant medication can reduce the chance of postoperative seizures and is particularly recommended for large AVMs, AVMs in temporal or parietal locations, and those presenting with seizures.
3. Cerebral edema can be controlled by careful surgical technique and diligent blood pressure control in the perioperative period. Standard neurosurgical measures to control edema are applicable to AVM management.

Evidence and Outcomes

Surgical resection of brain AVMs is a highly effective treatment, with obliteration rates of 94–100% for patients with grade I–III lesions. In addition, surgical resection is associated with a marked reduction or elimination of seizures, with approximately 50–80% of patients seizure-free after resection. Overall operative morbidity and mortality from grade I–III AVMs is low in most series, whereas series of grade IV and V lesions have reported morbidity and mortality of up to 40%.

Treatment of unruptured brain AVMs remains an extremely controversial topic in cerebrovascular disease management. The most high-profile study addressing this topic, the Randomized Trial of Unruptured Brain Arteriovenous Malformations study, reported a 30.7% stroke and death rate in the interventional arm compared to 10.1% in the medical management arm of the trial over a mean follow-up of 33 months. This trial has been widely criticized and remains hotly debated in the literature. This study screened more than 1,700 patients to randomize 226 subjects. Treatment was not in keeping with the practice patterns in the United States because relatively few patients were treated with surgical resection and a substantial portion with embolization alone. In addition, the extremely short follow-up duration of 33 months has been criticized as inadequate when comparing an interventional risk, a one-time event, to a lifelong risk of hemorrhage. Nevertheless, the trial shows that intervention for unruptured brain AVMs does pose significant risk and should be carefully weighed against the lifetime risk of rupture, much as treatment decisions are approached for unruptured aneurysms. A decision analysis addressing smaller unruptured AVMs concluded that surgical intervention offered the greatest overall quality of life if the risk of major morbidity and mortality remained less than 7%.

Thus, the decision to treat an unruptured brain AVM is highly individualized, taking into account surgeon skill and experience and patient age, health, and life expectancy. The decision can only be made after a candid discussion between the patient and the surgeon and with a clear understanding by both parties of the risks and benefits. In this case, the patient was young, otherwise healthy, and had troubling seizures. Although the AVM was located in the motor cortex, there was a small margin of surrounding gliotic tissue, making resection feasible. The architecture of the AVM, with a large MCA feeding vessel, was favorable for preoperative embolization, thus reducing surgical risk. In addition, the superficial venous drainage made this case favorable for surgical resection. After surgery, the patient made an uncomplicated recovery and at last follow-up had a modified Rankin Scale score of 1 due to mild hand weakness, which was unchanged from his preoperative condition.

Further Reading

Brown RDJ, Wiebers DO, Forbes G, et al. The natural history of unruptured intracranial arteriovenous malformations. *J Neurosurg.* 1988;68(3):352–357. doi:10.3171/jns.1988.68.3.0352.

Lawton MT, Probst KX. Seven AVMs: Tenets and techniques for resection. 2014. http://public.eblib.com/choice/publicfullrecord.aspx?p=1643636

McInerney J, Gould DA, Birkmeyer JD, Harbaugh RE. Decision analysis for small, asymptomatic intracranial arteriovenous malformations. *Neurosurg Focus.* 2001;11(5):e7.

Mohr JP, Parides MK, Stapf C, et al. Medical management with or without interventional therapy for unruptured brain arteriovenous malformations (ARUBA): A multicentre, non-blinded, randomised trial. *Lancet.* 2014;383(9917):614–621. doi:10.1016/S0140-6736(13)62302-8.

Morgan MK, Winder M, Little NS, Finfer S, Ritson E. Delayed hemorrhage following resection of an arteriovenous malformation in the brain. *J Neurosurg.* 2003;99(6):967–971. doi:10.3171/jns.2003.99.6.0967.

Ondra SL, Troupp H, George ED, Schwab K. The natural history of symptomatic arteriovenous malformations of the brain: A 24-year follow-up assessment. *J Neurosurg.* 1990;73(3):387–391.

Spetzler RF, Martin NA. A proposed grading system for arteriovenous malformations. *J Neurosurg.* 1986;65(4):476–483. doi:10.3171/jns.1986.65.4.0476.

Spetzler RF, Ponce FA. A 3-tier classification of cerebral arteriovenous malformations: Clinical article. *J Neurosurg.* 2011;114(3):842–849. doi:10.3171/2010.8.JNS10663.

Unruptured Eloquent Arteriovenous Malformation Presenting with Arm Weakness

Adeel Ilyas, Dale Ding, Matthew J. Shepard, and Jason P. Sheehan

23

Case Presentation

A 38-year-old female with no past medical history presents to the emergency department with sudden-onset left arm weakness. In the emergency department, the patient has a simple partial seizure, with shaking of her left arm that promptly resolves after receiving a loading dose of phenytoin. She reports that 2 days prior, she presented to an outside medical facility with a headache and was prescribed pain medication. The patient does not routinely take any medication, including oral contraceptives. Detailed neurologic examination, including fundoscopic examination, by the neurosurgeon reveals only weakness of the left upper extremity.

Questions

1. What is the differential diagnosis?
2. What are the appropriate diagnostic images to obtain?
3. What is the appropriate timing of this diagnostic workup?

Assessment and Planning

The neurosurgeon suspects the presence of a right-sided space-occupying intracranial lesion, localized to the region of the primary motor cortex. The differential diagnosis includes arteriovenous malformation (AVM), cavernous malformation, other dural or pial arteriovenous fistulae, ruptured distal middle cerebral artery aneurysm, and cortical venous thrombosis. An ischemic stroke should be considered in any patient with acute-onset weakness. However, this diagnosis is less likely given the patient's young age, reversible seizure symptoms, and the absence of additional medical comorbidities.

AVMs and cavernomas have an incidence of less than 1% annually, although AVMs are diagnosed at a slightly higher frequency than cavernomas. Both vascular malformations may present with seizures or hemorrhage; however, hemorrhage is the most common presentation of AVMs, whereas seizure is the most common presentation of cavernomas. A focal neurological deficit may occur secondary to rupture of an AVM or cavernoma. In addition, AVMs, particularly large lesions, can present with progressively worsening neurological deficit secondary to chronic vascular "steal."

In addition to the neurological examination, the physical examination should focus on skin lesions because brain AVMs are associated with several multiorgan conditions, including hereditary hemorrhagic telangiectasia (i.e., Osler–Weber–Rendu syndrome) and Sturge–Weber syndrome. Obtaining family history may also be useful because both AVM and cavernous malformations have familial forms.

Diagnostic workup should begin with a brain computed tomography (CT) without contrast to identify intracranial hemorrhage. Vascular imaging with either CT or magnetic resonance angiogram should be obtained to identify the lesion. In the current case, a brain CT without contrast demonstrated right frontal lobe edema and scattered subarachnoid hemorrhage overlying the convexity (Figure 23.1A). This hemorrhage was likely the etiology of the patient's headache, and the subsequent edema may have caused the seizures.

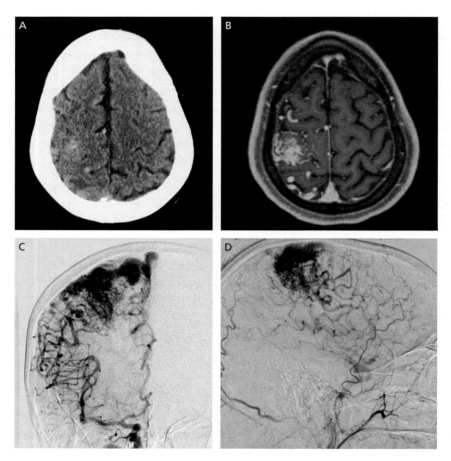

Figure 23.1 (A) Axial noncontrast cerebral CT scan exhibiting right frontal lobe edema and scattered subarachnoid hemorrhage overlying the convexity. (B) Subsequent T_1-weighted post-contrast MRI revealed a right frontal AVM spanning the central sulcus. Anterior–posterior (C) and lateral (D) cerebral angiography confirmed a 3.8 × 3.4 × 2.5 cm AVM being fed by branches of the middle cerebral, pericallosal, and callosomarginal arteries with superficial cortical drainage into the superior sagittal sinus.

Brain magnetic resonance imaging (MRI) revealed a right frontal AVM spanning the central sulcus (Figure 23.1B). MRI is useful to anatomically localize the lesion and guide treatment. In addition, hemosiderin deposition can be appreciated on the gradient echo sequence, indicating prior rupture. Digital subtraction catheter angiography (DSA) remains the gold standard for AVM evaluation and should be obtained in all suspected cases. DSA is a dynamic study that enables the neurosurgeon to more accurately identify feeding vessels, determine transit times into the draining vein(s), and detect associated angioarchitectural features (e.g., prenidal and intranidal aneurysm, intranidal fistula, venous stenosis, and venous varix). In the current case, DSA confirmed a right frontoparietal AVM, measuring $3.8 \times 3.4 \times 2.5$ cm (volume 16.2 cm^3), fed by branches of the middle cerebral, pericallosal, and callosomarginal arteries, with exclusively superficial venous drainage into the superior sagittal sinus (Figures 23.1C and 23.1D). The AVM spanned eloquent regions including the primary motor and sensory areas.

Oral Boards Review—Diagnostic Pearls

1. The most common presentation of a brain AVM is hemorrhage, and a vascular malformation should be suspected in any young patient who presents with a spontaneous intracranial hemorrhage. Seizures are the second most common presentation of AVMs. Persistent neurologic deficits in AVM patients may be secondary to chronic vascular steal and are more commonly observed in large AVMs.

2. DSA is the gold standard for AVM evaluation, and it characterizes angioarchitectural features (e.g., prenidal or intranidal aneurysm, intranidal fistula, venous stenosis, and venous varix identification of feeding vessels) and provides hemodynamic information. DSA is particularly useful when the diagnosis of an AVM is unclear based on noninvasive imaging. Pure arterial malformations or developmental venous anomalies can mimic an AVM. Compared to an AVM, these disparate lesions will have only an arterial or venous component, respectively, without evidence of arteriovenous shunting.

3. Whereas the Spetzler–Martin (SM) grading system was designed for predicting outcomes of AVM resection, the Virginia Radiosurgery AVM Scale (VRAS) better predicts AVM patient outcomes after stereotactic radiosurgery (SRS). A lower VRAS score portends a better chance of a favorable outcome as defined by AVM obliteration and no post-treatment hemorrhage or permanent complications following treatment.

Questions

1. How do these clinical and radiographic findings influence surgical planning?
2. What are potential treatment options?

Decision-Making

Embolization, microsurgery, and SRS are employed, alone or in combination, in the treatment of AVMs with the primary goal of nidal obliteration, thereby eliminating the risk of hemorrhage. Each of these modalities has its merits and drawbacks. Microsurgery affords immediate obliteration but incurs substantial neurological morbidity for AVMs in eloquent brain regions. For small to medium-sized (<3 cm in maximal diameter) AVMs localized to critical regions of the brain, SRS is generally the preferred treatment due to its relatively favorable complication profile. Embolization may be used as a neoadjuvant therapy prior to either approach, although it may decrease the obliteration rate when performed prior to SRS.

When evaluating the role of intervention in the management of an AVM, the risk of hemorrhage predicted by the natural history is weighed against risks and likelihood of achieving obliteration related to the chosen treatment modality. Prior AVM rupture has been shown to increase the risk of subsequent hemorrhage. In this case, the presence of symptomatic AVM hemorrhage as well as the patient's young age yield a cumulative lifetime hemorrhage risk of greater than 50%. Therefore, intervention is warranted. Given the AVM's eloquent location and large size, SRS is an ideal treatment modality.

Radiosurgical outcomes for this AVM are most reliably predicted by the VRAS. This simple, reliable scoring system predicts AVM patient outcome after SRS and utilizes three factors: history of prior hemorrhage (unruptured = 0 points, ruptured = 1 point), AVM volume (<2 cm³ = 0 points, 2–4 cm³ = 1 point, >4 cm³ = 2 points), and eloquent or noneloquent location of the AVM (noneloquent = 0 points, eloquent = 1 point). Patients with a VRAS score of 0, 1, 2, 3, and 4 have probabilities of a favorable outcome (defined as AVM obliteration and no post-treatment hemorrhage or permanent complications) of 83%, 79%, 70%, 48%, and 39%, respectively.

Questions

1. How effective is SRS treatment of AVM in eliminating seizures?
2. What further imaging study may be useful in planning the SRS approach?
3. What is the timing of surgical intervention?

Surgical Procedure

SRS for the treatment of AVMs can be accomplished with the Gamma Knife (GK), CyberKnife, linear accelerator, or proton beam. These approaches differ not only in their means of energy generation but also in their reliance on frame-based versus frameless systems. In this case, GK was used.

After close inpatient observation and a discussion of treatment approaches, the patient was discharged home with a plan to return in 3 weeks for treatment. Prior to the day of GK radiosurgery, the patient was evaluated in clinic for her preoperative assessment. On the day of the procedure, a Leksell G frame was applied to the patient's head under a combination of local anesthesia and conscious sedation. The patient then underwent DSA and MRI, which were used to complement one another during treatment planning (Figure 23.2). GammaPlan software was used to devise a single matrix overlay

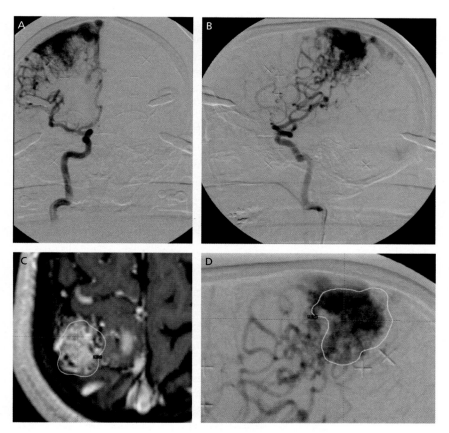

Figure 23.2 In a Leksell G stereotactic frame, the patient underwent repeat cerebral angiography for Gamma Knife planning. Representative anterior–posterior (A) and lateral (B) arterial phase angiograms are shown. (C) The GammaPlan software was used to devise a single matrix overlay using 20 isocenters to cover the nidus in a highly conformal fashion.

using 20 isocenters to cover the nidus in a highly conformal fashion. The AVM nidus was treated with a prescription dose of 16 Gy to the 50% isodose line (maximum dose of 32 Gy). The target volume was 9.32 cm³.

Oral Boards Review—Management Pearls

1. There is no perfectly defined algorithm for the management of AVMs. Small to medium-sized superficial AVMs located in noneloquent cortex are usually best treated with microsurgical resection. The AVM is typically shaped like a cone that tapers toward the nearest ventricle. A wide exposure is critical to identify feeding arteries, which are ligated early, and en passage vessels, which are preserved. The draining vein(s) should be left intact until the final stages of resection, when the nidus has been devascularized.

2. SRS depends on accurate alignment of preoperative imaging studies with the position of the patient during the procedure. For frame-based stereotaxy, as is used in GK SRS, the Leksell G frame should be affixed so that the borders of

the AVM nidus can be targeted. A sufficient number of fiducials, as is used in frameless approaches (e.g., CyberKnife), should be placed such that the region of interest is adequately covered.

3. Large AVMs may be managed with staged SRS using either a dose- or volume-staged approach. The outcomes for volume- versus dose-staged SRS are not considerably different, although volume-staged SRS may have a higher obliteration rate, whereas dose-staged SRS may have a lower risk of complications. Incompletely obliterated AVMs that have shrunken after the initial SRS procedure can be treated in a single session with repeat SRS.

4. The results of A Randomized Trial of Unruptured AVMs study and the Scottish Audit of Intracranial Vascular Malformations prospective AVM co-hort study have rendered the management of unruptured AVMs a highly controversial topic. Both studies reported significantly worse outcomes after intervention, compared to conservative management, for unruptured AVMs at interim follow-up. In general, SM grade I and II AVMs are favorable for intervention, whereas SM grade IV and V AVMs, particularly those without hemorrhagic presentation, should be monitored without treatment. SM grade III AVMs are heterogeneous, and their management depends on patient and nidal factors, although many can be safely and successfully treated with SRS.

Pivot Points

1. If the patient had presented with AVM rupture, she would be a candidate for acute or subacute intervention because the risk of subsequent hemorrhage is elevated compared to that for an unruptured AVM.

2. Both microsurgery and SRS for AVMs can improve seizure outcomes. Therefore, patients with AVM-associated seizures are reasonable candidates for treatment, and seizure control may be higher with surgical resection than with SRS.

Aftercare

The vast majority of patients are discharged home within a few hours after GK radiosurgery, following removal of the stereotactic frame. Patients are followed clinically and radiologically with MRI every 6 months after GK radiosurgery for 2 years and then yearly thereafter. Once AVM obliteration is diagnosed on follow-up MRI, catheter angiography is performed to confirm obliteration. Even after obliteration has been achieved, long-term clinical follow-up is important because some delayed post-SRS complications can have latency periods of up to several years.

In this case, the patient developed perilesional inflammation and edema consistent with radiation-induced changes (RICs), which was associated with mild and temporary worsening of her preoperative seizures 10 months following SRS. This adverse radiation effect was managed with a course of corticosteroids for several weeks, as well as adjustment of her anticonvulsant medication, with complete resolution of edema

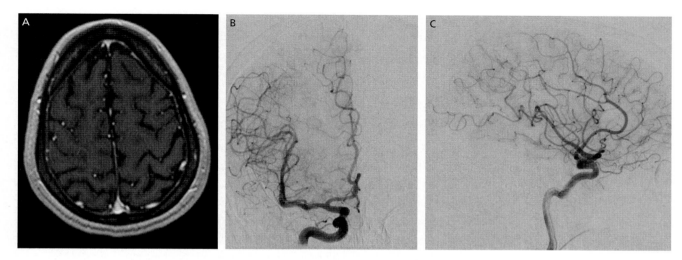

Figure 23.3 Two years following Gamma Knife radiosurgery, axial T_1-weighted post-contrast MRI showed resolution of the right frontal nidus (A), which was confirmed on subsequent cerebral angiography. Representative anterior–posterior (B) and lateral (C) arterial phase angiograms are shown.

on follow-up MRI. At 2-year follow-up, the patient underwent a diagnostic angiogram, which showed complete obliteration of the AVM (Figure 23.3). Her weakness had resolved, she denied any new-onset sensory disturbances, and her seizures were well controlled with anticonvulsant medication. The patient had been seizure-free for 1 year (Engel class IA outcome).

Complications and Management

Compared to microsurgical resection, one of the disadvantages of SRS for the treatment of AVMs is the time interval from intervention to obliteration, which can vary over a span of 1–3 years. During this latency period, the patient remains at risk for AVM hemorrhage, although this risk appears to be reduced compared to that of an untreated AVM. The most common adverse radiation effects after SRS for AVMs are RICs, which are evident as perinidal T_2-weighted hyperintensities on MRI. RICs are categorized as radiologic (any neuroimaging evidence), symptomatic (associated with neurological symptoms), and permanent if there is neurologic decline without recovery. Approximately one-third of AVM patients who undergo SRS will develop some form of RIC, and the rates of symptomatic and permanent RICs are approximately 10% and 3–4%, respectively. Less common post-SRS complications include delayed cyst formation, which occurs in approximately 3% of cases, and radiation-induced cavernoma or tumor development, both of which are extremely rare. Of note, the latency period for post-SRS cyst formation typically exceeds 5 years, highlighting the importance of long-term surveillance.

The vast majority of symptomatic RICs can be managed with medical therapy alone, usually including corticosteroids. Other therapies, such as glycerol infusions, bevacizumab, pentoxifylline, and vitamin E, have also been used in patients who do not respond to corticosteroids. Patients who develop new or worsening seizures related to RICs are treated with anticonvulsants. The majority of post-SRS cysts can be observed with serial imaging. However, surgical intervention should be considered for enlarging cysts or those causing new or worsening neurological symptoms. Superficial cysts requiring intervention should generally undergo fenestration or resection, whereas deep-seated cysts may be managed with shunt placement or stereotactic aspiration.

Oral Boards Review—Complications Pearls

1. Deep AVM location, larger AVM volume, and higher SRS dose are risk factors for symptomatic RICs after SRS. Patients with unruptured AVMs who undergo SRS are more likely to develop radiologic RICs which may or may not be symptomatic.

2. Routine and long-term follow-up are critical in AVM patients treated with SRS because both the benefits and complications of this modality manifest in a delayed fashion. The typical time periods are obliteration (60–80% of patients) in 2 or 3 years, RICs (radiologic in 30–35%, symptomatic in 10%, and permanent in 3% or 4% of patients) in 6–18 months, and cyst formation (3% of patients) in greater than 5 years. Medical therapy with corticosteroids is the first-line treatment for symptomatic RICs, and associated seizures should be managed with anticonvulsants.

3. Most patients who develop post-SRS cysts can be managed conservatively. Patients with enlarging or symptomatic cysts should be evaluated for surgical intervention, including resection, fenestration, stereotactic aspiration, or shunting.

Evidence and Outcomes

Several studies have shown that SRS is an effective treatment option for patients with small to medium-sized AVMs located in deep or eloquent brain regions. Although the SM grade was developed to stratify the operative risk of surgically treated AVMs, it has been shown to correlate with SRS outcomes as well. SRS outcomes can be predicted with VRAS or the modified radiosurgery-based AVM score, which is a weighted score comprising patient age, AVM volume, and AVM location (dichotomized as superficial vs. deep). In the current case, the AVM had a SM grade of III and a VRAS of 4.

Specifically regarding primary motor and somatosensory cortex AVMs, we analyzed a cohort of 134 patients who underwent SRS, with median radiologic and clinical follow-up durations of 64 and 80 months, respectively. The most common presenting symptoms were seizure and hemorrhage in 40% and 28%, respectively. Pre-SRS embolization was performed in 34%, the median AVM volume was 4.1 cm^3, and the median margin dose was 20 Gy. Obliteration was achieved in 63%, which was higher for AVMs less than 3 cm^3 (80%) compared to those greater than 3 cm^3 (55%). A lack of prior embolization ($p = 0.002$) and a single draining vein ($p = 0.001$) were independent predictors of obliteration in multivariate analysis. The annual post-SRS hemorrhage risk in the latency period prior to obliteration was 2.5%, and the overall rates of transient and permanent SRS-related morbidity were 14% and 6%, respectively.

In addition, SRS of AVMs improves seizure outcomes in the majority of patients, although many remain on anticonvulsant medications. Seizure control (abolition or reduction of seizures) is achieved in approximately 70% of patients with AVM-associated seizures after SRS, although seizure freedom is generally reported in less than half of patients. Patients with obliterated AVMs have been found to have more favorable seizure outcomes, and approximately one-third of patients are able to be weaned off of their pre-SRS anticonvulsant medications.

Further Reading

Al-Shahi R, Bhattacharya JJ, Currie DG, et al. Prospective, population-based detection of intracranial vascular malformations in adults: The Scottish Intracranial Vascular Malformation Study (SIVMS). *Stroke*. 2003;34(5):1163–1169.

Ding D, Starke RM, Kano H, et al. Stereotactic radiosurgery for Spetzler–Martin grade III arteriovenous malformations: An international multicenter study. *J Neurosurg*. 2017;126(3):859–871. doi:10.3171/2016.1.JNS152564.

Ding D, Starke RM, Kano H, et al. Radiosurgery for unruptured brain arteriovenous malformations: An international multicenter retrospective cohort study. *Neurosurgery*. 2017;80(6):888–898. doi:10.1093/neuros/nyx181.

Ding D, Starke RM, Quigg M, et al. Cerebral arteriovenous malformations and epilepsy, Part 1: Predictors of seizure presentation. *World Neurosurg*. 2015;84(3):645–652. doi:10.1016/j.wneu.2015.02.039.

Ding D, Yen C-P, Xu Z, Starke RM, Sheehan JP. Radiosurgery for primary motor and sensory cortex arteriovenous malformations: Outcomes and the effect of eloquent location. *Neurosurgery*. 2013;73(5):816–824. doi:10.1227/NEU.0000000000000106.

Ilyas A, Chen C-J, Ding D, et al. Radiation-induced changes after stereotactic radiosurgery for brain arteriovenous malformations: A systematic review and meta-analysis. *Neurosurgery*. 2018;83(3):365–376. doi:10.1093/neuros/nyx502.

Przybylowski CJ, Ding D, Starke RM, et al. Seizure and anticonvulsant outcomes following stereotactic radiosurgery for intracranial arteriovenous malformations. *J Neurosurg*. 2015;122(6):1299–1305. doi:10.3171/2014.11.JNS141388.

Starke RM, Kano H, Ding D, et al. Stereotactic radiosurgery for cerebral arteriovenous malformations: Evaluation of long-term outcomes in a multicenter cohort. *J Neurosurg*. 2017;126(1):36–44. doi:10.3171/2015.9.JNS151311.

Yen C-P, Sheehan JP, Schwyzer L, Schlesinger D. Hemorrhage risk of cerebral arteriovenous malformations before and during the latency period after GAMMA knife radiosurgery. *Stroke*. 2011;42(6):1691–1696. doi:10.1161/STROKEAHA.110.602706.

Carotid Cavernous Fistula Presenting with Vision Loss

Rajeev D. Sen, Louis Kim, and Michael R. Levitt

24

Case Presentation

A 57-year-old female with a past medical history of rheumatoid arthritis presents with 1 month of pain, decreased vision, and difficulty moving the left eye. This was accompanied by bulging of both eyes. She has no history of trauma. Detailed examination by the ophthalmologist revealed a visual acuity of 20/400 in the left eye and elevated intraocular pressures in both eyes, 27 mm Hg in the right and 30 mm Hg in the left. There was no afferent pupillary defect in either eye. There was a partial right abducens nerve palsy.

Questions

1. What is the most likely diagnosis?
2. What is the classic triad of symptoms?
3. What is the pathophysiology of vision loss in this entity?
4. What is the most commonly affected cranial nerve?
5. What are the typical findings on magnetic resonance imaging?

Assessment and Planning

Given the clinical presentation, the most likely diagnosis was a carotid cavernous fistula (CCF). Other entities on the differential include cavernous sinus thrombosis, neoplasm within the cavernous sinus, inflammatory pseudotumor, and Graves ophthalmopathy. There are two anatomical types of CCFs. Direct or type A CCFs typically result from trauma to the cavernous carotid artery or an inherent weakness in the vessel wall, such as a cavernous carotid aneurysm. Indirect CCFs are vascular shunts between meningeal branches of the external carotid artery (ECA) and/or internal carotid artery (ICA) and the cavernous sinus. In contrast to the direct type, indirect CCFs are low-flow malformations that are further subcategorized into type B involving meningeal branches of the ICA, type C involving those of the ECA, and type D involving those of both ICA and ECA. Between the major types, direct CCFs comprise approximately 75% of CCFs.

Direct CCFs can present with rapidly progressive symptoms due to the high velocity of blood flow through the ICA. Most commonly, this involves chemosis, proptosis, vision loss, ophthalmoplegia, and headache. Indirect CCFs may also present in a similar fashion, or they may present with cerebral venous congestion-type symptoms of

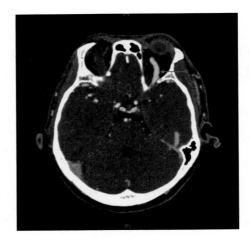

Figure 24.1 Presenting computed tomography angiogram demonstrating a markedly dilated left superior ophthalmic vein (arrow).

headache, confusion, and intracranial hemorrhage. Although a proportion of CCFs close spontaneously, timely diagnosis and intervention are imperative to minimize permanent deficits, most importantly vision loss.

Imaging studies that may suggest a diagnosis of CCF are computed tomography angiography (Figure 24.1) and magnetic resonance angiography. In addition to proptosis, engorged, tortuous vessels (specifically the superior ophthalmic vein) may be observed. The extraocular muscles may also be enlarged. The radiographic gold standard for diagnosis, however, remains a diagnostic cerebral angiogram (Figure 24.2). This will reveal shunting of blood from the carotid artery into the cavernous sinus manifested by early and rapid opacification of the cavernous sinus, petrosal sinuses, and/or ophthalmic veins.

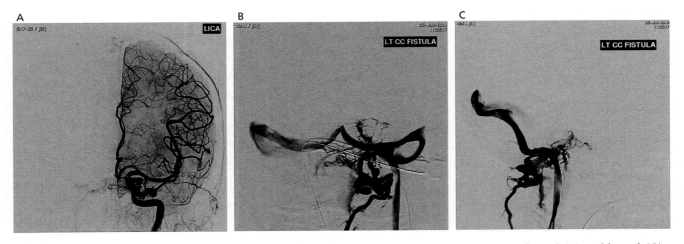

Figure 24.2 Preoperative catheter angiography with frontal (A) and selective venous views, frontal (B) and lateral (C), demonstrating the indirect left CCF.

Questions

1. What are the classic imaging findings for CCFs?
2. What are the distinct endovascular approaches to treat CCFs?

Oral Boards Review—Diagnostic Pearls

1. The classic triad for CCFs consists of chemosis, pulsatile proptosis, and ocular bruit.
2. Direct CCFs tend to have more rapid onset and progression of symptoms due to their high flow state.
3. Angiography maneuvers can assist in the characterization of CCFs.
   a. Huber maneuver: In the lateral view, the ipsilateral vertebral artery is injected while compressing the affected carotid artery. This reveals the upper extend of the fistula and whether there are multiple fistulous openings.
   b. Mehringer–Hieshima maneuver: Inject the affected carotid at a slow rate of approximately 2 or 3 mL/second while compressing the same carotid below the catheter tip. This provides a controlled injection allowing for clear identification of the fistula.

Decision-Making

The goal of treatment is to obliterate the fistulous connection between the carotid artery and the cavernous sinus, normalizing venous and intraocular pressures.

Some indirect, low-flow CCFs thrombose spontaneously and can be observed, assuming that the patient is clinically stable with normal intraocular pressures. A passive adjunct to observation involves compression of the ipsilateral cervical carotid artery using the contralateral hand. This maneuver decreases arterial inflow and increases venous drainage. Radiosurgery is another option for indirect CCFs either alone or in conjunction with endovascular treatment. However, due to the delay of several years in obliteration of the CCF, radiosurgery is rarely used. In contrast to indirect CCFs, direct CCFs are high-flow malformations and when symptomatic can lead to rapid deterioration. Clinical indications for emergent treatment in either direct or indirect CCFs include signs of venous hypertension such as epistaxis or otorrhagia, diplopia or headache, diminishing visual acuity, or stroke. Angiographic findings that suggest the need for emergent treatment include the presence of a pseudoaneurysm, cortical venous reflux, and thrombosis of venous outflows. Generally, urgent treatment is recommended.

Endovascular embolization remains the gold standard for management of CCFs. Two approaches are used either alone or in tandem: transarterial and transvenous. Direct CCFs are typically treated using the transarterial route. Indirect CCFs are often difficult to approach transarterially given the numerous small meningeal feeding vessels. Furthermore, ECA–ICA anastomoses as well as ECA supply to cranial nerves make the risk of arterial embolization unacceptably high. Although there are exceptions to this, such as indirect CCFs caused by trauma that commonly have large, single feeding arteries and type C indirect CCFs that involve only ECA feeders, the mainstay for treating indirect CCFs is via the transvenous approach.

Questions

1. What are the indications for emergent intervention for direct CCFs?
2. Which unique indirect CCFs can be treated transarterially?

Surgical Procedure

As mentioned previously, the transarterial route is more commonly employed for treatment of direct CCFs, whereas transvenous embolization is employed for indirect CCFs (Figure 24.3). In either case, arterial access is obtained in the usual fashion and can be done through the femoral or radial arteries. The patient is heparinized to maintain an activated clotting time of at least 250 seconds. A guiding catheter is advanced into the cervical ICA, and a microcatheter is navigated through the fistula into the cavernous sinus. There are several effective options for occlusion of the cavernous sinus. Detachable platinum coils can be easily controlled and adjusted for optimal placement within the cavernous sinus. However, due to the septations of the cavernous sinus, coils can collect within a single compartment, leading to incomplete obliteration of the sinus. This can cause backflow of venous blood into cortical veins, resulting in intraparenchymal hemorrhage, or into the superior ophthalmic vein, resulting in vision loss. To circumvent this risk, coils may be used in combination with liquid embolization material.

The two main liquid embolic agents are *N*-butyl cyanoacrylate (NBCA) and ethylene vinyl alcohol copolymer (Onyx). NBCA polymerizes rapidly and is highly effective with regard to cavernous sinus obliteration. However, it must be quickly deployed before it hardens; thus, it does not allow for angiographic monitoring during injection. Onyx, on the other hand, can be injected slowly. Furthermore, due to its viscous

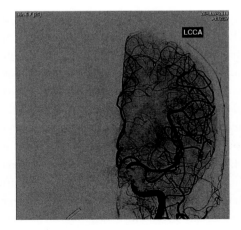

Figure 24.3 Direct postoperative catheter angiography after transvenous coil embolization demonstrating complete occlusion of the left CCF with a patent left internal carotid artery.

nature, Onyx improves penetration through the cavernous sinus septations. The major risk involved with liquid embolic agents is backflow into the arterial system, leading to embolic stroke, or into the superior ophthalmic vein. For this reason, coils are typically deployed prior to the use of liquid agents.

In the case of indirect CCFs, in addition to arterial access, transfemoral venous access is obtained and a guide catheter is advanced into the internal jugular vein. Typically, the cavernous sinus is accessed by navigating a microcatheter through the inferior petrosal sinus. However, if the inferior petrosal sinus is not accessible, alternative pathways to the cavernous sinus include the contralateral inferior petrosal sinus, the facial vein, and (via direct percutaneous puncture) the superior and ophthalmic veins.

More recently, stents have been used in the cavernous ICA across the fistula. Neoendothelialization along the stent results in exclusion of the cavernous sinus from the arterial circulation. Although stents have been shown to be highly effective for treatment of direct CCFs, successful deployment can be technically challenging due to the tortuous course of the cavernous carotid.

Questions

1. Why is it difficult to treat indirect CCFs using the transarterial route?
2. What are the major differences between the two liquid embolic agents, Onyx and NBCA?

Oral Boards Review—Management Pearls

1. Direct CCFs can be approached via the transvenous or the transarterial route. On the other hand, it is often only feasible to approach indirect CCFs through the venous system given the difficulty of catheterizing small meningeal feeders.
2. Indirect CCFs require embolization of the venous side to ensure no recruitment of new arterial feeders.
3. The balloon occlusion test to evaluate dependence on the ipsilateral carotid circulation can be falsely positive due to a vascular steal effect. The patient may develop neurologic deficits after carotid occlusion due to the fistula stealing retrograde flow as opposed to true dependence on carotid perfusion.

Pivot Points

1. If endovascular intervention fails to completely occlude the fistula while maintaining patency of the ICA, ipsilateral carotid occlusion is indicated, assuming the patient passes a balloon occlusion test.
2. If the patient cannot tolerate carotid occlusion and endovascular intervention fails, open surgery is possible and involves bypass and carotid occlusion in the case of direct CCFs or cavernous sinus packing in the case of indirect CCFs.

Aftercare

After completion of the procedure and withdrawal of catheters, hemostasis is typically achieved using a sealing device for the arterial site and manual pressure for the venous site. It is recommended that the patient lie flat for up to 6 hours in the case of venous access. Patients can be monitored in the intensive care unit during the first night for close neurological monitoring.

Ophthalmological evaluation is imperative in the acute post-procedure time period to formally assess and document the patient's visual acuity and extraocular movements. More important, persistently elevated intraocular pressures can be a sign of failure of the procedure. In patients who develop cranial neuropathies, it may be beneficial to initiate a short steroid course such as dexamethasone 4 mg every 6 hours for 5 days.

Assuming successful completion of the fistula and that no further complications arise, the patient should expect a relatively brief hospital course. Upon discharge, the patient should be counseled on the fact that clinical improvement can take anywhere from several hours up to 6 months. Patients who develop cranial nerve palsies should be informed that the deficit is likely transient; however, they should also be made aware of the possibility of permanent dysfunction. They should be scheduled for appropriate angiographic and ophthalmologic follow-up imaging.

Questions

1. How soon should patients expect improvement in their symptoms?
2. What is the purpose of post-procedure steroids?

Complications and Management

The major limitation to isolated coil embolization is partial occlusion of the cavernous sinus. As mentioned previously, this can result in redirection of venous blood flow into cortical veins or the superior ophthalmic vein, causing devastating hemorrhagic infarcts or vision loss. The best way to avoid this complication is to use a combination of coils and liquid embolic agents. It is also possible for coils to herniate through the fistulous component of the ICA, contributing to partial cavernous sinus occlusion. In these cases, it may be beneficial to use a balloon-assisted technique in which a balloon catheter is inflated within the cavernous ICA to maintain coils within the cavernous sinus as they are deployed.

A unique complication associated with liquid embolic agents is microcatheter retention due to a glue-like effect after solidifying. This tends to occur more often with NBCA given its property of rapid polymerization. To prevent this, it is recommended that one withdraw the microcatheter immediately after reflux is seen or to use a detachable microcatheter. Onyx has a tendency to spread, increasing the risk of injection into unwanted parts of the circulation such as into the ICA or the superior ophthalmic vein. Reasonable solutions are to use a balloon to protect the ICA from retrograde flow and to coil the superior ophthalmic vein prior to Onyx injection.

Cranial nerve palsies are also a possible complication given their location within the cavernous sinus. Often, this complication is due to mass effect of the embolization material. Although a majority are transient, persistent palsies can greatly increase the morbidity of the procedure. Coils tend to have a higher rate of cranial nerve palsies due to their larger mass effect. A combination of coils and liquid agents may minimize mass effect while obtaining adequate occlusion of the cavernous sinus.

Questions

1. What are the risks of incomplete obliteration of the CCF?
2. Which are more likely to cause cranial neuropathies, coils or liquid agents?
3. How can injection of liquid agents into the superior ophthalmic vein be avoided?

Oral Boards Review—Complication Pearls

1. Coil embolization has higher rates of cranial neuropathies due to mass effect.
2. The major risks of using liquid embolic agents are retrograde injection via the superior ophthalmic vein, causing vision loss, and distal embolism of liquid embolic agent into the carotid arterial territory.

Evidence and Outcomes

Given the rarity of CCFs, there are limited data comparing approaches or techniques. Several large series have reported success using detachable balloon embolization of direct CCFs; however, such balloon devices for CCFs are no longer available in the United States. More current data on treatment of direct CCFs are sparse. One study reported on the treatment of 40 direct CCFs using either balloons or, more recently, coils and either the transvenous or transarterial route. The study reported a successful occlusion rate of 82%, with 37.5% of cases requiring multiple treatments.

A retrospective review of 135 cases of indirect CCFs reported a cure rate of 90% using the transvenous route. In this series, 30% of cases underwent two or more procedures. Another study also found higher cure rates for indirect CCFs with the use of both coils and liquid agents as opposed to coils alone.

Further Reading

de Castro-Afonso LH, Trivelato FP, Rezende MT, et al. Transvenous embolization of dural carotid cavernous fistulas: The role of liquid embolic agents in association with coils on patient outcomes. *J Neurointerv Surg*. 2018;10(5):461–462.

Ducruet AF, Albuquerue FC, Crowley RW, McDougall CG. The evolution of endovascular treatment of carotid cavernous fistulas: A single-center experience. *World Neurosurg*. 2013;80(5):538–548.

Ellis JA, Goldstein H, Connolly ES Jr, Meyers PM. Carotid-cavernous fistulas. *Neurosurg Focus.* 2012;32(5):E9.

Korkmazer B, Kocak B, Tureci E, Islak C, Kocer N, Kizilkilic O. Endovascular treatment of carotid cavernous sinus fistula: A systematic review. *World J Radiol.* 2013;5(4):143–155.

Lewis AI, Tomsick TA, Tew JM Jr. Management of 100 consecutive direct carotid-cavernous fistulas: Results of treatment with detachable balloons. *Neurosurgery.* 1995;36(2):239–244.

Miller NR. Dural carotid-cavernous fistulas: Epidemiology, clinical presentation, and management. *Neurosurg Clin North Am.* 2012;23(1):179–192.

Incidental Ethmoidal Dural Arteriovenous Fistula

Ilyas Eli, Robert Kim, Richard H. Schmidt, Philipp Taussky, and William T. Couldwell

25

Case Presentation

A 64-year-old right-handed male with past medical history notable for hypertension, hyperlipidemia, and tobacco use presented with symptoms of intermittent left lower facial numbness, headaches, and occasional nosebleeds. Neurological assessment was unremarkable, with intact cranial nerves II–XII and normal motor and sensory examinations. His intermittent left lower facial numbness was concerning for transient ischemic attacks, and the patient underwent imaging for further evaluation. Magnetic resonance imaging of the brain was notable for chronic microvascular disease without any evidence of cerebral infarction. Magnetic resonance angiography demonstrated an incidental ethmoidal dural arteriovenous fistula (eDAVF).

Questions

1. What is the differential diagnosis?
2. What are the presenting clinical symptoms of patients with eDAVF?
3. What further imaging modality should be obtained for definitive diagnosis?

Assessment and Planning

Digital subtraction angiography (DSA) is the gold standard for evaluation of most intracranial vascular lesions. DSA demonstrated a fistula fed by branches of the bilateral ophthalmic arteries, more prominent on the left (Figure 25.1).

eDAVFs, also termed anterior fossa or cribriform plate dural fistula, are extremely rare intracranial vascular malformations with a high risk of rupture based on cortical venous drainage. Unlike other DAVFs with drainage into the neighboring transverse, sigmoid, or superior sagittal sinus, eDAVFs most often drain directly into cortical veins because of the lack of a large venous sinus in the anterior skull base. Therefore, these fistulas are always categorized as Borden classification III or Cognard classification III and IV, making them high-grade DAVFs with a high risk of rupture due to thin-walled cortical venous involvement. eDAVFs may be diagnosed due to hemorrhage, visual symptoms, seizures due to parenchymal scar from remote hemorrhage, epistaxis, or headaches with nausea and vomiting; many are found incidentally.

Differential diagnosis for this lesion includes arteriovenous malformation, cavernous carotid fistula, and vascular tumors such as hemangiopericytoma.

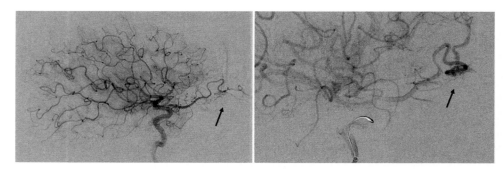

Figure 25.1 Internal carotid artery angiogram demonstrating eDAVF supplied by the ophthalmic artery supply and venous drainage into a cortical vein that drains into the superior sagittal sinus (arrows).

Oral Boards Review—Diagnostic Pearls

1. A detailed understanding of the anatomy is important for treatment.
   a. Arterial supply is most often from bilateral anterior ethmoidal dural branches of the ophthalmic arteries.
   b. Venous drainage is into frontal cortical veins, which drain into the superior sagittal sinus.
   c. eDAVFs can be associated with flow-related aneurysm and venous ectasias.
2. Preoperative DSA is essential for evaluation of eDAVFs.
3. Patients can present with symptoms related to frontal intracranial hematoma because these fistulas have a particularly high risk of hemorrhage. Other patient presentations include as an incidental finding, or with visual symptoms, seizures, epistaxis, or headaches.

A comprehensive understanding of the vascular anatomy using angiography is essential in assessing and planning treatment (Figure 25.2). Angiography often shows that the fistula's arterial supply originates from the anterior ethmoidal branches of the bilateral ophthalmic arteries. Other arterial supply may come from branches of the distal internal maxillary artery, superficial temporal artery, middle meningeal artery, cavernous internal carotid artery, or anterior cerebral artery. The venous drainage pattern is primarily into intracranial cortical veins (typically the frontopolar or orbitofrontal veins); however, drainage can also flow posteriorly into the posterior orbitofrontal or olfactory veins. Rare cases have drainage into the superior ophthalmic vein or inferior ophthalmic vein, which drain eventually into the superior sagittal sinus, inferior sagittal sinus, or cavernous sinus. Flow-related aneurysms and venous ectasia can be associated with these fistulas.

Questions

1. What is the arterial supply of an ethmoidal dural AVF?
2. What is the venous drainage pattern of ethmoidal dural AVF?
3. What is the risk of hemorrhage associated with ethmoidal dural AVF?
4. What are the treatment options for this type of fistula?

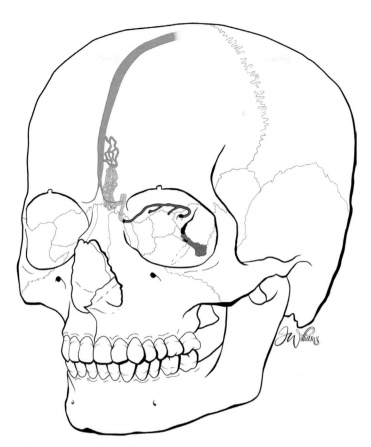

Figure 25.2 Illustration of an eDAVF.

Source: © Department of Neurosurgery, University of Utah.

Decision-Making

Because of their cortical venous drainage (Borden type III or Cognard types III and IV), eDAVFs have a high risk for hemorrhage and require treatment. The angioarchitectural heterogeneity of eDAVFs often requires neurovascular surgeons/interventionalists to tailor treatments for each patient. Currently, the treatment of choice for eDAVFs is either microsurgical disconnection or endovascular occlusion.

With their uncomplicated surgical anatomy, these lesions are traditionally managed through surgical disconnection of the fistula via a frontal cranial approach. Surgery is associated with a low morbidity rate and 100% rate of disconnection. Surgical approaches include pterional, orbitozygomatic, bifrontal, frontal, transfrontal sinus, or supraorbital craniotomy. These approaches enable interhemispheric exposure of the anterior skull base and the olfactory groove. Because of the cortical location of the fistula and noneloquent surrounding structures, microsurgery is considered relatively straightforward once adequate exposure is achieved. Arterialized veins typically arise through the floor of the cribriform plate and are usually easy to identify within the interhemispheric fissure. Vascular clips are used to occlude the fistulous flow across the arteriovenous system, and bipolar cautery is used to coagulate the draining vein, which effectively cures the eDAVF. Surgery should be favored in patients who have intracerebral hemorrhage because the surgical goal includes both hematoma evacuation and treatment of the fistula. Surgery should also be considered for patients with associated venous varices given the high risk of rupture and hemorrhage with this anatomical feature.

Endovascular treatment should be considered in patients with favorable angiographic anatomy, especially in those with surgical comorbidities. Endovascular embolization can be achieved via either transarterial or transvenous approach. The transarterial approach is generally preferred because it offers direct access to the fistulous site and because of the relative durability of the arterial walls compared with venous endothelium. In addition, the transarterial approach provides a shorter route to the fistula. The other option is the transvenous approach via the superior sagittal sinus, when a transarterial procedure fails or is not a feasible option. Endovascular glue is preferred to particle embolization because of its prolonged polymerization time and viscosity. One risk associated with endovascular treatment is vision loss resulting from embolization of the central retinal artery or branch of the ophthalmic artery. Embolization agents can also reflux into the intracranial circulation, causing remote strokes.

In our case, the patient underwent neuroendovascular treatment of the eDAVF. During the catheterization of the left ophthalmic artery, extravasation of contrast material was noted. Protamine sulfate was administered to reverse the patient's systemic heparinization. With the catheter remaining in this position, multiple attempts at coil embolization were made, but this resulted in coil and microcatheter herniation into the internal carotid artery. Repeat contrast injection of the vessel showed resolution of the extravasation. Given the difficulty of the endovascular attempt with the extravasation event, the procedure was aborted. Endovascular treatment was unsuccessful because of severe tortuosity of the feeding arteries, and the treatment attempt was complicated by vessel perforation and a small amount of resultant subarachnoid hemorrhage demonstrated on post-procedure noncontrast computed tomography. The patient's vision was not compromised.

Questions

1. What are the surgical options available for the treatment of eDAVFs?
2. How are eDAVFs obliterated surgically?
3. What are the two endovascular options utilized for embolization of eDAVFs?

Surgical Procedure

Plans were therefore made for a left frontal craniotomy via an eyebrow incision for occlusion of the fistula. The patient was pinned in the supine position with head extended. The left eyebrow incision was opened and dissected down to the calvaria. The left frontal sinus was marked out using neuronavigation. A craniotomy was performed, and the dura was exposed and then opened in a stellate fashion. Under the microscope, the frontal lobe was retracted, and an arterialized vein was readily identified within the interhemispheric fissure and traced back to its origin through the dura of the cribriform plate. The vein was then coagulated and clipped (Figure 25.3). The dura where the vein originated was coagulated. The distal aspect of the vein became dark blue and deflated, indicating successful fistula disconnection.

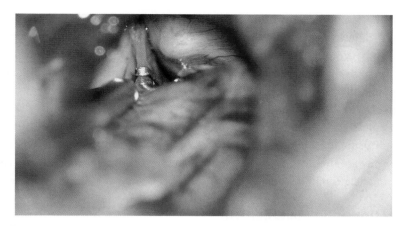

Figure 25.3 Intraoperative image demonstrating the vascular clip placed across the eDAVF.

Oral Boards Review—Management Pearls

1. Surgical disconnection is associated with 100% obliteration of the DAVF. Vascular clips are used to occlude the fistulous flow across the arteriovenous system, and bipolar cautery is used to coagulate the draining vein.
2. Endovascular treatment can be considered in patients with favorable angiographic anatomy.
3. Endovascular treatment can be achieved via a transarterial or a transvenous approach.

Pivot Points

1. Treatment of the eDAVF is recommended given its high propensity to hemorrhage. The choice between surgery and endovascular intervention depends on the angioarchitecture of the fistula and patient comorbidities.
2. If contrast extravasation is visualized during endovascular treatment, heparinization should be reversed, and the patient should be emergently referred for surgical treatment.
3. In surgical management of eDAVF with hemorrhagic presentation, hematomas and dilated cortical veins must be carefully manipulated to prevent rehemorrhage.

Aftercare

Aftercare of eDAVFs can differ substantially depending on the treatment modality, the initial presentation of the patient, and the presence or absence of periprocedural complications. Patients who undergo microsurgery or endovascular occlusion should be admitted to the neurocritical care unit for continuous arterial blood pressure monitoring and serial neurological examinations. This is especially important in cases in which the patient's initial presenting findings include intracranial hemorrhage to prevent rerupture, unless hemodynamically contraindicated. In addition, patients with progressively declining neurological deficit, seizure, cerebral edema, or vasospasm may require prolonged stay in the neurocritical care unit. Generally, patients who have undergone surgical resection of eDAVFs should undergo a postoperative angiogram prior to discharge to ensure complete obliteration of the fistulous connection. The absence of early venous drainage confirms the obliteration of the eDAVFs. Use of intraoperative indocyanine green may obviate the need for postoperative angiogram. Endovascular patients should receive frequent groin checks to ensure that no access site complications occur.

Complications and Management

Surgical Complications and Management

Complications that arise during the treatment of eDAVFs are often inherent to patient characteristics such as angioarchitecture of the eDAVF or to the type of procedure used to treat the fistula. In microsurgical disconnection, a low frontal or supraorbital craniotomy is often employed to expose the fistulous connection. The reported permanent complication rates from microsurgical disconnection of eDAVFs are very low, ranging from 0% to 20% depending on the patient's preoperative characteristics. These percentages are likely somewhat inaccurate due to the sheer rarity of the disorder. On the other hand, the success rates of occlusion have been reported to be 100% in almost all published case series. Despite the high success rate, potential complications should always be considered while attempting to obliterate the fistula via microsurgery. Upon exposure, patients with hemorrhagic presentation will often display blood clots around the fistula. Care must be taken to minimize the manipulation of the blood clots and cortical veins during exposure/disconnection, especially before vascular clip placement, to avoid bleeding under arterial pressure. In rare instances, a venous varix can be encountered with an even higher propensity to bleed. Adequate exposure and carefully executed proximal clipping will reduce the chances of complications such as intraoperative rupture.

Endovascular Complications and Management

Endovascular embolization may carry a higher potential risk profile compared with microsurgery and should be considered only in patients with favorable anatomy and surgical comorbidities. Complications such as vascular perforation or thromboembolic events can arise during the catheterization phase in tortuous arteries and veins and also during delivery of the embolisate. Occlusion of the major ocular arteries, including the central retinal artery or the ophthalmic artery, can occur because of migration of the embolisate. For example, a popular liquid embolic agent, Onyx, can reflux from the microcatheter during injection and potentially occlude the more proximally located central retinal artery. Microcatheter rupture and proximal migration of the Onyx embolisate resulting in acute retinal ischemia has also been reported. Occlusion of the central retinal artery can also occur during the catheter retrieval, as well as in cases of inadvertent dissection or vasospasm.

To circumvent complications that arise from arterial embolizations, transvenous approaches to eDAVFs have been suggested. The main advantage of a transvenous approach is that there is no concern for central retinal artery or ophthalmic artery occlusion. However, because of the inherent ectatic nature of the cortical draining veins, the transvenous approach carries a relatively risk of rupture during catheterization due to relatively thin draining veins.

Oral Boards Review—Complications Pearls

1. Postoperative monitoring of blood pressure and frequent neurological examination in the intensive care unit are recommended to prevent rerupture after treatment.
2. The risks of endovascular embolization include visual loss from reflux of embolic material into the central retinal artery and reflux into the intracranial circulation resulting in stroke.

Evidence and Outcomes

DAVFs account for approximately 10–15% of all vascular malformations, of which eDAVFs comprise 4–9%. Unlike DAVFs of the cavernous sinus, which predominantly affect females, eDAVFs have significant predilection for males of advanced age. Recently pooled data from 92 surgical cases of eDAVFs indicated that 80% of the cases involved males with a mean age of 60 years. Because drainage almost always involves pial veins before they empty into the nearby venous sinus, almost all eDAVFs are classified as Borden III or Cognard III, with high potential for hemorrhage from the pressurized venous channels. In addition, venous tortuosity or venous ectasia was found frequently, with the reported rate of up to 100%. These factors combine to play a role in the propensity of eDAVFs to hemorrhage in 50–84% of patients at presentation.

The surgical obliteration rate of eDAVFs has been nearly 100% in all clinical series performed. A pooled study of various clinical series demonstrated that eDAVF obliteration was achieved via a surgical approach in 100% (92/92) of patients. Some of the most important rationales behind the advocacy of surgical management for eDAVFs were (1) the near 100% efficacy and (2) the lack of associated visual complications secondary to arterial perforations or embolysate reflux. Therefore, surgery was considered the gold standard of eDAVF treatment.

Endovascular options have been historically avoided when treating eDAVFs because of the potential risk of visual complications; however, with advancements in endovascular techniques and technologies, more cases of eDAVFs are being treated with endovascular embolization with success. The success rate associated with the transarterial approach varies widely from 22% to 100%, often in small case series. In a multiple-center, retrospective study evaluating 24 patients with eDAVFs, 11 patients were treated microsurgically and 11 endovascularly. Seven of the 11 patients treated with an transarterial endovascular approach were cured, whereas 4 of the 11 patients failed the initial embolization therapy, eventually requiring open microsurgery. In a study of 4 patients who underwent transvenous embolization of eDAVF, a 100% rate of occlusion was achieved via the transvenous route; however, 1 patient had already failed a transarterial embolization attempt because of microcatheter rupture, resulting in retinal ischemia and acute vision loss. In light of this, one must carefully weigh the morbidity of microsurgery against the risk of vision loss with the endovascular approach.

Further Reading

Abrahams JM, Bagley LJ, Flamm ES, Hurst RW, Sinson GP. Alternative management considerations for ethmoidal dural arteriovenous fistulas. *Surg Neurol.* 2002;58(6):410–416.

Agid R, Terbrugge K, Rodesch G, Andersson T, Soderman M. Management strategies for anterior cranial fossa (ethmoidal) dural arteriovenous fistulas with an emphasis on endovascular treatment. *J Neurosurg.* 2009;110(1):79–84.

Cannizzaro D, Peschillo S, Cenzato M, et al. Endovascular and surgical approaches of ethmoidal dural fistulas: A multicenter experience and a literature review. *Neurosurg Rev.* 2018;41(2):391–398.

Gross BA, Moon K, Kalani MY, et al. Clinical and anatomic insights from a series of ethmoidal dural arteriovenous fistulas at Barrow Neurological Institute. *World Neurosurg.* 2016;93:94–99.

Lawton MT, Chun J, Wilson CB, Halbach VV. Ethmoidal dural arteriovenous fistulae: An assessment of surgical and endovascular management. *Neurosurgery.* 1999;45(4):805–811.

Limbucci N, Leone G, Nappini S, et al. Transvenous embolization of ethmoidal dural arteriovenous fistulas: Case series and review of the literature. *World Neurosurg.* 2018;110(4):e786–e793.

Martin NA, King WA, Wilson CB, Nutik S, Carter LP, Spetzler RF. Management of dural arteriovenous malformations of the anterior cranial fossa. *J Neurosurg.* 1990;72(5):692–697.

Tahon F, Salkine F, Amsalem Y, Aguettaz P, Lamy B, Turjman F. Dural arteriovenous fistula of the anterior fossa treated with the Onyx liquid embolic system and the Sonic microcatheter. *Neuroradiology.* 2008;50(5):429–432.

Transverse Sinus Arteriovenous Fistula Presenting with Tinnitus

John F. Morrison and Adnan H. Siddiqui

26

Case Presentation

A 53-year-old male is followed in the neurology clinic for chronic headaches and left-sided tinnitus. The headaches are characterized as migraines that are vascular in semiology with symptoms of vertigo. He averages one headache per week which he manages conservatively with acetaminophen. The left-sided tinnitus is described as a continuous, low-pitched, mechanical sound and is more noticeable when the surrounding environment is quiet, such as at night.

Several months before evaluation in the neurosurgery clinic, he visited the emergency department with a more severe headache. During this visit, magnetic resonance imaging (MRI) and magnetic resonance angiography (MRA) of the brain demonstrated a serpiginous area of parenchymal susceptibility in the left occipital lobe.

Questions

1. What is the differential diagnosis?
2. What are the next appropriate imaging examinations?
3. Is further outpatient evaluation or emergency admission warranted?

Assessment and Planning

The clinical presentation of dural arteriovenous fistulas (AVFs) varies widely, with signs or symptoms ranging from headache to cranial nerve deficit, exophthalmos, ophthalmoplegia, facial pain, pulsatile tinnitus, and hemorrhage. Evaluation of vascular headaches is uncommon for neurosurgeons and often undertaken by the primary care physician or a neurologist. Commonly, an MRI is obtained and sometimes this may demonstrate engorged or ectatic veins or thrombus within a vessel. Given the described imaging findings in our patient, concern for an arteriovenous malformation or AVF remains high.

Dural AVFs are most commonly classified by the Borden or Cognard classification system. Each system is based on an angiographic evaluation of the pattern of venous drainage and the extent of reflux to adjacent structures, such as draining veins or cortical parenchyma. Borden type I is arterial drainage only to a dural venous sinus, type II is arterial drainage to a dural venous sinus or cortical venous vein but with cortical reflux, and type III is drainage with cortical reflux only. Cognard type I is arterial drainage only to a dural venous sinus; type IIa is arterial drainage to a dural venous sinus, with retrograde venous reflux but without cortical venous reflux; type IIb is arterial drainage to a dural venous sinus, without dural venous reflux but with cortical venous drainage reflux; type IIa+b is arterial drainage to a dural venous sinus with reflux to the dural venous sinus and the cortical vein; type III is arterial drainage to a cortical vein; type IV is arterial venous drainage to a cortical vein with venous ectasia; and type V is a spinal dural venous fistula.

A detailed understanding of the arterial and venous anatomy of the fistula is imperative for treatment planning. Advanced MRA and computed tomography angiogram or angiography (CTA) technologies that allow temporal resolution, such as MRA time-resolved angiography with interleaved stochastic trajectories (TWIST) or four-dimensional (4D) CTA, may demonstrate the arteriovenous shunting in dural AVF. However, they are inadequate for treatment planning and best reserved for initial diagnosis or post-treatment radiographic surveillance. To devise a treatment strategy, all patients with suspicion of an AVF should undergo digital subtraction angiography (DSA). For a transverse sinus fistula, a complete six-vessel cerebral angiogram (internal carotid artery, external carotid artery, and vertebral artery on each side) is necessary because the arterial supply can arise from any or multiple arterial sources. Likewise, an extended venous phase during each angiographic injection helps one appreciate the underlying angioarchitecture, physiology, and flow dynamics of the fistula.

With conservative management, Borden type I dural AVFs may involute spontaneously, remain stable, or progress to type II. Whereas type I fistulas are usually observed, treatment modalities for higher grade lesions include endovascular or open surgical approaches. The goal of each of these approaches is to disrupt the fistulous connection at the arterial–venous interface, thus disconnecting the arterial supply from the venous drainage. Although stereotactic radiosurgery has been proposed as an alternative, this treatment is still investigational or used for salvage in most centers.

In the current case, the angiogram displays a dural–meningeal branch feeding the left transverse sinus directly with cortical, but not parenchymal, venous reflux (Figure 26.1).

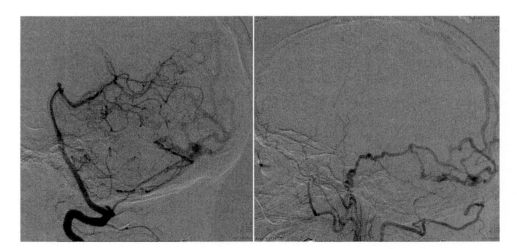

Figure 26.1 Lateral (left) and anteroposterior (right) left vertebral artery injections showing occipital artery, posterior auricular artery, middle meningeal artery, and posterior meningeal artery branches supplying the left transverse sinus.

Questions

1. What type of fistula is this? What Cognard grade? What Borden grade?
2. What are the treatment options?
3. What is the timing of treatment?
4. How should this lesion be approached (transarterial/transvenous/combined)?

Oral Boards Review—Diagnostic Pearls

1. Physical examination for subtle findings:
   a. Cranial nerve deficits: The most commonly involved cranial nerves are III, IV, VI, and VII, and these are readily evident on neurological examination.
   b. Conjunctivitis and exophthalmos: Venous hypertension can lead to increased venous pressure within the globe and orbit.
   c. Audible bruit: A retroauricular or orbital bruit may be auscultated with a stethoscope.
2. MRI and CTA may not display smaller, dural-based fistulas.
3. Cerebral DSA with a six-vessel injection is necessary for the vast majority of dural AVFs. A complete, long venous phase during the study also helps one to understand the angioarchitecture.

Decision-Making

Low-grade AVFs, Borden type I, have a low risk of hemorrhage or development of features indicating progression to a higher grade. Management can be conservative with symptomatic relief of headaches and radiographic surveillance with temporally resolved CTA or MRA; however, if symptoms are intolerable, surgical treatment may become necessary. Higher grade lesions have an increased risk of hemorrhage and should be managed with upfront endovascular, microsurgical, or combined treatment.

Endovascular treatment can be approached via transarterial, transvenous, or combined routes. Because the ultimate goal is to disconnect the fistula's arterial supply from the venous pouch, the transarterial approach may be insufficient, in which case a venous approach to embolize the fistulous sac becomes necessary. In the current case, combined microsurgical exposure of the feeding artery and selective arterial catheterization for transarterial injection of liquid embolic agent was undertaken in the hybrid operating room (Figure 26.2). This approach was chosen due to the extreme tortuosity of the proximal feeding artery and distal nature of the fistulous connection. The hybrid operating suite allows for open surgical procedures to be performed and combined with endovascular studies, and it is ideal for difficult cases that may require both approaches.

Questions

1. How does venous involvement change the surgical plan?
2. What is the hemorrhage risk?
3. What alternatives could have been selected?

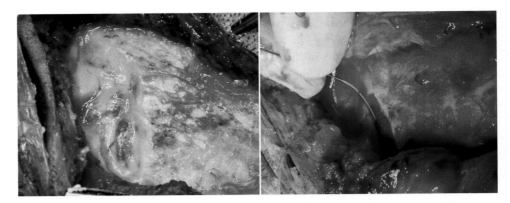

Figure 26.2 Intraoperative images demonstrating skeletonization of the extremely tortuous middle meningeal artery (left) and direct selective microcatheterization of the vessel (right).

Surgical Procedure

The procedure is performed in the neurointerventional biplane suite and can be conducted under conscious sedation or general anesthesia. We prefer conscious sedation because it allows the patient to be examined during the procedure for neurovascular changes and reduces the risks associated with general anesthesia. For patients requiring general anesthesia because of anxiety or continued motion, which makes intraprocedural visualization around the skull base more difficult, we typically perform neurophysiological monitoring, including electroencephalography, electromyography, and somatosensory evoked potentials.

The overarching goal of the procedure is to inject a liquid embolic agent at the fistulous arteriovenous connection point, filling the fistulous sac while avoiding reflux to feeding arteries or arterial anastomoses or embolus to the venous system. A planning diagnostic angiogram is necessary prior to the interventional procedure because understanding the vascular anatomy is paramount for a successful procedure. We routinely perform 3D rotational DSA and high-definition/high-speed digital angiography (≥15 frames per second [fps] as opposed to 3 fps on standard digital angiography). We utilize a 3D workstation for reconstruction of these studies to aid in our planning. This allows for determination of optimal working views of the biplane arms during the intervention, as well as an appreciation of adjacent arteries or veins at risk for injury or inadvertent occlusion during injection of the embolic agent. The main concern during planning is identifying dangerous intracranial anastomoses around the skull base whose embolization can lead to stroke as well as arterial supply to cranial nerves. In the case of transverse sigmoid junction fistulae, the main concerns are embolization into the anterior inferior cerebellar artery or posterior inferior cerebellar artery vessels as well as through tentorial branches into the internal carotid artery. The concerns of embolization through the middle meningeal artery are inadvertent occlusion of the petrosal branch, which supplies the geniculate ganglion (presenting itself with facial nerve palsy), the ascending pharyngeal branches (which can cause lower cranial nerve palsies with risk of impaired swallowing), or the ophthalmic artery via the lacrimal branch (which can cause blindness). Also of importance is protection the airway which can be compromised by embolization of the lower cranial nerves, sometimes necessitating post-procedure placement of a tracheostomy or gastrostomy tube.

The patient is taken to the neurointerventional suite and positioned supine on the angiography table. Conscious sedation is induced, and transfemoral or radial access is obtained with a 6 Fr sheath. The parent vessel of the artery supplying the fistula is selected. Extracranial and intracranial runs are obtained in anteroposterior (AP) and lateral planes, and working views are selected.

Selective microcatheterization of the artery supplying the fistula is undertaken, and an attempt is made to cross the fistula (if this cannot be accomplished, an alternative approach is chosen, such as a microsurgical cut-down or a transvenous approach). The "roadmap" function of the angiography software allows the previous injection run to be utilized to aid passage of the microwire and catheter. Microcatheter injection runs confirm placement of these devices at or close to the desired fistula connection point. Intraprocedural functional testing may be performed at this time with direct intra-arterial administration of sodium amobarbital and lidocaine to ensure no direct supply to neurologically active structures, as noted previously.

The choice of a liquid embolic agent is often institutionally dependent. The most common agents are N-butyl cyanoacrylate and an ethylene vinyl alcohol copolymer (Onyx). We typically use Onyx for treatment of an AVF or arteriovenous malformation. Onyx comes in ready-to-use vials containing the copolymer in two formulations, Onyx 18 and Onyx 34. These are then dissolved in dimethyl sulfoxide (DMSO) in various concentrations (6.0%, 6.5%, or 8.0%) with micronized tantalum powder for radiopacity. Onyx 18 is less viscous than Onyx 34; as the concentration increases, the viscosity of the Onyx also increases, allowing for more or less distal penetration with the embolic agent. Lower viscosity formulations are useful for deeper penetration in low-flow fistulas, whereas higher viscosity formulations are useful to create a primary, proximal plug. In the presented case, we completed the entire procedure with Onyx 34.

The microcatheter is pre-injected with DMSO to fill the catheter's dead space slowly, never exceeding a rate greater than 0.16 mL per minute, which can result in vasotoxicity. Onyx is then injected slowly under live fluoroscopy. Pausing after each incremental injection and obtaining angiographic runs via the guide catheter help assess the status of the placement of the embolic agent, as well as the status of adjacent vessels or draining veins. Complete obliteration of the fistula sac is necessary or the fistula may recur. Following completion of the embolic injections, final AP and lateral images are obtained, as well as other views and/or a 3D angiogram to assess the occlusion (Figure 26.3).

Oral Boards Review—Management Pearls

1. Complete occlusion of the fistulous connection and fistula sac is necessary; otherwise, a high risk of recurrence exists.
2. Slow injection of the liquid embolic agent allows for controlled occlusion of the feeding arteries and filling of the fistulous sac. Furthermore, appropriate selection of the concentration and viscosity of the embolic agent diminishes the risk of venous embolism during injection.

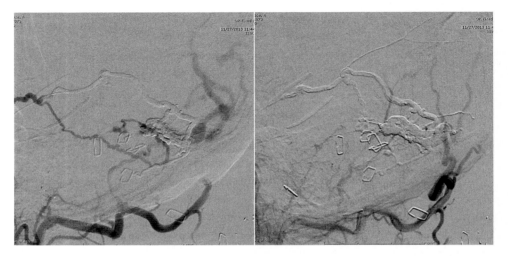

Figure 26.3 Intraoperative images demonstrating anteroposterior (left) and lateral (right) injections following fistula occlusion with Onyx liquid embolic agent.

Pivot Points

1. If a patient presents with a hemorrhage, the management of acute issues, such as mass effect, is necessary. Unless the patient is experiencing acute herniation, preoperative vascular imaging including DSA can be extremely important to avoid intraprocedural complications.
2. Evidence of venous reflux or ectasia represents an increased risk of future hemorrhage and should be addressed promptly.

Aftercare

Following successful endovascular treatment (complete or near-complete fistula occlusion), the patient is admitted to the neurointensive care unit for observation during the first 24 hours. Rapid changes in intracranial hemodynamics place the patient at an increased risk of periprocedural intracerebral hemorrhage; therefore, close monitoring is essential.

For transfemoral access, the patient is kept at bed rest and the leg is immobilized for 2 hours if an access site closure device is used or for 6 hours if the site is clamped. For radial access, we apply a pressure dressing, which is gradually lessened following a 2-hour period. We perform routine neurovascular examinations of the access site, monitoring for hematoma and distal pulses.

As with most endovascular procedures, periprocedural antibiotics are not administered. Antiepileptics or steroids are neither necessary nor indicated. Procedural pain tends to arise from the femoral or radial access site or the head. Headache is attributed to dural ischemia and typically self-limiting. In the acute setting, pain can usually be controlled with acetaminophen.

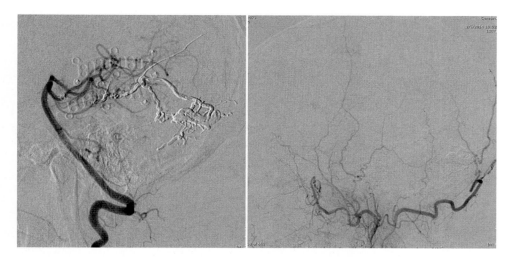

Figure 26.4 Follow-up angiogram at 6 months demonstrating lateral (left) and anteroposterior (right) vertebral artery injection with complete occlusion of the arteriovenous fistula.

There is follow-up in the clinic at 4 weeks. A follow-up 4D CTA or MRA TWIST is obtained at 3 months. We routinely perform a follow-up angiogram at 6 months, as in this case, in which the angiogram demonstrated durable complete occlusion (Figure 26.4).

Complications and Management

The most frequent complications involved in endovascular treatment of AVFs of the transverse sinus include inadvertent migration of the embolic agent; microcatheter retention; vessel injury; post-procedural venous hemorrhage; and the intrinsic risks of endovascular treatment, such as catheter-related stroke or access site dissection, hemorrhage, or infection.

Inadvertent injection of Onyx into a critical collateral vessel is managed by cessation of the embolic injection. The road map can be re-created with a new angiographic run and embolic injection can be resumed, which almost always results in injection into a different vessel. A thorough understanding of extracranial to intracranial anastomoses is necessary to avoid inadvertent injection of embolic material into the posterior circulation. Injection of embolic agent to the venous system may result in a pulmonary embolism. Although the volume of embolic material is typically small, it has been reported to result in significant hemodynamic changes and hypoxemia. However, this is extremely rare in the setting of dural AVFs, which are much lower flow lesions than arteriovenous malformations with direct arteriovenous high-flow fistulae. Complications can be avoided through careful selection and slow injection of the embolic agent. Management is conservative and with medical hemodynamic support (volume resuscitation, oxygen supplementation, and vasopressors).

One technique utilized to prevent venous embolization of the liquid embolic agent to central veins is transvenous access and balloon occlusion of the transverse sinus. This limits the outflow, allowing for hardening of the liquid embolic agent in the fistulous sac.

Another advantage is the prevention of occlusion of the draining sinus by protecting the lumen during liquid embolic placement within its walls, which is typically where the venous pouch and fistulae occur. Although in most cases with cortical venous reflux, the sinus is nonfunctional and occlusion is well tolerated, in a small number of cases, the sinus is still a key part of venous drainage of the brain and the patient may develop a venous hemorrhagic infarction after occlusion of the sinus. Careful review of venous drainage of the brain is critical for avoiding this complication; thus, the initial diagnostic angiographic runs should include both fistulous venous drainage and the later phase cortical venous drainage, which can also reveal whether the vein of Labbé drains functional tissue (in which case the origin must be preserved) or flows retrograde (and may be safely occluded).

The occurrence of catheter retention during embolic injection has been reported. If unable to free the catheter by gently pulling it, gentle traction at the access site and ligation of the catheter at the skin may be necessary. More recently, manufacturers have developed microcatheters with detachable tips that allow for the retained portion of the catheter to be included in the embolic plug. Limiting the amount of Onyx reflux proximal to the catheter tip reduces the risk of catheter retention.

As with any intracranial endovascular intervention, vessel injury can occur during arterial access in the form of flow-nonlimiting or flow-limiting dissections, which may require intraprocedural administration of a loading dose of dual antiplatelet agents and acute stenting of the dissected vessel. Injury may occur with a transvenous approach as well, and even more so when crossing a thrombosed segment. If injury occurs, it will be noted by contrast extravasation. Careful placement of detachable coils and liquid embolic should be used to rapidly address this event and prevent further hemorrhage.

Post-procedural venous hypertension and hemorrhage occur because of rapid changes in intracranial hemodynamics and venous drainage. Likewise, venous thrombosis can propagate and involve further venous sinuses, affecting the venous drainage of the brain more profoundly. This can be avoided with maintenance of adequate intravascular volume. Signs of hemorrhage, such as changes in mental status or new focal neurologic deficit, warrant an emergent head CT scan. Parenchymal hemorrhage due to venous thrombosis may be managed conservatively through systemic anticoagulation with an intravenous heparin infusion; however, larger or expanding hemorrhages may require surgical evacuation.

Procedure-related stroke is rare, and it is avoided with meticulous technique. Ensuring that any air bubbles are released from the system (pressure bag, stopcock, copilot, and catheter) before or during use is imperative. The use of a "double-flush" technique allows for continuous infusion while using a wire or contrast material and helps offset the risk of thrombus formation within or along the tip of the guide catheter. Vigilance of post-procedural neurovascular checks ensures early detection of periprocedural stroke. An emergent CT perfusion imaging stroke study and/or MRI diffusion-weighted imaging–fluid-attenuated inversion recovery helps clarify the cause of new post-procedural deficits. Management is dependent on time of detection. In most cases, there is no contraindication to intravenous thrombolytic therapy with tissue plasminogen activator, although a mechanical thrombectomy may be performed for large-vessel occlusions.

Groin site complications also are rare. Careful attention to vessel caliber prior to use of the closure device and to the formation of a groin hematoma or device failure during closure helps avoid escalating severity of complications. For closure device failure, the application of pressure for at least 20 minutes manually (if anticoagulation therapy has not been instituted) or with a clamp is necessary. Increased frequency of neurovascular and vital sign monitoring is required. Likewise, obtaining serial complete blood counts is indicated to detect an occult or retroperitoneal hemorrhage. For cases with further concern, a CT scan of the abdomen and pelvis is warranted and, if necessary, a consultation with a vascular surgeon should be held.

Oral Boards Review—Complications Pearls

1. A thorough understanding of the angioarchitecture, including the sinus anatomy and fistula point, venous ectasia, and any associated aneurysms, is necessary for selection of the proper approach.
2. Avoiding sacrifice of draining sinuses prevents complication risk.
3. Knowledge and avoidance of arterial anastomoses between the extracranial and intracranial circulation prevent unintentional arterial embolus leading to neurological deficit.
4. Knowledge of arterial supply to cranial nerve ganglia and avoiding their occlusion comprise the main strategy to avoid cranial nerve deficits.

Evidence and Outcomes

Early efforts to understand dural AVFs focused on classification of angioarchitecture and determination of hemorrhage risk. In 1996, based on a large series of 98 patients, it was determined that venous drainage patterns were the most significant factor for elevated risk of hemorrhage or neurologic deficit.

More recently, efforts to understand the natural history of dural AVFs have been described. A tendency for increased hemorrhage risk for higher grade (Borden II or III) lesions or evidence of venous outflow resistance has been reported. Based on a literature review and multicenter chart review that identified 16 studies with 328 patients with intracranial hemorrhage, outcome following AVF hemorrhage was investigated. Patients were included regardless of whether they had received treatment. At 12-month follow-up, mortality was 4.7%, and poor outcome (modified Rankin Scale score $\geq$3 and Glasgow Outcome Scale score $\leq$3) was 8.3%.

A 2017 case series described the experience with endovascular treatment in 36 patients with Cognard type I–IIb dural AVFs. The study differentiated sinus-preserving and sinus-occluding treatment with respect to the extent of liquid embolic invasion of the draining sinus. Sinus-occluding therapies had a higher rate of definitive treatment compared to sinus preserving (93% vs. 71%, respectively) but had a significantly higher complication rate (33% vs. 0%, respectively).

Acknowledgments

We thank Paul H. Dressel for preparation of the figures and W. Fawn Dorr and Debra J. Zimmer for editorial assistance.

Further Reading

Borden JA, Wu JK, Shucart WA. A proposed classification for spinal and cranial dural arteriovenous fistulous malformations and implications for treatment. *J Neurosurg.* 1995;82:166–179.

Chen CJ, Lee CC, Ding D, et al. Stereotactic radiosurgery for intracranial dural arteriovenous fistulas: A systematic review. *J Neurosurg.* 2015;122:353–362.

Cognard C, Gobin YP, Pierot L, et al. Cerebral dural arteriovenous fistulas: Clinical and angiographic correlation with a revised classification of venous drainage. *Radiology.* 1995;194:671–680.

Ertl L, Bruckmann H, Kunz M, Crispin A, Fesl G. Endovascular therapy of low- and intermediate-grade intracranial lateral dural arteriovenous fistulas: A detailed analysis of primary success rates, complication rates, and long-term follow-up of different technical approaches. *J Neurosurg.* 2017;126:360–367.

Gross BA, Du R. The natural history of cerebral dural arteriovenous fistulae. *Neurosurgery.* 2012;71:594–602.

Piechowiak E, Zibold F, Dobrocky T, et al. Endovascular treatment of dural arteriovenous fistulas of the transverse and sigmoid sinuses using transarterial balloon-assisted embolization combined with transvenous balloon protection of the venous sinus. *AJNR Am J Neuroradiol.* 2017;38:1984–1989.

Youssef PP, Schuette AJ, Cawley CM, Barrow DL. Advances in surgical approaches to dural fistulas. *Neurosurgery.* 2014;74(Suppl 1):S32–S41.

Large Temporal/Insular Cavernous Malformation Presenting with Headaches

Xiaochun Zhao, Claudio Cavallo, Evgenii Belykh, and Peter Nakaji

27

Case Presentation

A 21-year-old male presented with a 2-week history of nausea and vomiting along with worsening headaches and slurred speech for 1 week. Computed tomography (CT) scan showed a large, well-circumscribed hematoma in the left temporal–insular region with heterogeneous radiological findings (Figure 27.1).

Questions

1. What is the workup for an atypical hematoma of this type?
2. What laboratory tests should be considered for an intracranial hemorrhage?

Assessment and Planning

A few diagnoses should be included in the differential for a well-circumscribed hemorrhage with atypical features and a heterogeneous pattern on CT scan in a young patient. Intratumoral hemorrhage should be considered given the substantial mass effect, and magnetic resonance imaging (MRI) should be performed if there is a clinical and radiological suspicion. Partially thrombosed giant aneurysm can be another possible cause to include in the differential diagnosis because it shares similar radiological features. CT angiography (CTA) and cerebral angiography should be performed.

Blood coagulation studies such as platelet count, bleeding time, prothrombin time, partial thromboplastin time, and international normalized ratio should be considered as well for a young patient with intracranial hematoma. In addition, these laboratory studies should be routinely done preoperatively, and the use of antiplatelet or anticoagulant medications should also be investigated.

In this patient, the MRI scan showed a non-enhancing, heterogeneous, round lesion in the left temporal lobe interspersing with hemorrhagic components (Figure 27.2). The insular portion of the lesion extended medially into the posterior part of the internal capsule, and the right thalamus was displaced medially. A developmental venous anomaly was identified at the medial–posterior portion of the lesion. The angiogram did not reveal any aneurysm (Figure 27.3). All blood tests were shown to be within normal limits. Cavernous malformation was considered the most likely diagnosis.

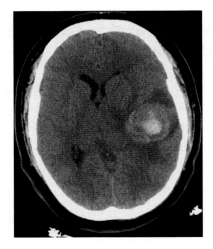

Figure 27.1 Preoperative CT scan showed a left temporal–insular round mass in high density with heterogeneous texture, which indicates hemorrhage.

Oral Boards Review—Diagnostic Pearls

1. Cavernous malformation is a vascular lesion with a heterogeneous pattern on MRI and usually negative findings on cerebral angiogram.
2. CTA and angiogram are necessary for the diagnosis to rule out other cerebrovascular lesions.
3. The coexistence of a cavernous malformation and a developmental venous anomaly is common.

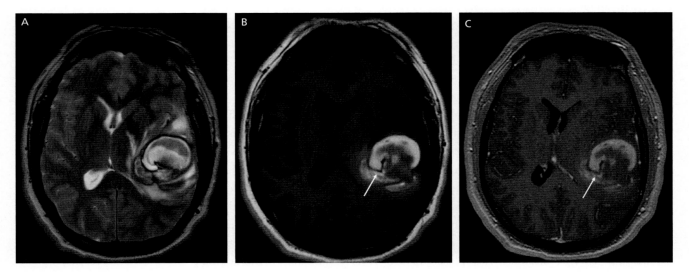

Figure 27.2 (A) MRI-T$_2$, (B) MRI-T$_1$, and (C) MRI-T$_1$ with contrast demonstrated a heterogeneous, well-circumferential lesion in the left temporal–insular region. The lesion was non-enhancing and contained a hemorrhagic compartment. A developmental venous anomaly was identified at the posterior–medial margin of the lesion (arrows).

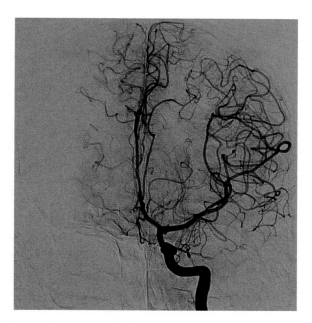

Figure 27.3 Angiograph was negative for any aneurysm.

4. Susceptibility-weighted imaging MRI (SWI-MRI) is a novel neuroimaging technique that is particularly useful for cavernous malformations because it is sensitive blood products such as deoxyhemoglobin and hemosiderin. SWI-MRI has a higher resolution compared to routine $T_2{}^\star$-weighted gradient-recalled echo images for detection of cerebral microbleeds.

Questions

1. What is the next best step in management?
2. What is the anatomical significance of a lesion in this area?

Decision-Making

Cavernous malformations are often asymptomatic. Acute symptoms may indicate either seizure or a hemorrhagic episode with a rapid increase in mass effect. Cavernous malformations in the temporal and insular regions in particular can present with a variety of symptoms, including seizure, language dysfunction, and motor or sensory deficits, depending on the anatomical location.

Surgical removal of a cavernous malformation is reasonable for patients with symptomatic presentation as long as the risk of surgical morbidity is lower than that of the natural history. Acute symptoms such as seizure or motor function deterioration usually indicate compression or irritation caused by acute hemorrhage. When there is a large or compressive hematoma, surgery should be performed to prevent permanent damage, and in the case of seizure, resection is often curative. The choice of surgical approach depends on the location of the lesion and the neural or neurovascular structures at risk of injury intraoperatively. For this patient, surgery was felt to be indicated given the size and symptoms of the lesion, and regular preoperative tests were carried out.

In terms of anatomical significance, cavernous malformations in the temporal and insular regions are bordered medially by critical structures such as the basal ganglia and the internal capsule. The claustrum is part of the external capsule and can be considered as the lateral limit of the basal ganglia. The surgical dissection should be stopped if the claustrum is encountered.

Lateral and medial lenticulostriate arteries are one of the most common causes of either ischemic or hemorrhagic events. They are also vulnerable during the resection of intrinsic lesions in the temporal and insular regions. Lateral lenticulostriate arteries are branches of middle cerebral artery, and medial lenticulostriate arteries are branches of anterior cerebral artery. Together, they provide blood supply to the basal ganglia. It is challenging to identify and follow these arteries given their large number (2–13 branches) and small size (80–1,400 μm).

Questions

1. What approaches can be used for lesions in the temporal–insular region?
2. What are the advantages and disadvantages for each approach?

Surgical Procedure

The trans-temporal approach or the trans-sylvian trans-insular approach can be used for intra-axial lesions in the temporal–insular region. The trans-temporal approach includes transgression of the superior or middle temporal gyrus, which can result in damage of language-related areas in the dominant hemisphere. The trans-sylvian approach involves sylvian fissure dissection to expose and create a cortical window in the surface of the insula or temporal operculum. The trans-sylvian approach provides a short and straight surgical trajectory, and it has been associated with better postoperative outcomes compared to the trans-temporal approach for basal ganglia hemorrhages. However, the risk of vascular damage during the dissection of the sylvian fissure should be considered.

For this patient, a temporal craniotomy for the trans-sylvian trans-insular approach was performed with the assistance of neuronavigation. The dura was opened in a cruciate fashion, the distal sylvian fissure was dissected, and an entry point was immediately identified because of the hemosiderin stain. A small cortical window was fashioned, and the lesion was encountered by visual identification of the hemosiderin discoloration of the brain. The hematoma was evacuated, and the lesion was circumferentially dissected out, while the developmental venous anomaly was meticulously preserved. Once the dissection was completed, the surgical cavity was fully inspected and hemostasis was achieved.

Oral Boards Review—Management Pearls

1. Surgical removal of a cavernous malformation is indicated symptomatic patients; however, surgical risks may lead to conservative management in some.
2. Hemosiderin stain in the cortical parenchyma can facilitate the identification of the lesion.
3. Careful inspection of the surgical cavity after lesion removal can prevent hemorrhage from residual.

Pivot Points

1. For deep-seated cavernous malformations in the brain parenchyma, localization can be difficult; intraoperative ultrasound can be used as a supplementary adjunct to assist in localizing the lesion.
2. Cavernous malformations with a more medial location may affect the basal ganglia and involve branches of the lenticulostriate artery. Surgical resection might be challenging, and a piecemeal resection is considered a safer method of debulking in such cases.

Aftercare

A good outcome is anticipated for a patient with cavernous malformation. An immediate postoperative CT scan is necessary to rule out postoperative hemorrhage. Antiepileptic medications should be continuously administered and then gradually tapered off during the next 3–6 months.

The patient recovered well postoperatively. His symptoms were improved, and he was discharged on postoperative day 3. He had no new deficits, and no seizures at delayed follow up.

Complications and Management

Complications and risks related to the surgical procedure vary based on the location of the lesion. For large cavernous malformations in the temporal–insular region, complications are associated with violation of deeper structures such as the internal capsule and lenticulostriate artery branches.

Intraoperative adjuncts can be used to identify the location of the internal capsule when it is medially displaced because of a substantial mass effect. Neuronavigation is essential to guide and delineate the area of surgical resection. Intraoperative subcortical electrical stimulation is recommended for mapping the internal capsule. Lateral lenticulostriate arteries are also at risk intraoperatively, and any injury might lead to

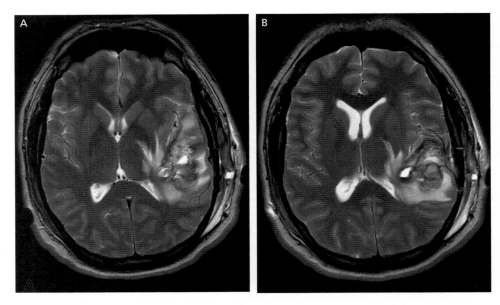

Figure 27.4 Postoperative MRI scan showed gross total resection of the cavernous malformation with preservation of the developmental venous anomaly.

subsequent ischemic strokes. Manipulation or violation of either the internal capsule or the lateral lenticulostriate arteries may lead to transient focal neurological deficits that are usually treated with postoperative rehabilitation and induced hypertension.

Oral Boards Review—Complications Pearls

1. Possible complications from the resection of a cavernous malformation are related to the location of the lesion.
2. Focal neurological deficits after resection of insular cavernous malformation can result from damaging deep structures, including the basal ganglia and lenticulostriate arteries.

Evidence and Outcomes

Excellent outcomes without any new neurological deficits should be the goal for all patients with cavernous malformations. Most preoperative symptoms may resolve after extensive rehabilitation. Postoperative MRI scan is effective for evaluating the presence of any residual. Annual MRI scan should be obtained for 2 or 3 years to detect recurrence.

In our patient, postoperative MRI scan showed that a gross total resection of the lesion was achieved (Figure 27.4). All symptoms improved postoperatively. He receives routine clinical follow-up.

Acknowledgment

We thank the staff of Neuroscience Publications at Barrow Neurological Institute for assistance with manuscript preparation.

Further Reading

Amin-Hanjani S, Ogilvy CS, Ojemann RG, et al. Risks of surgical management for cavernous malformations of the nervous system. *Neurosurgery*. 1998;42:1220–1227.

Bertalanffy H, Gilsbach J, Eggert H-R, et al. Microsurgery of deep-seated cavernous angiomas: Report of 26 cases. *Acta Neurochir*. 1991;108:91–99.

Duffau H, Capelle L, Lopes M, et al. The insular lobe: Physiopathological and surgical considerations. *Neurosurgery*. 2000;47:801–811.

Marinković S, Gibo H, Milisavljević M, et al. Anatomic and clinical correlations of the lenticulostriate arteries. *Clin Anat*. 2001;14:190–195.

Tatu L, Moulin T, Bogousslavsky J, et al. Arterial territories of the human brain cerebral hemispheres. *Neurology*. 1998;50:1699–1708.

Wang X, Liang H, Xu M, et al. Comparison between transsylvian–transinsular and transcortical–transtemporal approach for evacuation of intracerebral hematoma. *Acta Cir Bras*. 2013;28:112–118.

Wu A, Chang SW, Deshmukh P, et al. Through the choroidal fissure: A quantitative anatomic comparison of 2 incisions and trajectories (transsylvian transchoroidal and lateral transtemporal). *Neurosurgery*. 2010;66(6 Suppl Operative):221–229.

Yaşargil M, Von Ammon K, Cavazos E, et al. Tumours of the limbic and paralimbic systems. *Acta Neurochir*. 1992;118:40–52.

Small Cavernous Malformation Presenting with Medically Refractory Epilepsy

John R. Williams, Gabrielle A. White-Dzuro, Michael R. Levitt, and Andrew L. Ko

28

Case Presentation

A 31-year-old right-handed male presents to clinic for a second opinion of his medically refractory epilepsy. His seizures started 7 years ago and have continued despite multiple antiepileptic medications. He describes his seizures as twitching of the left face and arm, as well as temporary altered consciousness. He has had an extensive workup, including video electroencephalography (EEG) monitoring that showed right temporal predominance of his seizures. Magnetic resonance imaging (MRI) of the brain without contrast was done as part of the workup; it showed a heterogeneous $1.5 \times 1.3 \times 1.1$-cm mass in the right superior temporal lobe without significant surrounding edema (Figure 28.1). On examination, he is neurologically intact with no deficits.

Questions

1. What type of seizures does the patient suffer from?
2. What is the most likely diagnosis?
3. What is the most appropriate imaging modality?

Assessment and Planning

The neurosurgeon suspects that this patient's complex partial seizure disorder arises from a cerebral cavernous malformation (CCM). The differential diagnosis for this mass lesion includes a cavernous malformation, an arteriovenous malformation (AVM), a hemorrhagic contusion, or a hemorrhagic neoplasm. Given the classic "popcorn" or "mulberry" appearance on MRI, this lesion most likely represents a cavernous malformation.

MRI remains the most clinically useful, sensitive, specific, and diagnostic modality for cavernous malformations (Figure 28.1). It often shows a classic lobulated and variegated popcorn appearance with a rim of signal loss due to hemosiderin. T_2-weighted gradient echo or susceptibility-weighted sequences are more sensitive than T_1- or T_2-weighted images, which vary depending on the age of the blood products. If a recent hemorrhage has occurred, edema may be present. The lesions generally do not enhance, although it is possible.

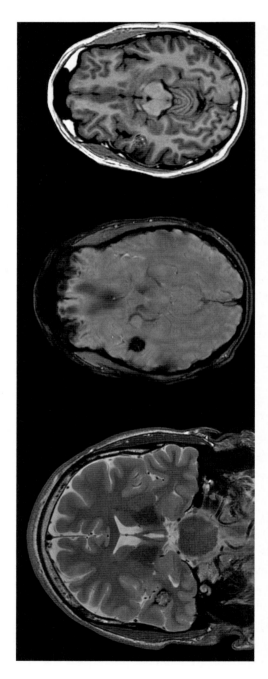

Figure 28.1 Preoperative MRI. (Left) Coronal T_2-weighted sequences demonstrate a mixed-intensity right superior temporal lesion with a hemosiderin ring. (Middle) Susceptibility-weighted sequences show greater sensitivity to blood products. (Right) T_1-weighted contrast-enhanced sequences demonstrate the heterogeneous nature of lesion enhancement.

Other workup for this patient will be determined based on the location of the lesion and the indication for surgical consultation. As mentioned previously, MRI is the most useful modality in diagnosis and surgical planning. Given the low-flow nature of these lesions, diagnostic cerebral angiography and other vascular imaging are expected to be negative, but they can be helpful to obtain to rule out an AVM or another high-flow lesion.

In this case, the patient presents with a lesion in his nondominant temporal lobe and medically intractable epilepsy; thus, further workup and discussion should be had about treatment options. The patient has already had video EEG, which suggested that his seizures arise from the nondominant temporal lobe, meaning they are most likely secondary to the lesion. Functional MRI or a Wada test should be completed to confirm the lack of language cortex on the right side.

Oral Boards Review—Diagnostic Pearls

1. Imaging is important to accurately diagnose the lesion.
   a. T_2 gradient echo with the classic "popcorn" pattern.
   b. Classically "angiographically occult." Venous flow is too slow to appear on CT angiography, MR angiography, or invasive angiography.
   c. Often seen in conjunction with developmental venous anomalies (DVAs), which will be apparent on venous phase angiography and/or T_1-contrasted MRI.
2. Presentation is usually determined by local irritation from blood products, most commonly headaches, seizure, or focal neurological deficit.
3. CCMs are a common cause of epilepsy. In patients presenting for consideration of epilepsy surgery, further workup including video EEG, functional MRI, and positron emission tomography scan may be completed.

Questions

1. What are the management options for this lesion?
2. What is the most appropriate timing for intervention in this patient?

Decision-Making

Options for management of these lesions include observation and surgical resection. Gamma knife radiosurgery has been studied; however, more recent data suggest outcomes with radiation therapy are equivalent to those associated with the natural history of the disease.

There are two separate approaches to CCMs—one in which the goal of surgical resection is the relieve epilepsy and the other in which surgery is performed to reduce the risk of CCM hemorrhage or improve a focal neurological deficit.

When considering surgery for medically refractory epilepsy (MRE), it is important to consider the goal of surgery and the likelihood of seizure freedom. Outcomes for seizure freedom are influenced by a variety of factors, including whether a patient has MRE, chronic epilepsy, or sporadic seizures. In a recent study that included 76 patients with CCMs and MRE, there was a seizure freedom rate of 88% at 2 years. In this study, MRE was more common in patients with temporal localization of CCMs, and in 84% of the cases, a more extensive resection was performed. Studies have shown that longer symptom duration is associated with worse seizure outcomes. It is believed that operating early decreases the likelihood of kindling and therefore prevents the development of an "epilepsy" syndrome.

Other reasons to resect a CCM are if there is an accessible lesion with a focal deficit that would be worsened by subsequent hemorrhage or if there is currently symptomatic hemorrhage. In these cases, it is important to consider the natural history of the lesion. Hemorrhage of these lesions is believed to be rare, with an annual rate of 0.5–1.1%. Several factors suggest an increased risk of hemorrhage, including age younger than 45 years, female gender, infratentorial location, and the presence of a dural venous anomaly. The risk of hemorrhage is highest in patients whose lesions have characteristics of prior hemorrhage on imaging.

As mentioned previously, gamma knife radiosurgery is a controversial option. In a retrospective series of 96 patients who underwent gamma knife for high surgical-risk cavernous malformations, the annual rate of hemorrhage decreased from 3.06% pretreatment to 1.4% during the first 3-year latency interval and 0.16% thereafter. Four patients developed new location-dependent neurological deficits, and 3 patients had edema-related headaches; all of these patients recovered fully.

Surgical Procedure

Microsurgical resection of a cavernous malformation is a major procedure carried out under general anesthetic with a Foley catheter and duplicate intravenous access in place. Based on the location of the lesion, intraoperative neuromonitoring including somatosensory evoked potentials (SSEPs) and motor evoked potentials (MEPs) can alert the surgeon to ischemia during resection. Intraoperative electrocorticography (ECoG) can also be used to help determine the extent of resection in cases of MRE. In this case, given the location of the lesion within the temporal lobe and years of intractable epilepsy, the operative strategy included planning for an extended lesionectomy, intraoperative corticography, and potential tailored anterior temporal lobectomy with resection of mesial structures if evidence of independent mesial temporal epileptiform activity was seen on ECoG.

Patients are positioned based on the location of the lesion. For the lesion in question, the patient is placed supine with his head turned toward the left, away from the lesion. Preoperative imaging for stereotactic intraoperative navigation can be used to localize the CCM. A curvilinear incision is made, beginning at the zygomatic arch, 1 cm anterior to the tragus, and arcs to the midline behind the hairline. After skin incision, the scalp and temporalis muscle are mobilized forward as a myocutaneous flap. Using stereotactic navigation, a craniotomy is planned to allow access to the lesion as well as to allow for an anterior temporal lobectomy. The dura is tacked up circumferentially, and hemostasis is obtained. The dura is then opened with a C-shaped incision based just superior to the sylvian fissure. The superior temporal gyrus and middle temporal gyrus are identified and confirmed with intraoperative neuronavigation. Intraoperative ultrasound can be used in addition to navigation to further confirm the location of the lesion and identify the best trajectory for resection. In patients undergoing epilepsy surgery, further invasive monitoring including ECoG may be completed at this stage. Electrode coverage over the lesion and perilesional cortex is ensured, and subtemporal electrodes are also used to cover mesial temporal structures. If independent spiking activity is visualized from the mesial temporal lobe structures, a complete temporal lobectomy can be performed in addition to resection of the lesion.

The microscope is brought into the field, and circumferential dissection of the cavernous malformation is performed. As discussed previously, the extent of resection will be based on the indication for surgery. If the goal of surgery is a reduction in seizures, most advocate removal of the surrounding hemosiderin ring. If lesion removal is the goal, or the lesion is located adjacent to an eloquent structure, then the hemosiderin-stained cortex can be preserved.

DVA identification and avoidance is critical. In CCMs primarily diagnosed on noncontrast MRI, either CT angiography or contrasted T_1 sequences should be obtained to identify nearby DVAs. DVAs drain normal brain tissue, and inadvertent resection or injury may result in venous infarction; thus, DVAs associated with CCMs should be preserved during resection.

If used, MEPs and SSEPs are monitored throughout the surgery. In case of changes during resection, immediate cessation of further resection is important to prevent permanent neurological deficit. After irrigation, the dura is closed with running 4–0 sutures, and the bone flap is replaced with titanium plates and screws. Temporalis muscle, galea, and skin are then closed in a sequential fashion using a combination of sutures and staples.

Oral Boards Review—Management Pearls

1. The following are indications for surgery:
   a. Recurrent bleeding with progressive neurological deficits
   b. Seizures or intractable epilepsy
2. In patients with epilepsy, intraoperative ECoG can be performed to determine the extent of resection.
3. DVA identification and preservation prevents inadvertent venous infarction.

Pivot Points

1. If the goal of surgical resection is to reduce the risk of subsequent hemorrhage, then a lesionectomy is all that is required. However, if the goal of surgery is to reduce seizures related to the CCM, then resection of the lesion, hemosiderin ring, and possibly mesial temporal lobe structures should be performed, especially if ECoG demonstrates epileptiform activity.
2. Many lesions can be removed nearly en bloc. However, careful inspection of the resection cavity after lesion removal often leads to the discovery of

> additional lesion in pockets of cortex or in difficult-to-visualize areas. The entire lesion must be removed to ensure reduction in hemorrhage risk (and seizure frequency, if applicable).

Aftercare

In the immediate postoperative setting, imaging and serial examinations should be obtained to assess for treatable, postoperative complications. A postoperative head CT is obtained to evaluate for any immediate postoperative hemorrhage. Small postoperative hemorrhages require additional imaging to confirm stabilization and may require a longer period of time in an inpatient setting for observation, whereas an unexpected, larger hemorrhage with significant mass effect often requires immediate return to the operating room for evacuation. Serial, frequent neurological exams in an intensive care setting are part of the standard of care for patients having craniotomies for CCM resection. Serial exams can shed light on evolving postoperative issues, such as delayed hemorrhage or edema with mass effect, seizure, or venous thrombosis.

Blood pressure should be controlled to avoid delayed hemorrhage from instrumented blood vessels in the operative field. In patients with epilepsy, antiepileptic medications should be continued indefinitely until seizure freedom on medication has been established. In the absence of preoperative seizures, antiepileptic medications are often administered in the postoperative period because manipulation of the cortex is an independent risk factor for seizure. A short course of high-dose corticosteroids, such as dexamethasone, can help prevent secondary neurologic injury resulting from edema and treat common postcraniotomy symptoms including headache and nausea.

After discharge, the patient's incision site should be checked 1 or 2 weeks postoperatively. Repeat MRI should be obtained no sooner than 3 months after surgery to allow time for resolution of iatrogenic blood products, which may obscure the extent of resection. If completely resected, the risk of hemorrhage is thought to be negligible. However, persistent hemosiderin staining prevents radiographic confirmation of gross total resection. Frequency of follow-up and imaging can be reduced over time if patients remain stable clinically and radiographically.

Complications and Management

Risk of postoperative hemorrhage is lower with CCMs than with other high-flow vascular malformations such as AVMs, and postoperative hypotension is not usually required. Complete surgical resection is necessary because residual cavernous malformation would have continued risk of hemorrhage and seizure. Repeat resection may be necessary if residual lesion is seen on postoperative MRI or if rehemorrhage occurs in a previous CCM resection cavity.

One of the major risks in CCM resection is damage to structures surrounding the lesion. The most common complication of a temporal lobectomy (up to 22% in one study) is a visual field defect, usually a superior quadrantiopsia. However, some surgeons do not consider this a complication because they believe it to be an expected outcome of the surgery.

With a temporal lobectomy, nearby structures include the anterior choroidal artery and cranial nerve IV. With injury or spasm of the anterior choroidal artery, one can expect to find the triad of contralateral hemiplegia, contralateral hemisensory loss, and homonymous hemianopsia. Postoperative hemiparesis occurs at a rate of approximately 2%, with most being a mild permanent hemiparesis. The incidence of trochlear nerve palsy has been reported to be approximately 2% as well, the majority of which resolve spontaneously.

Oral Boards Review—Complications Pearls

1. Complete surgical resection of the lesion is necessary to decrease risk of hemorrhage and seizure.
2. Complications of a temporal lobectomy include visual field defect, anterior choroidal stroke, and cranial nerve IV palsy. Identification of relevant anatomy, preservation of the anterior choroidal artery, and avoidance of transgressing the medial pia mater can reduce the incidence of complications.

Evidence and Outcomes

Cavernous malformations are benign, low-flow vascular lesions that are commonly surrounded by a hemisoiderin-stained rim of tissue due to repeat microhemorrhages. They have an incidence of approximately 0.15–0.56 per 100,000 persons per year. The most common symptoms during presentation are headache, seizures, and focal neurologic deficits. Rupture rate in cohort studies has been reported to be between 0.5% and 3.1% per year, but it is commonly accepted to be between 0.5% and 1.1% per year. The risk of developing associated seizures has been reported to be 2.4% per year.

Most CCMs are supratentorial in location, with 10–23% in the posterior fossa and approximately 5% found in the spine. Approximately 50% of them are familial in origin and can be associated with mutations such as KRIT-1, which can be found more commonly in Hispanic patients. Multiple lesions are seen more commonly in familial forms. In patients with more than one lesion or a strong family history, the entire neuraxis should be imaged to assess for additional lesions.

CCMs are highly epileptogenic, and chronic epilepsy is one of the most common clinical manifestations of supratentorial lesions. Seizures and epilepsy occur in 40–70% of patients with CCMs, and it is believed that the epileptogenicity of CCMs depends on the location of the lesion more so than intrinsic epileptogenicity from the CCM.

Surgical resection is considered for cerebral and cerebellar CMs that are symptomatic and in noneloquent locations. Lesions causing seizure can be managed with antiepileptic medications initially, although progressive seizure or unacceptable functional disability with medical management are indications for surgery.

Further Reading

Englot DJ, Han SJ, Lawton MT, Chang EF. Predictors of seizure freedom in the surgical treatment of supratentorial cavernous malformations. *J Neurosurg.* 2011;115(6):1169–1174. doi:10.3171/2011.7.JNS11536.

Ruan D, Yu XB, Shrestha S, Wang L, Chen G. The role of hemosiderin excision in seizure outcome in cerebral cavernous malformation surgery: A systematic review and meta-analysis. *PLoS One.* 2015;10(8):e0136619. doi:10.1371/journal.pone.0136619.

Stapleton CJ, Barker FG 2nd. Cranial cavernous malformations: Natural history and treatment. *Stroke.* 2018;49(4):1029–1035. doi:10.1161/STROKEAHA.117.017074.

Upchurch K, Stern JM, Salamon N, et al. Epileptogenic temporal cavernous malformations: Operative strategies and postoperative seizure outcomes. *Seizure.* 2010;19(2):120–128. doi:10.1016/j.seizure.2009.11.006.

Ruptured Brainstem Cavernous Malformation

Stephan A. Munich and Jacques J. Morcos

29

Case Presentation

A 51-year-old female presented with a history of multiple cavernomas. Over many years, she has had symptoms of right-sided weakness that last for 1 or 2 weeks, followed by resolution after physical therapy. The offending lesion was thought to be a left frontal cavernous malformation (CM) (Figure 29.1), and this was resected by an outside neurosurgeon. Despite resection of this lesion, she had two more episodes of transient right hemiparesis. Repeat magnetic resonance imaging (MRI) revealed an increase in size of a left mesencephalic CM (Figure 29.2). She was transferred to our institution for management of this lesion.

Neurologic examination revealed near complete recovery from her most recent episode of right hemiparesis. Cranial nerve function was intact. Right upper and lower extremity strength was 4+/5. Left upper and lower extremity function was 5/5.

Questions

1. What are the genes associated with multiple CMs?
2. Which imaging modalities should be used (and which are not necessary) in the diagnostic workup?
3. Are the clinical features different for familial versus sporadic CMs? How about supratentorial versus infratentorial locations?

Assessment and Planning

The mesencephalic lesion has the classic radiographic "popcorn" appearance of a CM. This appearance is due to previous hemorrhage, a constant finding of CMs, which, combined with the deposition of hemosiderin, forms their characteristic appearance on MRI.

Cavernous malformations account for 10–15% of all vascular malformations of the nervous system. In both autopsy and radiographic studies, the incidence of CMs has been reported as between 0.3% and 0.5% of the general population. The majority of these occur in the supratentorial space, but approximately 15% of CMs occur in the brainstem.

Cavernous malformations occur in two forms: sporadic and familial. The sporadic form is discovered incidentally in 20–30% of cases, during investigation for unrelated symptoms. These typically occur as isolated lesions and may become symptomatic due

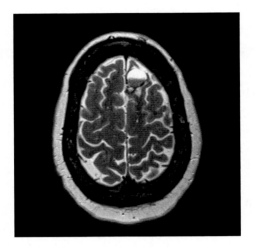

Figure 29.1 Axial T_2-weighted MRI demonstrating the resection cavity of a left frontal cavernous malformation.

to seizure or focal deficit due to enlargement secondary to hemorrhage. Due to variable definitions of CM hemorrhage (radiographic, symptomatic, etc.) across studies, the annual hemorrhage rate is typically estimated at 1–3%. However, one hemorrhage has been found to be a primary risk factor for a subsequent hemorrhage, with annual rates of rehemorrhage reported to range from 4.5% to 22.9%.

The familial form is characterized by three or more lesions and autosomal dominant inheritance with high but incomplete penetrance. Mutations of three loci have been found to be responsible for 96% of familial CM cases: the *CCM1* gene (chromosome 7q21), the *CCM2* gene (chromosome 7p13), and the *CCM3* gene (chromosome 3q26). The natural history of familial CMs is less well-defined. In a study of 59 members of six families, 61% of those harboring CMs were symptomatic, and the rate of development of a new lesion was 0.4% per patient per year. The incidence of symptomatic hemorrhage was 1.1% per lesion per year (6.5% per patient per year).

The risk of hemorrhage of brainstem CMs may be higher than that in other locations. In a large systematic review and meta-analysis of 25 studies, the annual incidence of hemorrhage of brainstem cavernomas was 2.8% (compared to 0.3% in non-brainstem locations), and the annual rate of rehemorrhage was 32.3% (compared to 6.3% in non-brainstem locations).

Oral Boards Review—Diagnostic Pearls

1. Cavernous malformations are occult on digital subtraction angiography and have a characteristic "popcorn" appearance on T_2 and gradient-echo MRI. However, imaging in the acute period in the presence of hematoma may obscure recognition of a thrombosed arteriovenous malformation (AVM). Therefore, the presence of a thrombosed AVM should be considered (albeit unlikely) even in the presence of these characteristic imaging findings.

2. Susceptibility-weighted, $T_2^\star$, gradient echo, or proton density MRI sequences exhibit high sensitivity in detecting CMs and often will reveal more lesions than can be revealed by enhanced T_1 sequences.

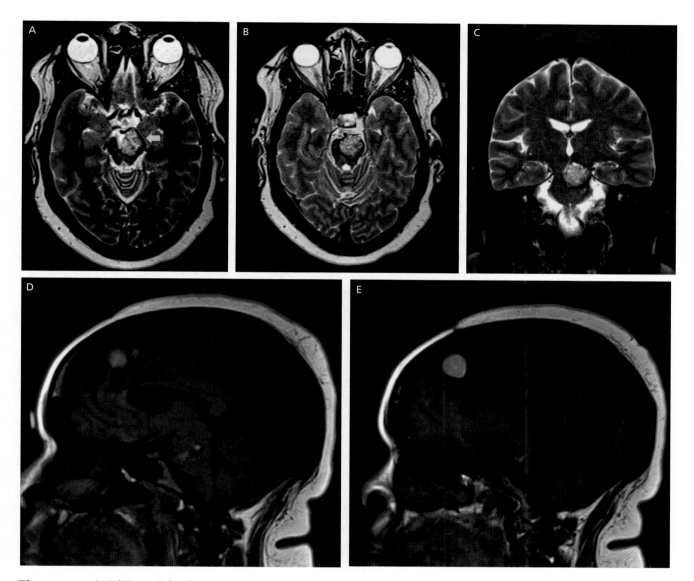

Figure 29.2 Axial T$_2$-weighted MRI demonstrating the intimate association of the cavernoma with the left posterior cerebral artery (A) and superior cerebellar artery (B) (arrows). Coronal T$_2$-weighted MRI (C) and sagittal T$_1$-weighted MRI (D and E) show the cavernous malformation located in the left mesencephalon and rostral pons.

3. Developmental venous anomalies (DVAs) are very frequently associated with CMs. It is postulated that DVAs play a significant etiological role in the formation of CMs, although exact pathophysiological mechanisms are not clear. The presence of a typical DVA with a "caput medusa" appearance reinforces the diagnosis of CM.

4. The clinical presentation of symptomatic CMs, particularly the familial/multiple lesions type, often mimics that of relapsing–remitting multiple sclerosis. This is because both diseases can present with spontaneous, repetitive attacks in the nervous system separated by space and time, resulting in cumulative deficits.

Questions

1. How does lesion location affect management?
2. What is the role of radiosurgery in the treatment of CMs?
3. What is the appropriate timing for resection of acutely ruptured CMs?

Decision-Making

The patient has a history of multiple CMs. Recently, she was clearly symptomatic from her left frontal CM—presenting with right hemiparesis and hemorrhage around that lesion. Given the symptomatic nature of the lesion and its superficial location, microsurgical resection is a relatively straightforward decision. However, the decision to operate on a brainstem CM should be made only with a firm understanding of safe entry zones, an appreciation of the distortion of fiber tracts due to the presence of the lesion, and a frank discussion with the patient regarding potential immediate and long-term morbidity. Although immediate postoperative morbidity is high (29–67%), long-term neurologic condition is the same or improved in as many as 89% of patients.

With a greater appreciation for anatomy and improvement in surgical microscopes, microsurgical techniques, instrumentation, and intraoperative navigation, lesions of the brainstem are no longer "off limits." The choice of approach depends primarily on an interplay of two pathoanatomical factors: (1) the location of eloquent fiber tracts and nuclei and (2) the location of the most superficial portion of the CM. These two factors may dictate two different surgical angles, and the eloquence of traversed brainstem tissue—if any—trumps all other factors.

Lesions of the midbrain are often most easily accessed using a trans-sylvian approach. For those in the ventral or ventrolateral aspect of the mesencephalon, a "half-and-half" (pretemporal, trans-sylvian) approach adds the ability to work on both sides of the oculomotor nerve. For lesions located laterally, a subtemporal approach may be all that is needed, with or without splitting of the tentorium, depending on exact rostrocaudal relation to the incisura. It would be unusual to require a more involved approach, such as an anterior petrosal or a posterior (presigmoid) petrosal approach. These are more likely to be used for pontine CMs not easily amenable to a retrosigmoid approach. Access to the dorsal and dorsolateral mesencephalon (i.e., posterior to the lateral mesencephalic sulcus) can be obtained using a supracerebellar infratentorial approach.

For brainstem CMs adjacent to the pial surface, a trajectory that accesses this point should be considered to avoid unnecessary injury to overlying mesencephalic fiber tracts. For those not approaching the pial surface, knowledge of and adherence to brainstem safe entry zones are critical to avoid neurologic morbidity. In the current case, a half-and-half (pretemporal, trans-sylvian) approach was used. As mentioned previously, the benefit of the pretemporal component of this approach is more anterolateral access to the lesion, which is where the lesion approached the pial surface. The lesion did not extend particularly superiorly. Therefore, the orbital rim and zygoma were not removed because there was no need to achieve an upward trajectory.

A subtemporal approach could have been used in this case. Although it would have also achieved an exposure of the superficial portion of the lesion, the axis of visualization of the deeper part would have been less favorable, given that the long axis of the lesion was more in the anterior–posterior direction than in the transverse direction. Furthermore, the approach requires temporal lobe retraction, which increases the risk of retraction injury and venous congestion. Retraction of the temporal lobe can be mitigated partially by placement of a lumbar drain. Additional risks associated with a subtemporal approach include ophthalmoparesis due to manipulation of cranial nerve (CN) III and CN IV.

The role of radiosurgery for the treatment of CMs remains unconvincing. Most reports suggest that radiosurgery is largely ineffectual in the durable treatment of CMs. Yet, reports from experienced radiosurgery centers have claimed its safety and efficacy in the reduction of rebleed rate for CMs located in areas of high surgical risk. They report annual rehemorrhage after stereotactic radiosurgery of 10.8–12.3% within the first 2 years after stereotactic radiosurgery and 0.8–1.1% thereafter. Many would counter-argue that these results are simply a reflection of the natural history of CMs that are well known to exhibit temporal clustering of bleeding episodes. Adverse effects of radiation were observed in 13% of patients.

Questions

1. What are the different surgical approaches for ventral, ventrolateral, lateral, and dorsal midbrain CMs?
2. What associated structure must be preserved during the resection of CMs to prevent postoperative venous infarction?

Surgical Procedure

Resection of a brainstem CM necessitates an experienced surgical and anesthesia team. It is our preference to wait 2–4 weeks after an acute rupture before resection. By this time, the acute clot has liquefied, but adherent scar has not yet formed.

General anesthesia is used with monitoring of brainstem evoked potentials, somatosensory evoked potentials, motor evoked potentials, and appropriate cranial nerves. In this case, we monitored CNs III, IV, and VI. Stereotactic navigation can be extremely helpful in confirming the surgical trajectory, particularly when the CM is in a subpial location and will not be seen on the brainstem surface.

For the trans-sylvian and half-and-half approaches, the patient is positioned supine with the head turned approximately 20 degrees to the contralateral side. The pterional craniotomy is performed with particular attention to removal of the lesser sphenoid wing, thereby exposing the temporal tip. Critical to the half-and-half approach is a wide splitting of the sylvian fissure. The anterior bridging veins joining the sylvian venous system to the sphenoparietal sinus are coagulated and cut to permit mobilization of the temporal tip posteriorly (the sylvian veins are preserved).

Thorough arachnoid dissection commences, and the exposure can be seen to be centered on the oculomotor nerve at the depth. Continued arachnoid dissection through Liliequist's membrane exposes the basilar artery and ventral surface of the midbrain and pons (Figure 29.3). When the CM comes to the pial surface, discoloration can be seen on the brainstem surface, which directs the surgeon's entry into the lesion (Figure 29.4).

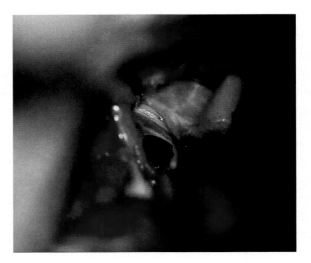

Figure 29.3 Left-sided "half-and-half exposure" demonstrating opening of Liliequist's membrane behind cranial nerve III.

When the lesion is completely subpial, there may be no discoloration at the surface, and brainstem safe entry zones must be utilized to gain access to the lesion.

In contrast to many supratentorial, cortical CMs, brainstem CMs are typically resected in a piecemeal fashion. Extracapsular dissection and en bloc removal are not tolerated in the brainstem due to the proximity of critical fiber tracts and brainstem nuclei. Similarly, whereas supratentorially, hemosiderin-stained perilesional brain is often removed in the interest of reducing epileptogenesis, this parenchyma is left in situ in the brainstem (Figure 29.5). Any associated DVA should be preserved.

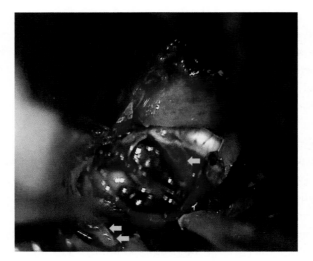

Figure 29.4 Visualization of the cavernous malformation following mobilization of the posterior cerebral artery (arrow) and duplicated superior cerebellar artery (double arrow).

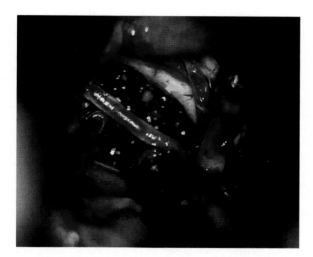

Figure 29.5 Coagulated cavernous malformation in situ. Coagulation of the lesion assists in shrinking the lesion to create surgical space as well as in identifying a dissection plane (arrow) between the lesion and the brainstem. The resection is carried out on either side of the superior cerebellar artery, which is seen coursing centrally over the cavernoma.

Following removal of the CM, the resection cavity should be inspected. In this particular case, in view of the size of the cavity, we used a 30-degree endoscope to inspect the entire surface of the cavity wall (Figure 29.6). It is essential to leave no residual CM because recurrence will be likely. Partial removal of a CM may be associated with a persistent (and possibly higher) risk of recurrent hemorrhage from the residual lesion. In ventral and ventrolateral mesencephalic CMs, the superior and superolateral aspect of the cavity must be thoroughly inspected because extension into the thalamus is possible.

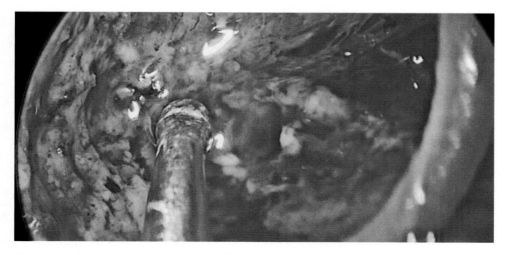

Figure 29.6 Endoscopic inspection of the resection cavity (using a 30-degree endoscope) demonstrating no residual lesion.

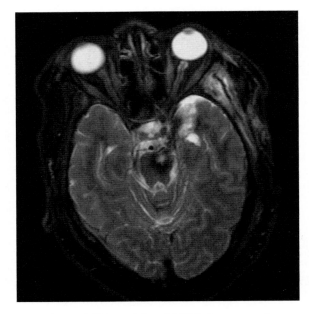

Figure 29.7 Postoperative axial T_2-weighted MRI demonstrating no residual cavernous malformation.

Oral Boards Review—Management Pearls

1. Complete resection of a CM is necessary to eliminate the risk of recurrent hemorrhage. Blood clots can easily mimic CM tissue; therefore, all suspicious tissue must be thoroughly inspected and resected if necessary.
2. Although there are conflicting data regarding resection of a DVA associated with a CM, most surgeons believe that preservation of the DVA is compulsory. The surgeon should proceed with the assumption that a DVA is present, even if one is not seen on MRI.

Pivot Points

1. If a midbrain CM extends into the thalamus, removal of the orbital rim may augment the surgical corridor by allowing a more inferior to superior trans-sylvian trajectory.
2. If a midbrain CM extends into the pons, removal of the petrous apex (anterior petrosectomy/Kawase approach) may augment the surgical corridor by allowing a more superior to inferior trans-sylvian trajectory.
3. Rarely, the presence of hemorrhage may obscure the recognition of a true AVM. Intraoperative discovery of a nidus and true AVM mandates a pivot to the basic principles of AVM surgery—occlusion of arterial inflow and preservation of venous outflow until all inflow has been occluded.

Aftercare

Resection of a brainstem CM, regardless of approach, is a delicate operation. The presence of pneumocephalus, hesitation to extubate the patient, and temporary disruption of arousal pathways often result in a delay in the return to baseline cognitive status and may result in prolonged intubation. During this time, it is critical to provide all routine and supportive intensive care unit measures (deep venous thrombosis prophylaxis, oral care, frequent position changes, etc.) to avoid postoperative medical complications.

Although there is no evidence to support immediate postoperative imaging, we elect to get an MRI as soon as possible (Figure 29.7). This allows assessment of the brainstem, particularly in terms of the presence of any infarct. Given the high periprocedural morbidity but low long-term morbidity, this radiographic assessment provides insight into prognosis and recovery of function.

Pharmacologic and mechanical deep venous thrombosis prophylaxis is started on postoperative day 1. Mobilization is begun as soon as possible. Assessments by physical and occupational therapy are essential for obtaining the appropriate rehabilitation needed to recover from the immediate postoperative deficits. Follow-up imaging with MRI is performed at 6 months and periodically thereafter. Recurrence of CMs in the brainstem is more likely than in less eloquent regions, as is residual CM after surgical resection.

Complications and Management

Injury to a DVA is the most feared complication of CM resection. This is amplified when operating on CMs of the brainstem. We believe the conflicting data in the literature regarding the importance of DVAs to be heavily influenced by reporting bias (i.e., surgeons not reporting the devastating complications associated with resultant venous infarction). Therefore, we take every measure to avoid disruption of the DVA. Should injury occur, postoperative care is supportive, including aggressive hydration, serial imaging to follow progression, and early mobilization and rehabilitation to promote recovery of any neurologic deficit.

Given the operative approaches and corridors needed to access the brainstem, retraction injury may occur. The risks of retraction injury to the temporal lobe during a subtemporal approach have been discussed previously. Retraction injury to the temporal tip during a half-and-half approach is also possible but generally well tolerated due to the thorough untethering resulting from a full sylvian fissure splitting. Retraction injury may result in neurologic deficit not attributable to the site of the offending pathology. It may be seen on postoperative imaging as fluid attenuation inversion recovery hyperintensity or restricted diffusion (when severe). Management of retraction injury is supportive, with measures to combat associated edema (steroids) or increased intracranial pressure (osmotic therapy).

Well known to neurosurgeons is the vulnerability of the oculomotor nerve. Simply its exposure, as in subtemporal, half-and-half, and trans-sylvian approaches to the brainstem, may result in a partial CN III palsy. Recovery of function is often spontaneous over time. Although there are no data to support the practice, many surgeons administer a short course of steroids to aid in recovery.

Complications related to arterial ischemia during brainstem surgery for CMs are rare. The mechanism is likely related to the injury of small perforator arteries.

Oral Boards Review—Complications Pearls

1. Assessment of patients' language dominance and lesion location is critical when considering surgical approaches to the brainstem. Avoidance of undue retraction on the dominant temporal lobe can prevent postoperative retraction injury and neurologic deficit.
2. Diffusion tensor imaging and tractography MRI, coupled with intraoperative navigation, may allow a more detailed understanding of brainstem fiber architecture and a safer planning of entry zones and surgical trajectories.

Evidence and Outcomes

As previously discussed, the natural history of brainstem CMs may be more ominous compared to that of their supratentorial counterparts. In summary, the rate of hemorrhage approaches 5% per person per year, and the rate of subsequent hemorrhage has been reported to range from 21% to 76%.

Prospective randomized controlled trials for the management of ruptured brainstem CMs are lacking. Although microsurgical access to the brainstem is a daunting proposition, in experienced hands, resection of CMs in this location can be performed with good long-term results (albeit with a high perioperative, temporary morbidity).

Recent guidelines, based on a systematic review of the literature, have recommended the following regarding brainstem CMs:

1. Surgery is not recommended for asymptomatic CMs, especially in eloquent, deep, or brainstem areas (class III, level B).
2. After reviewing the high risks of early postoperative mortality and morbidity and impact on quality of life, it may be reasonable to offer surgical resection of brainstem CMs after a second symptomatic bleed because those CMs might have a more aggressive course (class IIb, level B).

With knowledge of surgical approaches to the brainstem and brainstem safe entry zones, CMs of the brainstem can be resected with good long-term neurologic outcomes. As previously mentioned, immediate postoperative morbidity tends to be high (29–67%) but temporary, with long-term good neurologic outcome occurring in more than 80% of patients. Therefore, it is critical to have a detailed discussion with the patient and his or her family prior to surgical resection.

Further Reading

Akers, A, Salam RA, Awad IA, et al. Synopsis of guidelines for the clinical management of cerebral cavernous malformations: Consensus recommendations based on systematic literature review by the Angioma Alliance Scientific Advisory Board Clinical Experts Panel. *Neurosurgery.* 2017;80(5):665–680.

Cavalcanti DD, Preul MC, Kalani MY, Spetzler RF. Microsurgical anatomy of safe entry zones to the brainstem. *J Neurosurg*. 2016;124(5):1359–1376.

Giliberto G, Lanzino DJ, Diehn FE, Factor D, Flemming KD, Lanzino G. Brainstem cavernous malformations: Anatomical, clinical, and surgical considerations. *Neurosurg Focus*. 2010;29(3):E9.

Gross BA, Batjer HH, Awad IA, Bendok BR. Brainstem cavernous malformations. *Neurosurgery*. 2009;64:805–818.

Gross BA, Lin N, Du R, Day AL. The natural history of intracranial cavernous malformations. *Neurosurg Focus*. 2011;30(6):E24.

Taslimi S, Modabbernia A, Amin-Hanjani S, Barker FG 2nd, Macdonald RL. Natural history of cavernous malformation: Systematic review and meta-analysis of 25 studies. *Neurology*. 2016;86(21):1984–1991.

Spinal Dural Arteriovenous Fistula Presenting with Myelopathy

Vinayak Narayan and Anil Nanda

30

Case Presentation

A 36-year-old male who works as an elevator operator presents to the neurosurgery clinic with symptoms of mid-dorsal back pain and weakness of bilateral lower limbs. The symptoms have progressed gradually during the past month. He does not have leg pain, incontinence, or sexual dysfunction. Past medical and family history is unremarkable. Neurological examination reveals bilateral spastic paraparesis with 3/5 strength in all muscle groups. The deep tendon reflexes are brisk bilaterally, and the sensation is reduced in both lower limbs. His rectal tone and perianal sensation are intact. There is no spinal deformity or focal tenderness. The rest of the general and neurological examination is within normal limits.

Questions

1. What is the differential diagnosis?
2. Where can the lesion be localized clinically and why?
3. What is the most appropriate imaging modality and why?

Assessment and Planning

The differential diagnoses of progressive bilateral spastic paraparesis includes spinal dural arteriovenous fistula (DAVF) or arteriovenous malformation (AVM), neoplasm (either extradural or intradural), autoimmune disease, infection, trauma, and prolapsed intervertebral disk. The lesion can be localized to the thoracic or lumbar spine, given the upper motor neuron signs and the bilateral symptoms without upper limb involvement. Prompt radiological workup should take place given the progressive symptoms and pathological reflexes. Magnetic resonance imaging (MRI) with and without contrast, as well as spinal MR angiography, can be helpful in further defining the pathology. In the current case, spinal MRI reveals multiple flow voids in serpentine fashion dorsal to the spinal cord extending from T9 to T11. There is no evidence of cord edema or hemorrhage (Figure 30.1).

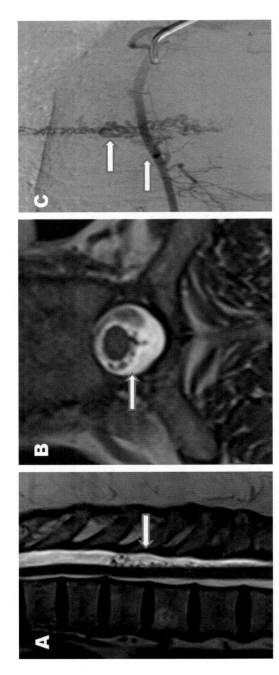

Figure 30.1 T$_2$-weighted MRI of the mid-thoracic spine in the sagittal (A) and axial (B) projections demonstrates multiple flow voids (arrows) suggestive of DAVF. (C) Spinal angiography demonstrates the fistulous connection between the segmental artery (bottom arrow) and the perimedullary venous plexus (top arrow).

Oral Boards Review—Diagnostic Pearls

1. A detailed clinical history of the progression of symptoms and neurological examination is very crucial in the accurate localization and diagnosis of the pathology.

2. Spinal DAVF can present with myelopathy, radiculopathy, subarachnoid hemorrhage, spontaneous hematoma, and/or symptoms due to steal phenomenon.

3. The following are clinical characteristics of spinal arteriovenous malformations:

   a. Type 1: AVF located between a dural branch of spinal ramus of radicular artery and an intradural medullary vein. It is more common in the fifth and sixth decades and most often presents clinically with progressive myelopathy with associated sensory involvement. Although acute exacerbation of symptoms is not uncommon, hemorrhage is relatively rare.

   b. Type 2: Intramedullary glomus malformation with a compact nidus within the substance of the spinal cord. Myelopathy and radiculopathy are not rare. It is more common in individuals younger than age 40 years and may manifest with intramedullary or subarachnoid hemorrhage.

   c. Type 3: Extensive AVM often extending into the vertebral body and paraspinal tissues. It is a common cause of acute neurologic deficit in the pediatric population due to hemorrhage and steal phenomenon.

   d. Type 4: Intradural perimedullary AVF. It is more common in adults and commonly manifest as progressive myelopathy due to venous hemodynamic changes and rarely manifest as acute neurologic deficit secondary to rupture of feeding vessel aneurysm.

4. Spinal AVF can be extradural/intradural and ventral (small/medium/large shunts)/dorsal (single/multiple feeders).

5. Prolapsed intervertebral disk usually affects the lumbar/cervical region, resulting in nerve root compression causing characteristic radicular pain in the involved dermatome with or without neurologic deficit.

6. The common intramedullary spinal cord lesions are ependymoma, astrocytoma, and hemangioblastoma. Ependymoma is commonly located in the low spinal cord/conus region, whereas astrocytoma is predominantly located in the mid- to upper spinal cord. The common clinical manifestation is progressive myelopathy with sensory involvement, with rare acute neurologic worsening.

7. Spinal angiography is the gold standard investigation for the diagnosis of spinal vascular malformations.

A spinal vascular lesion is suspected. Because MRI does not provide sufficient information, a thorough spinal angiogram should be performed. This should include evaluation of the aortic arch, the descending aorta, the abdominal aorta, the pelvic vasculature including the iliac arteries and the median sacral artery, the vertebral arteries, the thyrocervical trunk, and the deep and ascending cervical arteries in addition to injection of the segmental arteries at each spinal level. An anastomosis of a dural branch of a radicular artery (very rarely a radiculomedullary artery) and a radiculomedullary vein should be looked for in a suspected case of dural fistula. Both arterial and venous phase studies are important because prolonged imaging in the venous phase of the angiogram may be necessary to diagnose fistulas with slower flow (e.g., type 1).

Questions

1. How do these clinical and radiological findings influence the management?
2. What is the goal of treatment?
3. What are the two treatment approaches, and what are the advantages and disadvantages of each?

Decision-Making

Myelopathy secondary to DAVF can be caused by venous hypertension, congestion of the spinal cord, or by the mass effect by the dilated epidural vein. Making the correct diagnosis, localizing the lesion, and characterizing the precise anatomy of the DAVF are the key steps prior to treatment. Progressive myelopathy is more in favor of intradural DAVF, whereas associated radiculopathy or spontaneous hematoma may suggest an extradural location.

In most scenarios irrespective of location, the goal of treatment is the disruption of the abnormal arteriovenous shunting between feeding arteries and draining veins, thus relieving venous congestion and restoring normal spinal cord blood flow. Both endovascular and surgical options can be considered for most lesion types. In the case of type 1 spinal DAVF, advantages of surgical ligation include direct visualization of the draining vein, durable venous occlusion, and protection of normal spinal cord blood flow. Advantages of endovascular embolization are its minimally invasive nature, the ability to immediately treat the lesion upon angiographic diagnosis, reduced anesthetic and perioperative risks, and preservation of the structural integrity of the spinal column. In many institutions, the endovascular approach is attempted first, with surgical ligation is reserved for cases of failed embolization. Most studies report a comparable clinical response to both treatment types. In the current case, the patient is referred for spinal angiography and embolization at the time of diagnosis.

Questions

1. What are the critical structures to preserve during spinal DAVF embolization?
2. In which situations should embolization be abandoned in favor of surgical ligation?

Surgical Procedure

Endovascular therapy for spinal vascular malformations should be performed with the patient under general anesthesia and with controlled respiration. Transfemoral arterial access is obtained, the patient is fully heparinized, and a complete diagnostic spinal angiogram is performed if the location of the lesion has not been previously identified. Once the lesion has been fully characterized, and the locations of critical spinal arteries such as the anterior spinal artery (ASA) and the posterior spinal artery (PSA) are known, embolization may proceed if deemed safe and feasible. Selective and superselective catheterization of the feeding artery are performed with a hydrophilic microcatheter.

Different embolic agents are available to treat spinal cord vascular malformations, and there are different opinions regarding the best embolic agent. The choices include polyvinyl alcohol (PVA) and microspheres (of polyacrylamide and gelatin), liquid adhesives, and embolic coils. The occlusive effect of PVA and microspheres tends to be temporary and is frequently associated with recanalization. Coil embolization is often used only for large fistulas, and it rarely provides durable results. For most spinal DAVF embolizations, glue or Onyx is used. Both are liquid embolic agents that provide permanent arterial occlusion. Onyx is a cohesive polymer whose main advantage is precise control of the injection by building a proximal plug of embosylate followed by distal penetration of the lesion. Disadvantages of Onyx include increased procedural time from incremental embolization. Glue (such as *N*-butyl cyanoacrylate) is an adhesive whose main advantage is near-immediate vessel occlusion. Disadvantages of glue include the inability to precisely control the distal penetration of the agent and the need for rapid catheter removal once reflux occurs around the catheter tip to prevent adhesion of the catheter into the vessel.

Regardless of the agent chosen, closure of the fistula requires embolization of at least a portion of the feeding artery proximal to the fistula, the fistula itself, and a limited portion of the proximal draining vein as well. After embolization, control angiography after embolization should be performed on the contralateral segmental artery at the same level as the feeding pedicle and on segmental arteries two levels above and below on both sides to rule out collateral circulation reconstituting the fistula. An angiogram of the segmental artery supplying the anterior spinal artery may show immediate improvement of the spinal cord circulation. The catheters are then withdrawn, and femoral arterial closure is performed.

Oral Boards Review—Management Pearls

1. Superselective catheterization and direct access to the pathology are the key steps for successful obliteration.
2. Extradural AVFs are treated almost exclusively by the endovascular approach, whereas intradural AVFs may be managed by endovascular or surgical approaches.

Pivot Points

1. If the arterial supply of a spinal DAVF shares the same segmental artery as a critical spinal cord artery (e.g., the ASA or PSA), embolization may be of higher risk. Surgical ligation should be considered in such cases, especially if the microcatheter is not navigated substantially distal to the origin of such an artery.

2. Once a single arterial feeder is found, the remainder of the diagnostic spinal angiogram must be performed to ensure that no additional feeders (or lesions) are present.

3. If embolic agent is not visualized all the way into the fistulous pouch, the fistula should not be considered cured, and surgical ligation should be performed to ensure durable fistulous disconnection.

Aftercare

After embolization, the patient is admitted to a neurosurgical intensive care unit for serial neurological examinations. Corticosteroids are occasionally administered but have not been shown to substantially improve outcome after spinal DAVF embolization. Continuous heparinization for 24–48 hours postoperatively is considered in patients with large DAVF or pre-existing venous edema to prevent progressive venous thrombosis and consequent neurological worsening.

Serial follow-up angiograms are indicated to monitor for lesion progression. If complete occlusion of the lesion was achieved, a follow-up spinal angiogram or MRI is often repeated at 3 months, and if unchanged, an angiogram is obtained at 1 year and occasionally at 3 years. If complete treatment of the lesion was not achieved, angiographic follow-up is based on clinical grounds. Progression or recurrence of neurological symptoms warrants repeated angiographic imaging.

Complications and Management

The clinical complications of the endovascular treatment of spinal DAVFs can be attributed to procedural error, incomplete obliteration, and recanalization of fistula. The most important periprocedural complication is neurological deterioration secondary to inadvertent occlusion of important vessels (e.g., the ASA or PSA). Occlusion of the ASA or PSA and subsequent spinal cord infarction may arise from improper placement or accidental displacement of the microcatheter, incorrect choice of embolic agent, unexpected reflux of liquid embolic material into the proximal artery or into newly opened unexpected collateral supply to the spinal cord, and fundamentally incomplete understanding of the lesion's angioarchitecture. Superselective catheterization and liberal diagnostic angiography to evaluate the complete angioarchitecture of lesion are the other safe techniques that can be employed to prevent many of these complications.

Other complications include dissection of segmental arteries supplying the fistulous branches, vessel perforation by the wire or catheter, vessel perforation secondary to increased pressure while embolizing, vessel rupture as a result of a glued-in catheter, and catheter retention. Dissection of segmental arteries supplying fistulous branches rarely results in neurological deficit, but it does eliminate the possibility of endovascular treatment and requires subsequent surgical ligation. Catheter retention and vessel rupture can be avoided by careful injection of embolic agent. Access site complications may warrant urgent referral to vascular surgery for further management.

Incomplete obliteration of intradural AVFs may result in later recurrence of the lesion because of recruitment of collateral arterial feeders, which may be more difficult to deal with at a later time. Embolization with liquid embolic agents (rather than particles or coils) is associated with much lower rates of recanalization.

Oral Boards Review—Complications Pearls

1. Complications can be the direct consequences of embolization techniques, failed obliteration, or recanalization.
2. Careful preoperative angiographic assessment, especially of the arterial feeders and the nature of the arteriovenous shunt, choice of embolic material, and selective catheterization technique are the important factors in complication avoidance.
3. Groin hematoma, vascular dissection, and thrombosis may need careful observation/urgent vascular surgery referral depending on the scenario.

Evidence and Outcomes

Various studies have analyzed the procedural outcome after endovascular embolization or open surgery in spinal DAVF. Both approaches are noted to be effective at halting progressive congestive myelopathy and obliterating abnormal fistulous connections. The advantages of the endovascular approach are its less invasive nature, shorter hospital stay, early mobilization, good clinical response with excellent outcome, and minimal major or permanent morbidity in safe hands. Surgical approaches have a higher likelihood of immediate fistula disconnection and should be considered in patients with low perioperative morbidity or in cases in which embolization fails.

Further Reading

Brown PA, Zomorodi AR, Gonzalez LF. Endovascular management of spinal dural arteriovenous fistulas. *Handb Clin Neurol.* 2017;143:199–213.

Cesak T, Adamkov J, Poczos P, et.al. Multidisciplinary approach in the treatment of spinal dural arteriovenous fistula: Results of endovascular and surgical treatment. *Acta Neurochir (Wien).* 2018;160(12):2439–2448. doi:10.1007/s00701-018-3672-z.

Day AL, Turkmani AH, Chen PR. Spinal arteriovenous fistulae: Surgical management. *Handb Clin Neurol.* 2017;143:189–198.

Kiyosue H, Matsumaru Y, Niimi Y, et al.; JSNET Spinal AV Shunts Study Group. Angiographic and clinical characteristics of thoracolumbar spinal epidural and dural arteriovenous fistulas. *Stroke.* 2017;48(12):3215–3222.

Krings T, Lasjanias PL, Rodesch G, et al. Imaging in spinal vascular disease. *Neuroimaging Clin North Am.* 2007;17:57–72.

Liu A, Gobin P, Riina H. Endovascular surgery for vascular malformations of the spinal cord. *Oper Tech Neurosurg.* 2003;6:163–170.

McDougall CG, Deshmukh VR, Fiorella DJ, et al. Endovascular techniques for vascular malformations of the spinal axis. *Neurosurg Clin North Am*. 2005;16:395–410.

Narvid J, Hetls SW, Larsen D, et al. Spinal dural arteriovenous fistulae: Clinical features and long-term results. *Neurosurgery*. 2008;62:159–166.

Niimi Y, Berenstein A, Setton A, et al. Embolization of spinal dural arteriovenous fistulae: Results and follow-up. *Neurosurgery*. 1997;40:675–682.

Spetzler RF, Detwiler PW, Riina HA, et al. Modified classification of spinal cord vascular lesions. *J Neurosurg*. 2002;96(2 Suppl):145–156.

Ruptured Spinal Arteriovenous Malformation

Brandon D. Liebelt, Michaela H. Lee, Peter Nakaji, and Robert F. Spetzler

31

Case Presentation

A 37-year-old male presents to the emergency department with acute-onset mid-thoracic back pain and paraparesis. The patient has no significant past medical or surgical history and no history of trauma. There is no family history of spinal disease or of neurovascular malformations. The patient recalls some mild gait instability during the preceding 6–9 months. Physical examination findings revealed normal cranial nerves and intact upper extremity strength, reflexes, and sensation. Lower extremity strength was markedly decreased, with proximal muscle groups affected more than distal. Sensation to light touch and pinprick was reduced through the lower extremities and lower abdomen below the umbilicus. Hyperreflexia was present in the lower extremities.

Questions

1. What is the differential diagnosis and most likely diagnosis for this patient given his presentation?
2. What imaging studies should be ordered?

Assessment and Planning

The patient presents with symptoms of acute-onset back pain with associated lower extremity neurologic deficit. In the setting of nontraumatic acute onset of severe back pain with associated neurological deficits, the neurosurgeon should consider spinal cord or cauda equina pathology, including either intramedullary pathology or extramedullary or extradural lesions compressing the spinal cord. In the absence of trauma, the differential should include spinal vascular malformations, vascular spinal tumors, disc herniation in the thoracic or lumbar spine, and pathologic spinal fracture. Spinal vascular malformations are a diverse group of disorders comprising spinal dural arteriovenous fistula, true spinal cord arteriovenous malformations, and cavernous malformations. The acute onset of spontaneous severe back pain should cue the possibility of a spinal vascular malformation and associated spinal subarachnoid hemorrhage.

Spinal vascular malformations make up approximately 4% of all primary intraspinal masses, with 80% occurring between ages 20 and 60 years. Intramedullary spinal arteriovenous malformations (AVMs) account for approximately 15% of all spinal vascular malformations and most commonly present with rupture leading to subarachnoid hemorrhage, as in the current case.

Oral Boards Review—Diagnostic Pearls

1. Classification scheme for spinal vascular malformations
   a. Type 1: Dural AVM (dural arteriovenous fistula [AVF])—occurs in nerve root sleeve, comprises 80% of spinal vascular malformations in the adult, and presents with progressive lower extremity myelopathy
      i. Type 1a: Single arterial feeder
      ii. Type 1b: Multiple arterial feeders
   b. Type 2: Spinal glomus AVM (intramedullary AVM)—15–20% of spinal vascular malformations
   c. Type 3: Juvenile spinal AVM (extradural–intradural)—occupies spinal cord and involves vertebral body and occasionally associated muscle and skin
   d. Type 4: Perimedullary AVM (AVF)—direct fistula between anterior spinal artery and draining vein
2. Modified classification of spinal vascular malformations
   a. Extradural AVF
   b. Dorsal intradural AVF
   c. Ventral intradural AVF
   d. Extradural–intradural AVM
   e. Intramedullary AVM
   f. Conus AVM

Magnetic resonance imaging (MRI) of the spinal axis should be performed with and without contrast. In patients with spinal AVMs, a focal vascular malformation may be visualized at least partially within the spinal cord parenchyma (Figure 31.1). Patients with spinal dural AVFs (type 1) may or may not be apparent on MRIs. Dilated serpiginous vessels may be visible in the intradural space, particularly on T_2 sequences. There may also be evidence of venous congestion and hypertension in the spinal cord, seen as signal hyperintensity on both T_2 and inversion recovery (short T_1 inversion recovery or fluid-attenuated inversion recovery) sequences.

A formal spinal angiogram is mandatory for definitive and accurate diagnosis of a spinal vascular malformation (Figure 31.2). A spinal vascular malformation may be seen on angiogram even in the setting of a normal spinal MRI scan. For this reason, it may be indicated to obtain a spinal angiogram with a normal MRI scan if a high degree of clinical suspicion is present. For type 1 spinal vascular malformations, angiography should be meticulous and encompass all dural feeders of the neuraxis, including all radicular arteries, internal and external carotid arteries, thyrocervical trunks, internal iliac arteries, and the median sacral artery (if present).

Myelography may be a helpful adjunct if a patient has a contraindication to MRI scanning. Computed tomography (CT) myelogram, similar to MRI, would reveal serpiginous vessels in the intradural space. If CT myelogram is utilized, performing the study in both supine and prone positions will help prevent missing subtle findings associated with these malformations.

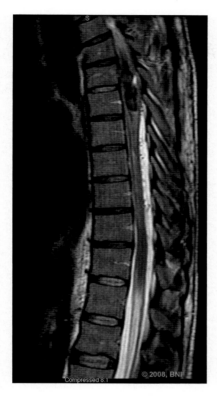

Figure 31.1 A sagittal T$_2$ MRI of the thoracic spine shows an intraparenchymal hematoma within the spinal cord at the top of the image and dilated vasculature dorsal to the spinal cord below.

Questions

1. What are the different types of spinal vascular malformations? What classification schemes exist for their categorization?
2. What are the differences in clinical presentation between spinal dural fistulas and intrinsic spinal AVMs?
3. What is the appropriate radiographic workup for spinal vascular malformations?

Decision-Making

Treatment options for spinal vascular malformations include open surgery for resection or exclusion of the malformation, endovascular occlusion, radiotherapy, or a combined approach. In the setting of an intramedullary AVM, endovascular embolization serves as a useful preoperative adjunct in the treatment of these complex lesions in select cases. Blood supply typically originates from single or multiple dilated anterior spinal artery feeders, but the posterior spinal arteries can also contribute (Figure 31.3). Spinal AVMs can further have either a compact or a diffuse nidus. Careful judgment must be applied when selecting which patients to embolize preoperatively because the small caliber of

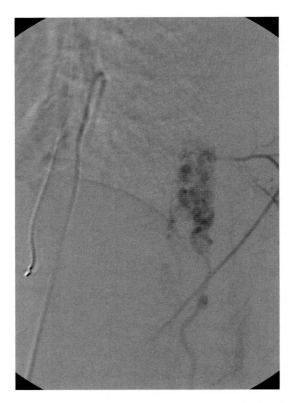

Figure 31.2 A spinal angiogram with selective injection at the level of the lesion shows an AVM nidus with draining veins exiting below.

vasculature of feeding arteries near the spinal cord and lesion makes them prone to vasospasm, potentially leading to inadvertent embolization of normal vessels and unsuccessful treatment. Furthermore, the lack of collateral supply of certain regions of the spinal cord predisposes these regions to ischemic complications should inadvertent vasospasm or vessel occlusion occur.

Surgical resection, particularly in the setting of a ruptured lesion, remains the mainstay of treatment for intramedullary AVMs. Unique features of each case will dictate the most suitable treatment strategy with regard to possible preoperative embolization and surgical goals. In the setting of a ruptured spinal cord AVM, the presence of hematomyelia may help define dissection planes around the lesion and help guide surgical removal. A pial dissection strategy to remove the extramedullary component of the AVM while leaving the intramedullary component has been described. By removing the superficial component of the AVM, disconnecting surface vessels, and respecting the pial plane, neurologic function can be maximally preserved while feeding and draining vessels are devascularized (Figure 31.4).

Questions

1. Which type of spinal vascular malformation is most suitable for endovascular therapy alone?
2. What surgical principles apply to treatment of spinal cord AVMs extending deep to the pia?

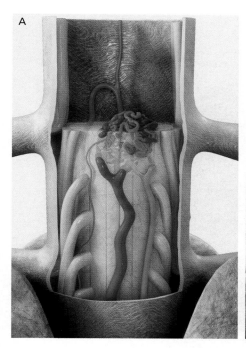

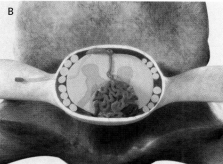

Figure 31.3 (A) Coronal cutaway view of a compact AVM nidus within the spinal cord with vascular contribution from both anterior and posterior circulation arteries and a dorsal draining vein. (B) Axial view of the AVM nidus in the dorsal spinal cord fed by an anterior spinal artery that feeds from a left radicular artery.

Surgical Procedure

Consideration for adjunctive preoperative embolization should be given to devascularize major feeding vessels if it can be safely performed. Surgical resection of intramedullary spinal cord AVMs is typically performed in the prone position through a midline approach. The patient can be placed on standard gel chest rolls or a Wilson frame. Neuromonitoring is essential throughout the procedure and should include both somatosensory evoked potential and motor evoked potential monitoring. An arterial line should be placed for tight control of blood pressure and strict monitoring to prevent hypotension during the procedure.

Careful preoperative review of the spinal angiogram and attention to the spinal anatomy on CT or X-rays should be performed prior to surgery. Localization is a critical step in the procedure and should be performed with radiography; thoracic levels are particularly challenging to localize, and special attention should be given to the number of ribs and the number of lumbar vertebrae because variations in normal anatomy can be encountered. Preoperative embolization material may serve as a useful fluoroscopic landmark for localization of the correct level at surgery. In cases with a compact nidus, a laminectomy or laminoplasty is performed. With diffuse AVMs, the lesion frequently favors one side. In this case, the approach should be tailored to maximize the exposure through the additional removal of bone on the ipsilateral side, such as via a costotransversectomy. This maneuver may leave the spine unstable, however, sometimes necessitating a fusion.

The dura is opened and sutured to the muscle, as opposed to draping suture over the edge of the wound, in order to maximize the width of the dural opening. If access to the

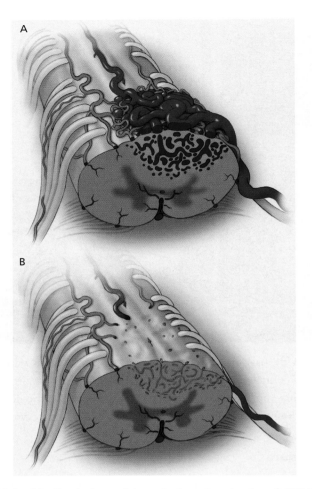

Figure 31.4 (A) An idealized view of the spinal cord and a dorsal AVM that is illustrated with both surface and intraparenchymal components. (B) Removal of the AVM at the surface leads to devascularization of the intraparenchymal component, which is not the case with brain AVMs.

lateral or ventrolateral cord is necessary for resection of the spinal cord AVM, the dentate ligaments can be sectioned.

The location of a spinal cord AVM also dictates the goals of surgery. Cervical location is more favorable for aggressive resection given more its extensive collateral blood supply than for thoracic and lumbar lesions. Resection of these lesions can be achieved either through circumferential dissection (especially within a gliotic plane or hematoma) or with a pial dissection technique. The senior author prefers performing microsurgical resection by sacrificing arterial supply prior to interrupting venous drainage, similar to cranial AVMs; however, others have had success with resection of these lesions with retrograde dissection from the venous side. A pial dissection strategy, potentially leaving residual AVM within the parenchyma of the spinal cord, affords the possibility of superior neurologic outcomes by leaving the spinal cord undisturbed. Remnants of AVM within the cord parenchyma do not behave in the same fashion as cranial AVMs with regard to a high risk of rupture of residual AVM. Partial resection of spinal cord AVMs can afford better outcomes through less surgical morbidity. Long-term follow-up of these patients showed persistent obliteration of AVM in 83% of patients and stability in those with residual AVM postoperatively.

After resection of the AVM is complete, an intraoperative catheter angiography or indocyanine green videoangiography is performed to assess the completeness of resection. Closure is performed in typical fashion with watertight dural closure. The dural closure can be performed with a prolene, Nurolon, or Gore-Tex suture; the integrity of the dural closure is evaluated with the Valsalva maneuver. The remainder of the wound is closed in standard fashion, with reattachment of the posterior elements if a laminoplasty is preferred.

Oral Boards Review—Management Pearls

1. Spinal cord AVMs can be safely resected with the use of the pial dissection technique, preventing transgression into spinal cord parenchyma and preserving neurologic function.
2. Although endovascular treatment of intramedullary AVMs has been described, its predominant use is as a surgical adjunct in preoperative devascularization of major feeding vessels.
3. Postoperative spinal angiography is essential to confirm complete removal of these lesions. Intraoperative angiography should be utilized in select cases.

Pivot Points

1. If a patient presents with symptoms suggestive of a spinal vascular malformation, meticulous spinal angiography including all neuroaxis vessels should be performed.
2. Endovascular embolization is an effective adjunct in managing intramedullary spinal cord AVMs and should be utilized in select cases prior to surgical resection.
3. If an area of AVM nidus is within a critical functional area of the spinal cord, a remnant may be purposefully left unresected to preserve neurological function. Unlike in cranial AVM surgery, residual nidus does not seem to lead to substantially worse outcomes.

Aftercare

Patients are typically kept flat in bed overnight, and the incision is monitored in the postoperative period for spinal fluid leak. Postoperative spinal angiography is necessary for confirmation of complete removal. Residual AVM can be addressed either in the early postoperative period by return to the operating room or by observation if the residual AVM was expected and left in the cord parenchyma in order to preserve neurologic function. Spinal angiography should be utilized to monitor the lesion for any changes beginning at 1 year postoperatively.

Complications and Management

Transient neurological decline following surgery for spinal cord AVMs can occur from manipulation of the spinal cord, similar to intramedullary surgery for spinal cord tumors. Tight blood pressure maintenance, especially avoidance of hypotension, ensures adequate perfusion of the spinal cord in the immediate postoperative period. If significant or unexpected decline occurs after surgery, urgent spinal MRI should be performed to rule out postoperative hematoma.

Spinal fluid leak and pseudomeningocele can occur and should be addressed promptly to prevent meningitis. Immediate re-exploration of the wound with attempt to primarily repair the leak is preferable. A lumbar drain may be used for several days after surgery to aid in wound healing.

Spinal instability can be encountered in the postoperative period, particularly if the facet joint and pedicle are resected during the approach without supplemental instrumentation. The cervical and lumbar spine are more prone to destabilization than are the thoracic segments. Spinal CT and dynamic standing radiographs can diagnose instability or kyphosis across the surgical site. Laminoplasty may help maintain stability if surgery is performed across multiple segments. When instability or postoperative kyphosis are encountered, reoperation for instrumented fusion is indicated.

Recurrence or changes to residual spinal AVM should be monitored for with spinal angiography beginning at 1 year. Recruitment of additional vessels may be an indication for additional surgery, attempted endovascular treatment, or close monitoring and should be managed on a case-by-case basis given the complexity of these rare lesions.

Oral Boards Review—Complications Pearls

1. Spinal fluid leak and pseudomeningocele should be addressed promptly with early surgical re-exploration and attempted primary repair.
2. Patients should be monitored with spinal angiography immediately after surgery and at 1, 3, 5, and 10 years post-procedure to assess for morphological change or recurrence of the lesion.
3. Spinal stability should be considered when choosing an approach. Instrumented fusion may be indicated either during the initial surgery or if instability or kyphosis develops postoperatively.

Evidence and Outcomes

Spinal cord vascular malformations are rare entities, with few published case series documenting outcomes and discussing appropriate classification systems based on anatomy and pathophysiology.

As discussed previously, a combination of endovascular and surgical management is useful in most cases. Successful endovascular treatment of an intramedullary AVM has been reported, but surgical resection remains the mainstay of therapy with or without adjuvant embolization. Gross total resection rates have been documented between 80% and 92%, with high rates of symptomatic control. Dysesthetic pain symptoms are a frequent side effect of surgical management, and they may be mitigated by medications such as gabapentin.

Further Reading

Abecassis IJ, Osbun JW, Kim L. Classification and pathophysiology of spinal vascular malformations. *Handb Clin Neurol.* 2017;143:135–143.

Boström A, Krings T, Hans FJ, Schramm J, Thron AK, Gilsbach JM. Spinal glomus-type arteriovenous malformations: Microsurgical treatment in 20 cases. *J Neurosurg Spine.* 2009;10:423–429.

Ducruet AF, Crowley RW, McDougall CG, Albuquerque FC. Endovascular treatment of spinal arteriovenous malformations. In: Spetzler R, Kalani M, Nakaji P, eds. *Neurovascular Surgery* . 2nd ed. New York: Thieme; 2015. doi:10.1055/b-003-122312.

Kim LJ, Spetzler RF. Classification and surgical management of spinal arteriovenous lesions: Arteriovenous fistulae and arteriovenous malformations. *Neurosurgery.* 2006;59(5 Suppl 3):S195–S201.

Martin NA, Khanna RK, Batzdorf U. Posterolateral cervical or thoracic approach with spinal cord rotation for vascular malformations or tumors of the ventrolateral spinal cord. *J Neurosurg.* 1995;83(2):254–261.

Velat GJ, Chang SW, Abla AA, Albuquerque FC, McDougall CG, Spetzler RF. Microsurgical management of glomus spinal arteriovenous malformations: Pial resection technique. *J Neurosurg Spine.* 2012;16(6):523–533.

Ruptured Conus Medullaris Arteriovenous Malformation

Michaela H. Lee, Brandon D. Liebelt, Peter Nakaji, and Robert F. Spetzler

32

Case Presentation

A 30-year-old female presents to the emergency room with worsening headaches and back pain radiating down both legs. Upon further questioning, she reports difficulty climbing stairs and urinary retention for the past several weeks. She had attributed this to the increased dose of narcotics that she was taking for her back and leg pain. She has no significant past medical or surgical history. On examination, she has nuchal rigidity, diminished but present rectal tone, perianal numbness, absent ankle jerk reflexes bilaterally, and mild weakness of her lower extremities. Noncontrast head computed tomography (CT) shows mild diffuse subarachnoid hemorrhage. CT angiogram (CTA) of the head was negative for any intracranial vascular pathology. Her lumbar spine magnetic resonance imaging (MRI) is shown in Figure 32.1.

Questions

1. What is the likely diagnosis?
2. What additional imaging is needed?
3. What are the pathophysiological mechanisms that contribute to the clinical presentation?

Assessment and Planning

Based on the lumbar spine MRI that show serpiginous vascular flow voids in the spinal canal centered at T12–L1, the differential diagnosis includes spinal arteriovenous malformation (AVM) or spinal arteriovenous fistula (AVF) that likely ruptured, causing the subarachnoid hemorrhage on the head CT. Complete spinal MRI should be done to confirm that there is no other pathology at other levels. The gold standard for evaluation of any spinal vascular lesion is a spinal angiogram (Figure 32.2).

Historically, spinal vascular malformations have been categorized under multiple classification schemes that evolved with the advancement of imaging techniques, particularly with the introduction of spinal arteriography. The Spetzler classification system divided spinal vascular malformations into four categories: type I—dural AVFs; type II—glomus AVMs; type III—juvenile AVMs; and type IV—pial AVFs. The modified

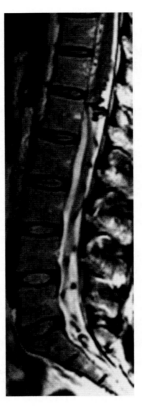

Figure 32.1 Sagittal T_2 lumbar MRI demonstrating vascular flow voids at the thoracolumbar junction extending superiorly and inferiorly along the cauda equina and filum terminale.

Spetzler classification system was proposed to reflect a more accurate understanding of the anatomy, angioarchitecture, and pathophysiology of these lesions and optimize their treatment. The six categories are as follows: extradural AVFs, intradural dorsal AVFs intradural ventral, extradural–intradural AVMs, intramedullary AVMs, and conus medullaris AVMs.

Based on the MRI and spinal angiogram for this presenting case, the diagnosis is a conus medullaris AVM. Spinal vascular malformations are not common in general, accounting for 3% or 4% of all intradural spinal cord lesions, and conus medullaris AVMs are even more rare.

Conus medullaris AVMs are considered to be in a separate subcategory due to their complex angioarchitecture and unique location. They consist of multiple direct shunts from both the anterior spinal artery (ASA) and the posterior spinal artery (PSA) and sometimes even radicular arteries that drain into both anterior and posterior venous plexi forming a complex vascular network at the level of the conus (Figure 32.3). The shunts and draining veins can be very large. They can also involve multiple glomus-like niduses that are usually extramedullary and pial or intramedullary. The vascular network can also extend along the entire filum terminale.

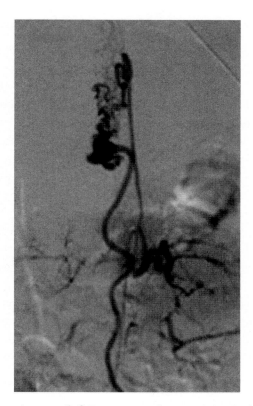

Figure 32.2 Spinal angiogram (left L2 segmental artery injection) demonstrating supply to both the anterior spinal artery and a conus medullaris AVM. A large draining vein is also seen.

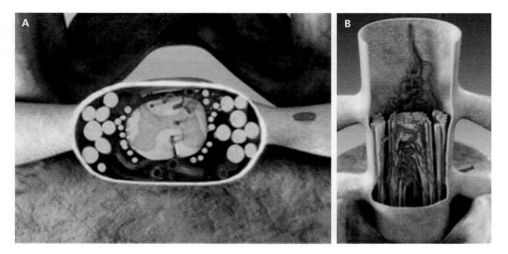

Figure 32.3 Artist's rendition of a conus AVM from axial (A) and posterior (B) views demonstrating a complex vascular network of multiple arteriovenous shunts from the ASA and PSA and large dilated draining veins at the level of the conus medullaris.

Oral Boards Review—Diagnostic Pearls

1. Physical examination and clinical findings, such as ascending progressive myelopathy, can be very important in making the diagnosis of a spinal vascular malformation that may not always be readily apparent on MRI. The initial differential can be wide, including degenerative spinal stenosis, demyelination, inflammation/infection, and tumor, but if the clinical presentation does not correlate with the imaging, spinal vascular malformations should also be included, necessitating spinal angiography.

2. Vascular flow voids of enlarged perimedullary veins on T_2-weighted MRI with cord fluid-attenuated inversion recovery hyperintensity should prompt a spinal angiogram.

3. The gold standard for any spinal vascular malformation is a spinal angiogram. CTA and MR angiography (MRA) can be useful adjuncts.

4. Neurologic decline will progress if patients are not diagnosed accurately and treated.

5. Although usually insidious in onset, some patients can present with acute loss of neurologic function. Prompt recognition and expedited imaging workup can be critical to potential recovery.

Patients with conus medullaris AVMs frequently present with slow, progressive myeloradiculopathy. Because these lesions are intimately involved with both the spinal cord and the nerves of the cauda equina, they can present with both upper and lower motor symptoms secondary to both venous congestion and mass effect from engorged veins on the nerve roots, respectively. Bowel and bladder dysfunction is also very common in this patient population, and baseline urodynamic status should be obtained. The neurological decline is usually stepwise and insidious. Acute subarachnoid hemorrhage (as in this case) is rare, as is intraparenchymal hemorrhage, or ischemia from vascular steal syndrome, which is more common in other types of spinal AVMs.

Questions

1. What is the goal of management?
2. How do these clinical findings and radiographic findings influence the surgical approach and plan?
3. How does a preoperative spinal angiogram aid surgical planning?

Decision-Making

The goal in the management of conus medullaris AVMs is obliteration of the AVM in order to prevent further neurological deterioration and ideally achieve functional recovery. Myelopathy secondary to venous congestion can be reversible, but if left untreated chronically, it can cause irreversible ischemia and damage. Therefore, early treatment is advocated. The patient in this case has progressively worsening symptoms as well as an acute hemorrhage and needs definitive treatment as soon as possible. Conus medullaris AVM angioarchitecture can be quite complex, requiring a multimodal approach with preoperative endovascular embolization followed by surgical resection.

Preoperative spinal angiography allows identification of both the ASA and the PSA and the precise level and location of the arterial supply as well as the venous drainage. Superselective angiography can then be performed for embolization of arterial feeders to facilitate surgical resection and reduce intraoperative blood loss. However, if a feeding segmental artery also supplies the ASA or the PSA, endovascular embolization may not be a feasible option due to high risk of spinal cord ischemia.

The majority of spinal vascular lesions can be approached surgically with a posterior or posterolateral approach with the patient positioned prone. There is an increased risk of injury to the anterior spinal artery and suboptimal dural closure with cerebrospinal fluid (CSF) leak with anterior approaches, so these are rarely used. A laminectomy or laminoplasty can be performed exposing one level above and one level below the AVM in order to access the lesion and identify normal parenchyma. In addition, a costotransversectomy or facetectomy can be added to allow more lateral exposure if the lesion extends cranially. If there is concern for instability, instrumented fusion can be done at the same time as resection surgery.

In the current case, a posterior approach would allow complete visualization and access to the vascular lesion. The selective spinal angiogram demonstrated that a segmental feeder supplied both the ASA and the AVM; therefore, due to the high risk of spinal cord infarct with reflux of embolic material, preoperative embolization was not attempted. The patient was taken to the operating room for a T11–L1 laminectomy, AVM resection, and laminoplasty.

Questions

1. How is a resection of spinal cord intramedullary/conus medullaris AVMs different from resection of cerebral AVMs?
2. What are the possible entry points when performing a myelotomy?
3. What additional intraoperative monitoring methods should be considered for conus medullaris AVM surgery?

Surgical Procedure

The patient is brought into the operating room and intubated under general anesthesia. A microscope with a filter for indocyanine green fluorescence (ICG) is sterily draped. An arterial line is placed by the anesthesiologist in order to monitor the patient's blood pressure at all times, with the goal of maintaining mean arterial pressure between 60 and 80 mmHg. Neurophysiological monitoring, including somatosensory and motor evoked potentials, is mandatory in these cases, and direct interfield stimulation should be available as needed. Once the patient is positioned prone, fluoroscopy is used to localize the level of surgery, and preoperative antibiotics and steroids are administered.

A midline lumbar incision is marked, and the surgical area is steriley prepped and draped. The incision is made sharply with a blade, and subperiosteal dissection is carried out in the usual fashion. In a laminoplasty approach, the laminae are removed as one piece by making troughs on both sides, so the laminae can be replaced at the end of

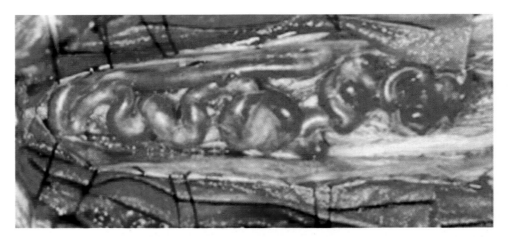

Figure 32.4 Intraoperative photo of conus medullaris AVM.

the case. The advantages of a laminoplasty include prevention of scarring and tethering of the dura, easier dissection in future surgeries, and protection of the neural elements.

After achieving a bloodless field, the dura is opened carefully in a linear fashion and tacked up with sutures. If possible, the dura and arachnoid are opened separately to prevent leakage of blood into the subarachnoid space. The arachnoid is then tacked to the dura with hemostatic clips (Figure 32.4).

ICG angiography is performed to visualize the angioarchitecture of the malformation prior to any sharp dissection and can be repeated throughout the case as needed to evaluate the progress of the resection. If necessary, the spinal cord can be further mobilized for better anterolateral visualization by transecting the dentate ligaments.

Conus medullaris AVMs typically contain a glomus-like nidus that is usually extramedullary and pial but can also extend into the parenchyma. Resection of the intramedullary component is similar to the microsurgical resection of intramedullary AVMs. Although a posterior midline myelotomy can be used to extirpate intramedullary AVMS, we advocate a pial dissection to identify, coagulate, and divide the feeding arteries and draining veins by staying at the pial surface and minimizing the disruption of the cord. The arterial feeders are divided at the entrance into the spinal cord instead of being followed into the parenchyma. Then, in coherence with tenets of AVM surgery, the arterial feeders are identified and divided before disconnecting the draining veins. This technique does require that the AVM has an extrapial component, but when done properly, it will devascularize the lesion sufficiently to alleviate the symptoms with less violation of the spinal cord.

Nevertheless, a midline myelotomy is sometimes necessary for evacuation of an intraparenchymal hematoma, drainage of a syrinx, and removal of AVMs entirely intramedullary with no extrapial component. The possible entry points include dorsal midline, dorsal root entry zone, between the dorsal and ventral nerve roots laterally, and anterior midline.

The conus medullaris AVM is unique because it is often intimately intertwined with functional nerve roots due to its location. Intraoperative electrophysiological monitoring, including direct stimulation, can help identify and avoid endangering nerve root function.

Once the large draining vein is clipped and ligated, a final intraoperative ICG angiography is performed to confirm obliteration of the AVM. The dura is closed in a watertight fashion, and suture line can be reinforced with fibrin glue. The laminae are replaced and secured with plates and screws. Intraoperative or postoperative spinal angiography should be done within 24 hours to confirm obliteration of the AVM.

Oral Boards Review—Management Pearls

1. A multidisciplinary approach with preoperative embolization (when feasible) and open microsurgical resection is favored for management of conus medullaris AVMs.
2. Intraoperative ICG can help identify arterial feeders and draining veins prior to resection and any residual vessels during the case.
3. Maintain frequent communication with anesthesia and electrophysiological teams to quickly identify any changes in blood pressure and intraoperative monitoring.
4. Unlike cranial AVM resection surgery, in situ disconnection of feeding arteries followed by draining veins, rather than subpial resection of the AVM nidus, is a useful approach for spinal AVMs, including those in the conus medullaris.

Pivot Points

1. In patients with extensive parenchymal involvement by the AVM nidus, radiosurgery can be considered instead of surgical resection to reduce the likelihood of postoperative neurological complications.
2. If a laminoplasty is not appropriate for the patient, consider closing the dura with a synthetic amniotic membrane graft to prevent tethering of the cord.

Aftercare

The patient should be transferred to the intensive care unit for serial neurologic examinations, and mean arterial pressure should be maintained greater than 85 mmHg for up to 3 days. Postoperative spinal angiography should be done to confirm obliteration of the AVM (Figure 32.5). It is not uncommon for the patient to have temporary worsening of neurological deficits, although most will improve with time. A short course of steroids can help during this period. In addition, bladder or bowel dysfunction often requires discharge with a Foley leg bag or straight catheterization schedule until resolution. Patients must be followed with serial imaging (MRI/MRA and spinal angiograms) for any recurrence and development of tethered cord or spinal instability.

In the current case, the surgery was uncomplicated, and the patient regained her strength and her myeloradiculopathy resolved several days postoperatively. She had some mild anesthesia in the lower sacral root distribution, and her urinary retention remained unchanged immediately after surgery, requiring straight catheterization. She

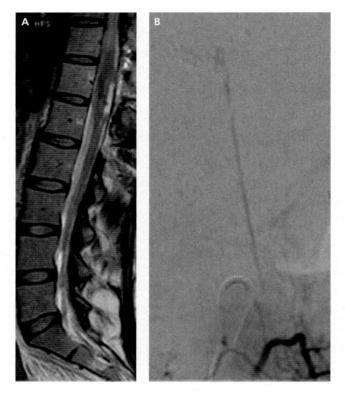

Figure 32.5 Postoperative sagittal T$_2$ lumbar MRI (A) and spinal angiogram (B) demonstrating obliteration of conus medullaris AVM.

was discharged home on postoperative day 4. Her repeat spinal angiogram at 6 weeks after surgery was stable with no residual, and her urinary retention resolved.

Complications and Management

Intraoperative monitoring is critical to identify ischemic insults to the spinal cord or nerve roots. If the surgeon is unsure whether a vessel is safe to coagulate and divide during surgery, the placement of a temporary aneurysm clip on the vessel followed by an observation period may allow the surgeon to prevent a potentially disastrous ischemic complication. Similarly, the use of electrophysiological stimulation in the operative field can be helpful in distinguishing dorsal from ventral nerve roots and to identify safe entry zones for myelotomy. Intraoperative angiography is useful for identifying residual AVM prior to surgical closure, to reduce the need for additional surgery, though this may be more difficult to perform in the prone position.

Postoperative hemorrhage, CSF leak, and pseudomeningocele are possible with any intradural spine surgery. It is important to achieve meticulous hemostasis and water-tight closure during the end of the case, which includes asking anesthesia to perform a Valsalva maneuver to test the dural suture line prior to closing. It is also reasonable to place a lumbar drain under direct visualization intraoperatively if a primary dural closure is not possible and/or to place the patient flat in bed for 24–72 hours postoperatively. However, if there is a persistent CSF leak, early re-exploration is advised.

Wound complications and infection can also occur. The risk can be reduced with 24-hour postoperative antibiotics, avoiding prolonged pressure on the incision with frequent turning of the patient when in bed, and judicious use of steroids. Finally, patients undergoing intradural spinal surgery are at risk for developing long-term complications such as tethered cord syndrome or spinal instability.

Oral Boards Review—Complications Pearls

1. Careful intraoperative identification and protection of functional nerve roots during surgery will aid in preserving and restoring their function postoperatively.
2. Any delayed or acute neurological exam change should warrant a prompt spinal MRI to evaluate for any postoperative hematoma, intraparenchymal hemorrhage, or worsening spinal cord edema.
3. A persistent CSF leak that has failed conservative measures requires a re-exploration surgery for definitive repair due to high risk of infection and meningitis.

Evidence and Outcomes

Unfortunately, the literature on conus medullaris AVMs is sparse at best, given the rarity of this lesion. For spinal AVMs in general, historical review reports severe disability within 3 years in untreated patients, and less than 10% are able to ambulate without assistance. In more recent literature, the largest case series to date regarding the treatment of conus medullaris AVMs demonstrated excellent long-term outcomes in a majority of patients, with 75% of non-ambulatory patients regaining the ability to walk after surgery. Pursuing aggressive treatment in this population with a multidisciplinary approach including embolization and microsurgical resection optimizes patient outcomes.

Further Reading

Bao YH, Ling F. Classification and therapeutic modalities of spinal vascular malformations in 80 patients. *Neurosurgery*. 1997;40(1):75–81.

Kim LJ, Spetzler RF. Classification and surgical management of spinal arteriovenous lesions: Arteriovenous fistulae and arteriovenous malformations. *Neurosurgery*. 2006;59(5 Suppl 3):S195–S201.

Rangel-Castilla L, Russin JJ, Zaidi HA, et al. Contemporary management of spinal AVFs and AVMs: Lessons learned from 110 cases. *Neurosurg Focus*. 2014;37(3):E14.

Wilson DA, Abla AA, Uschold TD, McDougall CG, Albuquerque FC, Spetzler RF. Multimodality treatment of conus medullaris arteriovenous malformations: 2 decades of experience with combined endovascular and microsurgical treatments. *Neurosurgery*. 2012;71(1):100–108.

Index

Page numbers followed by *f* and *b* refer to figures and boxes, respectively.

For the benefit of digital users, indexed terms that span two pages (e.g., 52–53) may, on occasion, appear on only one of those pages.